Gene Therapy

Gene Therapy

The use of DNA as a drug

Edited by

Gavin Brooks

BPharm, PhD, MRPharmS

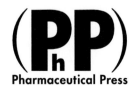

Pharmaceutical Press

Published by the Pharmaceutical Press
1 Lambeth High Street, London SE1 7JN, UK

© Pharmaceutical Press 2002

First published 2002

Text design by Barker/Hilsdon, Lyme Regis, Dorset
Typeset by Type Study, Scarborough, North Yorkshire
Printed in Great Britain by TJ International, Padstow, Cornwall

ISBN 0 85369 455 9

A catalogue record for this book is available from the British Library

*Front cover images courtesy of Dr Andrew Bicknell and Ms Liz
Pontin, School of Animal and Microbial Sciences, University of
Reading, UK*

For Katie and Lucy

Contents

Preface

It has been a decade since the first gene therapy trial was initiated in a human patient. Since that time, more than 3500 patients have been treated with gene therapy in over 300 studies for a variety of genetic disorders. The initial hype and promise that surrounded this technology have waned somewhat due to limited clinical success and especially following the recent death of Jesse Gelsinger in the USA as a direct result of gene therapy to treat a partial deficiency in ornithine transcarbamylase enzyme. However, despite these limitations, gene therapy still offers a real chance of recovery from certain diseases that are not treatable by conventional means. Indeed, the completion of the Human Genome Project, which will provide information on every human gene and their control sequences, coupled with the development of new gene delivery methods and vectors, will enable new gene therapeutics to be developed and suggest that gene therapy will take its rightful place in medicine within the next few years.

This book overviews the technology behind gene therapy and provides examples of how the approach is being used in clinical medicine to treat a variety of genetic diseases, including cancer, AIDS, cardiovascular disease and rheumatoid arthritis. The first two chapters focus on the structure of DNA and gene regulation and overview the modes of delivery of therapeutic DNA to its site of action. The Human Genome Project and its implications for treating human diseases is then described in detail. Each subsequent chapter is devoted to gene therapy of a specific disease or group of diseases and describes the aetiology of the disease, the limitations of current therapies and the potential of ongoing and future clinical gene therapy trials. The final chapter discusses the use of xenotransplantation for human organ transplants and considers the advantages and disadvantages of this technology from social, economic and ethical viewpoints.

This book provides scientists and those healthcare workers who are, or will in the future be, involved in gene therapy trials with a thorough background to the technology of the therapeutic approach and provides details on how it is being used clinically. It will also be extremely useful for undergraduate and postgraduate biomedical students with an interest in DNA and its therapeutic potential and will serve as an ideal reference source for those who have an interest in learning more about this exciting technology.

Gavin Brooks
July 2001

Acknowledgements

I would like to take this opportunity to thank all of my co-authors, without whose contributions this volume would not have been possible. In addition, I would like to extend my thanks to Paul Weller, Linda Horrell, Tamsin Cousins and other members of the Pharmaceutical Press for commissioning this book and for their help and support throughout the writing stages. I also would like to thank the following people for their continued interest and encouragement during all stages of producing this book: my parents, Jean and Colin Brooks; Kim, Jonathan, Ruth and Rebekah Gregory; Edna, Jimmie and Matthew King; Jane, Jeremy, Samuel and Joseph Bradford-King; Debbie, Adam, Ethan and Natalia King; Mel, Andy, Daniel and Kate Mercer; Nicky, Nick and Phoebe Busbridge; Lilly, Tom, Lorie and Natalia Robinson; Karen, Michael, Rachel and Paul Seckl; Richard, Memy, Oriana and Sebastian Vile; Dawn, Gabriel, Nathalie and Saskia Cozma; Julie, Renny and Zoe Shorter; Rachel Darren, Jessica, Samuel and Jacob Kenyon; Annie, William, Theo, Rory and Georgia Bird; Allie, Charlie, Tom and Hattie Foster; Deena Wells; and, Mark and Claire Ward. Finally, I would like to express my very special thanks to my wife, Anna, who, despite this project keeping us apart for long periods of time, never failed to give me her full support and understanding, and to my daughters, Katie and Lucy, for always bringing a smile to my face.

About the editor

Gavin Brooks obtained a first-class honours degree in pharmacy from the School of Pharmacy, University of London in 1984 and subsequently registered as a pharmaceutical chemist in 1985. In October 1985 he was awarded a Royal Pharmaceutical Society Postgraduate Research Fellowship to enable him to undertake a PhD degree in the areas of organic chemistry and pharmacology at the School of Pharmacy, University of London. Dr Brooks then joined the Imperial Cancer Research Fund Laboratories in London as a post-doctoral fellow in 1988 where he investigated the signal transduction mechanisms involved in the progression of normal melanocytes to malignant melanoma cells. Following a successful period at the ICRF, Dr Brooks was recruited, in January 1992, to the Department of Cardiovascular Research, the Rayne Institute, St Thomas' Hospital in London, where he established an active cardiovascular cellular and molecular biology laboratory and became recognised as an expert in the area of cardiac myocyte cell cycle control. In July 1997, he left St Thomas' to join the biopharmaceutical company Prolifix Ltd, as head of their cardiovascular programme. In January 1999, Dr Brooks returned to academia where he now is Reader in Cardiovascular Biology at the University of Reading. His current research interests focus on understanding the mechanisms that control physiological and pathophysiological cardiovascular cell growth. Dr Brooks is the author of over 90 peer-reviewed research papers, review articles and abstracts, and was the editor of *Biotechnology in Healthcare*, also published by the Pharmaceutical Press. He currently lives in south Oxfordshire with his wife, Anna, and their two daughters, Katie and Lucy.

Contributors

Sandra Amor BSc, PhD
Senior Scientist, Department of Neuroinflammation, Division of
Neuroscience, Imperial College of Medicine, Charing Cross Hospital,
Fulham Palace Road, London W6 8RF; and Senior Scientist,
Department of Immunobiology, BPRC, Lange Kleiweg 139, 2288 GJ
Rijswijk, The Netherlands

Katrina A Bicknell BSc, PhD
Postdoctoral Research Fellow, Cardiovascular Research Group, School
of Animal and Microbial Sciences, University of Reading,
Whiteknights, PO Box 228, Reading, Berks RG6 6AJ

Jan Bondeson MD, PhD, MSc, LicSc
Senior Lecturer and Consultant Rheumatologist, Department of
Rheumatology, University of Wales College of Medicine, Heath Park,
Cardiff CF14 4XN

Gavin Brooks BPharm, PhD, MRPharmS
Reader in Cardiovascular Biology, School of Animal and Microbial
Sciences, University of Reading, Whiteknights, PO Box 228, Reading,
Berks RG6 6AJ

Ian Dunham MA, DPhil
Group Leader, Human Genetics Group, The Sanger Centre,
Wellcome Trust Genome Campus, Cambridge CB10 1SA

Marc Feldmann MB BS, BSc, PhD, FRCPath, FRCP, FMedSci
Head of Cytokine and Cellular Immunology, Kennedy Institute of
Rheumatology Division, Imperial College School of Medicine,
1 Aspenlea Road, London W6 8LH

Sarah J Fidler BSc, MB BS, MRCP, PhD
Clinical Lecturer in GU Medicine, Department of Genito-Urinary
Medicine and Communicable Diseases, Division of Medicine, Imperial
College School of Medicine at St Mary's, Norfolk Place,
London W2 1PG

A John Frater BA, MB BS, MRCP
Clinical Training Fellow, Department of Genito-Urinary Medicine
and Communicable Diseases, Division of Medicine, Imperial
College School of Medicine at St Mary's, Norfolk Place,
London W2 1PG

Christine Kinnon BSc, PhD
Head of Molecular Immunology Unit, Institute of Child Health,
30 Guilford Street, London WC1N 1EH

Ravinder N Maini BA, MB, BChir, FRCP, FRCP(E), FMedSci
Director, Kennedy Institute of Rheumatology Division, Imperial
College School of Medicine, 1 Aspenlea Road, London W6 8LH

Myra O McClure PhD, FRCPath
Professor of Retrovirology and Honorary Consultant in GU Medicine,
Jefferiss Research Laboratories, Wright-Fleming Institute, Division of
Medicine, Imperial College School of Medicine at St Mary's, Norfolk
Place, London W2 1PG

Iain McNeish MRCP, PhD
ICRF Clinician Scientist, ICRF Molecular Oncology Unit, Imperial
College School of Medicine, Hammersmith Hospital, Du Cane Road,
London W12 0NN

Mehregan Movassagh BSc, MPhil
Postgraduate Research Student, Cardiovascular Research Group,
School of Animal and Microbial Sciences, University of Reading,
Whiteknights, PO Box 228, Reading, Berks RG6 6AJ

Michael J Seckl PhD, FRCP
Consultant Oncologist and Reader in Medical Oncology, Section of
Cancer Cell Biology, Imperial College School of Medicine,
Hammersmith Hospital, Du Cane Road, London W12 0NN

Paul A Smith BSc
Research Assistant, Department of Neuroinflammation, Division of
Neuroscience, Imperial College of Medicine, Charing Cross Hospital,
Fulham Palace Road, London W6 8RF

Adrian J Thrasher MB, PhD, MRCP(UK)
Reader in Molecular Immunology, Molecular Immunology Unit,
Institute of Child Health, 30 Guilford Street, London WC1N 1EH

Dharmesh J Vara BSc, MRPharmS
Postgraduate Research Student, Cardiovascular Research Group,
School of Animal and Microbial Sciences, University of Reading,
Whiteknights, PO Box 228, Reading, Berks RG6 6AJ

Graham J Wallace BSc
Research Assistant, Department of Neuroinflammation, Division of
Neuroscience, Imperial College of Medicine, Charing Cross Hospital,
Fulham Palace Road, London W6 8RF

Robin A Weiss PhD, FRS
Professor of Viral Oncology, Wohl Virion Centre, Windeyer Institute
of Medical Sciences, University College London, 46 Cleveland Street,
London W1P 6DB

1

An introduction to DNA and its use in gene therapy

Gavin Brooks

The discovery, almost 50 years ago, of the structure of deoxyribonucleic acid (DNA) by James Watson and Francis Crick (Watson and Crick, 1953) stands out as one of the most important scientific findings of the last millennium. Since DNA is so crucial to our existence and since small mutations in one or more genetic sequences can have devastating effects for the affected individual, it is essential that we fully understand how DNA controls life if we want to cure individuals who suffer from a genetic disease. The recent sequencing of the human genome (see Chapter 3) now offers us the very real possibility of identifying those genes responsible for a particular genetic disease. The identification of such genes might enable the defective gene to be replaced with a normal gene by gene therapy or gene transfer, thereby offering a possible cure for patients who suffer from such disorders.

The aim of this opening chapter is to provide the reader with an introduction to how DNA is synthesised in cells and to provide information on how the expression of specific genes encoded within that DNA is controlled. In addition, it serves as an introduction to the concept of using DNA as a drug to treat various genetic diseases and discusses some of the ethical, social and commercial issues surrounding the use of this technology. Subsequent chapters will deal more specifically with how DNA is delivered into body cells and tissues and is then used as a drug for the treatment of a variety of genetic disorders.

DNA and RNA molecules

DNA is the most important substance known to humanity since it carries within its structure the hereditary information that determines the structures of proteins – the essential elements that are the building blocks for all cells and tissues. DNA also provides the instructions for directing cells to grow and divide and sends the messages required by fertilised eggs to differentiate into the multitude of specialised cells that make up our bodies. Since Watson and Crick first published the double helical structure of DNA in 1953 (Watson and Crick, 1953), investigators have begun to understand more clearly how DNA controls the expression of genes and proteins within cells and consequently why one particular cell differentiates into one cell type, e.g. a brain cell, whilst another differentiates into a completely different cell type, e.g. a liver cell.

Chromosomes and chromatin

DNA is packaged within chromosomes in the nuclei of cells. Chromosomes are relatively large particles (a few micrometres in size) that are visible by light microscopy. Each chromosome is composed of a centromere from which protrudes four arms, each sealed by a telomere that helps to confer stability to the ends of the chromosome. Essentially, these structures can be regarded as assemblies of units made up of DNA, ribonucleic acid (RNA) and proteins, which are precisely duplicated during each cell division. The human somatic cell (i.e. any cell other than a gamete or germ cell precursor) contains 22 pairs of autosomal chromosomes and two sex-determining chromosomes – XX in the female and XY in the male. Since somatic cells contain two copies of each chromosome they are referred to as diploid; germ cells, on the other hand, contain only one chromosome partner from each pair and are referred to as haploid. When chromosomes become abnormal, for example due to the effects of certain drugs, X- or γ-radiations or other noxious agents, they can lead to the development of diseases such as cancer (see Chapter 5). Such chromosomal abnormalities can be detected by molecular biological analyses such as the polymerase chain reaction (PCR), that amplifies very rapidly minute amounts of DNA (in the form of complementary DNA or cDNA – see below) into larger quantities that can be used for analysis. Indeed, approaches such as PCR are used routinely in the diagnosis of such genetic disorders.

Chromosomes themselves consist of compactly folded mixtures of DNA and proteins called chromatin. Chromatin is composed of a string of DNA, approximately 1 m (metre) long and 0.2 nm wide, wound around a core of proteins called histones. Chromatin itself is composed of individually packaged units called nucleosomes which, by electron microscopy, appear as beads on a thin string. The human genome consists of approximately 3×10^7 nucleosomes, each of which measures about 11 nm in diameter and consists of two copies of four different histones, H2A, H2B, H3 and H4. Each nucleosome is wound round by a constant length of DNA and is separated from its neighbours by a length of DNA that is bound to a fifth histone protein called H1. Thus, although the core histone components of each nucleosome remain constant in each repeated unit, different sequences of DNA are wrapped around them. In this way, the cell can package very large amounts of DNA into a very small volume. In addition to histones, DNA also is covered with other proteins within the chromosome, including transcription factors, other structural proteins and various regulatory factors such as nuclear receptors (e.g. steroid receptors).

Base pairing

The DNA molecule is a double-stranded helix composed of two single-stranded monomers. Each strand is made up of nucleotides composed of a phosphosugar component attached to one of four different bases: the two purines, adenine (A) and guanine (G); and the two pyrimidines, thymine (T) and cytosine (C) (Figure 1.1). Each nucleotide is linked to its neighbours via covalent bonds made between the phosphates and sugars, forming a sugar–phosphate backbone. Each base has a specific, high affinity for only one other base, such that G recognises (base pairs with) C and A base pairs with T. The number of base pairs in a particular DNA sequence is used to record the size of that sequence. For example, the human insulin gene is ~1.5 thousand base pairs (kilobase pairs, kb) long, whereas the human dystrophin gene is more than 2000 kb long. It is estimated that there are three billion base pairs in the human genome, encoding 40 000–50 000 genes (see Chapter 3 for more details). The two strands of DNA are held together by non-covalent hydrogen bonding between the bases on each strand. Since base pairing is very specific, the nucleotide sequence of one strand can be deduced from, and is determined by, the other strand. Each strand of double-stranded helical DNA is directional, such that each has a 5′ and 3′ end; thus, the two strands are said to be complementary and antiparallel to one another (Figure 1.1). When a new DNA molecule is synthesised it always occurs in a 5′ to 3′ direction. Thus, the synthesis of the two strands of DNA occurs in opposite directions since the 5′ end of one strand is base paired with the 3′ end of the other (Figure 1.1).

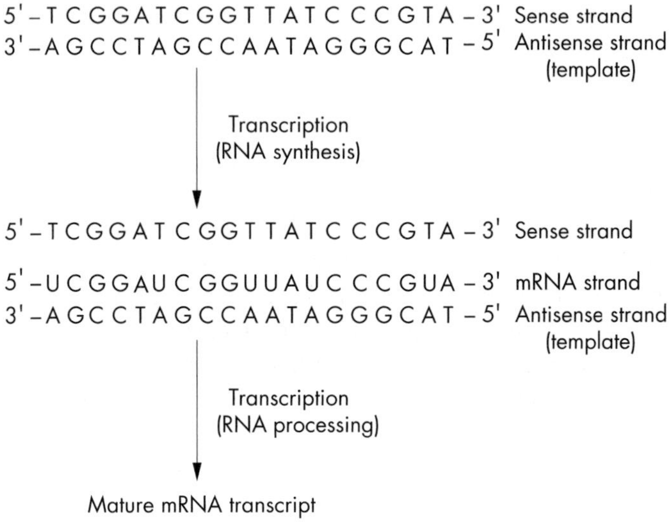

Figure 1.1 Schematic diagram to show how a hypothetical gene is transcribed from a double-stranded DNA sequence.

Transcription

Transcription is the process whereby a gene sequence within a DNA strand is copied into a messenger RNA (mRNA) molecule. The mRNA molecule (also referred to as the transcript) represents the sequence of a specific gene and is an intermediate product that serves as a template for the synthesis of a protein encoded for by that gene (the process called translation – see below). During transcription, one of the two strands of DNA, called the coding or sense strand, is copied into an mRNA molecule. The DNA sequence that is copied into an mRNA molecule is called a gene. Other RNA molecules also produced from DNA are used directly in the cell and are not translated into proteins (e.g. transfer RNA and ribosomal RNA). Not all DNA codes for RNA; in fact, the majority of the DNA in the genome does not code for anything specific and is called silent or nonsense DNA. Nonsense DNA is important, however, for separating gene sequences from each other. If individual genes were not separated in this way, problems could occur for the cell when it had to decide which protein to make, since specific recognition sequences found upstream (5′) of the transcribed gene would be lost in an adjacent gene sequence. The DNA strand that is antiparallel to the coding strand is called the non-coding or antisense strand and it is this strand that serves as the template for mRNA synthesis (since the antisense DNA strand determines the sequence of the sense strand, it also determines the sequence of the mRNA strand). By convention, the coding and mRNA strands are written from left to right, corresponding to the 5′ to 3′ direction. When a new protein is required by the cell, a portion of the coding strand of DNA is copied into a single-stranded RNA molecule by a process called transcription, which relies on complementarity of base pairing between DNA bases and RNA bases. The nucleotide sequence that is copied into RNA specifies an amino acid sequence from which a protein is ultimately produced by a process called translation. As is the case with DNA, RNA is made up of four different purine or pyrimidine bases on a phosphosugar backbone. Three of these bases (A, G and C) are identical to those found in DNA, but T is replaced by uridine (U) in RNA, where it base pairs with A (U is identical to T except that it does not have a methyl group on the basic ring). The cell can synthesise several different types of RNA, including mRNA, which corresponds to a nucleotide sequence that specifies an amino acid sequence (protein); ribosomal RNA (rRNA), which is the most abundant form of RNA and is important in protein synthesis; and transfer RNA (tRNA), which is involved in transporting amino acids to the site of translation on the ribosomes.

The process of RNA transcription proceeds as follows: RNA is copied (transcribed) from the non-coding strand of DNA (also referred to as the DNA template) and is synthesised in a 5′ to 3′ direction from the coding strand of DNA. Transcription of mRNA begins with the enzyme called RNA polymerase II recognising a specific sequence in the non-coding strand (called the initiation sequence), enabling it to bind to the 3′ end of the non-coding DNA strand. This attachment of RNA polymerase II is accompanied by a substantial conformational change in the DNA resulting in a local opening of the DNA duplex to enable the RNA molecule to be copied from the DNA template. Nucleotides are then recruited to the region and those complementary to the template are linked together to produce a new mRNA molecule that is complementary to the non-coding strand and identical to the coding strand of DNA, since its sequence has been determined by the base pairing of As to Us and Cs to Gs. Just as specific sequences are found in the DNA template that instruct RNA polymerase II to initiate transcription, so there are other sequences that instruct the enzyme to terminate the process such that the enzyme will be found at the 5′ end of the non-coding strand at the end of transcription. Once transcribed, the mRNA molecule is processed in the nucleus further by various splicing enzymes since not all of the copied mRNA molecule will code for a protein. The coding portion of the gene is located on one or more sections of the gene called exons (because these sections exit the nucleus into the cytoplasm). The regions located between the exons do not code for protein and are called introns (because they remain inside the nucleus; see Figure 1.2). The introns are excised from the mRNA molecule by the formation of loops, called lariats, that are then degraded in the nucleus. The 5′ and 3′ ends of the exon(s) also are not always coding sequences even though they form part of the mature mRNA molecule. Thus, the 5′ end of the exon becomes blocked by a 5′ to 5′ sugar–phosphate covalent bond called the RNA cap and the 3′ end of the exon has a string of repetitive As attached, known as the poly(A) tail. Indeed, mRNA commonly is referred to as poly(A)-rich RNA. Once processed in this manner, the mature mRNA molecule (now consisting only of exons) is transported into the cytoplasm of the cell where it is translated into protein (Figure 1.3).

Translation

Within a mature mRNA molecule, groups of three consecutive nucleotides form codons, each of which ultimately specifies one amino acid.

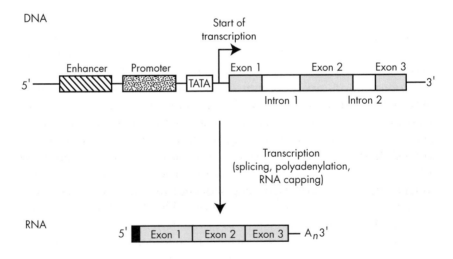

Figure 1.2 Hypothetical structure of a gene showing possible positions of enhancer, promoter, TATA box, exons and introns and subsequently how the mRNA molecule is modified prior to translation in the cytosol.

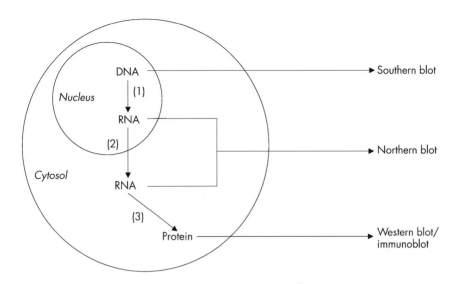

Figure 1.3   Schematic diagram to show where the processes of RNA synthesis (1), RNA processing (2) and translation (3) occur within a cell and the techniques used to identify DNA, RNA and protein species within a lysate prepared from such cells.

For example, the codon AUG encodes for methionine and the codon UGG encodes for tryptophan. It is the codons that form what is known as the genetic code, and since there are four nucleotides, there are a possible 4^3 (64) possible codons. However, only 20 amino acids (known as α-amino acids) are commonly found in proteins (there is a small number of other amino acids with important biological roles, e.g. the neurotransmitter γ-aminobutyric acid) and some amino acids are specified by more than one codon (e.g. serine is encoded by six different codons). In the process of translation, specific codons are recognised by tRNA molecules, each of which carries a specific amino acid and attaches this to the corresponding sequence on the mRNA molecule. Thus, the amino acid chain grows as directed by the codon sequence on the mRNA molecule. The translation process occurs on the ribosomes which bind the mRNA, tRNA, rRNA and ribosomal proteins together in a complex that allows the mRNA code to be read and translated into a polypeptide chain. Synthesis of the amino acid chain begins with the amino-terminal amino acid and finishes with the carboxyl-terminal amino acid and is encoded by the DNA coding sequence when read in the 5′ to 3′ direction.

Three of the 64 possible RNA codon combinations do not code for a specific amino acid. Instead these codons (UAA, UGA and UAG) serve as termination signals for protein synthesis. As soon as one of these codons is reached, the newly synthesised protein dissociates from the ribosomal complex and begins its function in the cell. In addition to the three termination codons, the AUG sequence (which encodes the amino acid methionine) can act as an initiation sequence for translation. Obviously, there will be many possible methionines encoded for within any particular protein and other sequences that are 5′ (upstream) of the actual initiation AUG sequence play a pivotal role in determining exactly which methionine residue will initiate protein synthesis.

Complementary DNA (cDNA)

cDNA is a double-stranded complementary DNA copy of a single-stranded mRNA molecule synthesised *in vitro* by reverse transcription. Since double-stranded DNA is more stable than single-stranded RNA, the cDNA molecule serves as a stable copy of a mature mRNA transcript (i.e. it contains exons only) and is useful for cloning procedures and other manipulations (including gene transfer) that require a stable product. Briefly, the mechanism of reverse transcription involves a three-step process. First, a strand of DNA that is complementary to the mRNA strand is synthesised using the enzyme reverse transcriptase and an oligodeoxythymidine primer that binds to the poly(A) tail of the mRNA sequence. Next, the mRNA strands of the mRNA–DNA hybrid are destroyed by the enzyme RNase H. The final step involves the generation of a DNA copy of the single-stranded DNA that was left following degradation of the mRNA strand. The final double-stranded DNA molecule is known as cDNA and represents a genetic sequence that lacks any introns. Thus, cDNAs are used routinely in cloning experiments where high expression of a particular gene product is required (e.g. in gene therapy).

Regulation of gene expression

Of the three billion base pairs that constitute the human genome, the majority are never transcribed into RNA (see Chapter 3). However, certain regions of the non-transcribed DNA have specific functions that instruct the cell to transcribe a specific gene. For example, RNA polymerases are instructed to attach to a short DNA sequence called the promoter that is upstream (5′) of the gene of interest (Figure 1.2). Although the promoter site is essential for instructing RNA polymerase where to start RNA synthesis, it is not sufficient by itself to permit the process to occur; other DNA sequences also are required. These additional DNA sequences are called enhancers and are recognised by specific protein molecules in the cell, e.g. transcription factors such as E2F and activator protein 2 (AP-2) (Figure 1.2). A factor that binds an enhancer is said to regulate gene transcription in a *trans*-regulatory manner and is referred to as a *trans*-activating factor, i.e. it is a protein produced from a gene that is physically distinct from the regulated gene (e.g. on a different chromosome). In contrast, the enhancer regulates gene transcription in a *cis*-regulating manner following the binding of a specific *trans*-acting protein. Activation of an enhancer results in an up to 1000-fold increase in the basal rate of transcription. Indeed, the effect of an enhancer on the rate of transcription is so strong that the effects still can be observed if it is placed at a distance several thousand base pairs from the transcription start site. Furthermore, enhancers are able to function in either orientation and therefore do not necessarily need to reside 5′ to a gene – they can be located within, or even downstream from, the transcribed region.

DNA sequences that are recognised by specific factors are commonly referred to as responsive elements, and all have regions, called consensus sequences, that are recognised by specific proteins. A consensus sequence is one that represents the bases most often found at a particular position in a DNA strand when a large number of similar DNA sequences are compared. Two common consensus sequences are the TATA box, which consists of seven nucleotides, five of which are invariant, and the CAAT box, which also contains invariant and variant nucleotides. Different enhancers have consensus sequences that are different for different regulatory proteins. For example, the glucocorticoid responsive element (GRE) has a consensus sequence that is different from the cyclic AMP responsive element (CRE), although a core consensus sequence for all eukaryotic enhancers has been identified as 5′-GTGAAG-3′.

Analysis of DNA

One of the most basic of all procedures in molecular biology is the purification of nucleic acid. Many different approaches can be used to study DNA and it is impossible to give an exhaustive list of all available methodologies here. However, a few of the routine procedures used are detailed below:

Preparation and purification of DNA

One advantage of studying DNA is that it is extremely stable. The stability of DNA is demonstrated by the fact that it can be extracted and purified from archival and even mummified remains that could be thousands of years old. The key step in isolating DNA is the removal of proteins which can be achieved by the sequential extraction of aqueous solutions of nucleic acids with phenol, then with phenol/chloroform and finally with chloroform alone. DNA is recovered from the extracted aqueous solution by precipitation with ethanol. Whilst this procedure produces good-quality DNA from cDNA preparations necessary for cloning, additional measures are required for preparation of DNA from cells and/or tissues, so that most of the protein in these cases is removed by digesting with proteolytic enzymes such as pronase or proteinase K prior to extraction with organic solvents. The above methods can be used to isolate DNA sequences that are >30 kb in length, although more commonly sequences of 10–30 kb are recovered.

Once isolated, the DNA preparation can be further purified either: by resuspending the precipitated DNA pellet in distilled water and re-precipitating with ethanol; by chromatography through Sephadex G-50 which separates high-molecular-weight DNA from smaller molecules; or by agarose gel electrophoresis. Although these techniques will not be discussed further here, details can be found in the References and suggestions for further reading section at the end of this chapter.

Detection of specific DNA sequences

Two of the most commonly used techniques for detecting the presence of a specific DNA sequence or gene in a preparation of genomic DNA are Southern blotting and the polymerase chain reaction (PCR).

Southern blotting

This method, which was first developed by Edward Southern in 1975, takes advantage of the fact that DNA fragments of different sizes can be separated in an electric field by agarose gel electrophoresis. The separated DNA fragments are then denatured within the gel in the presence of alkali, neutralised and then transferred and immobilised onto a nitro-cellulose or nylon filter. The DNA attached to the filter is then incubated (hybridised) to a ^{32}P-labelled cDNA or RNA probe that carries the sequence of the gene of interest. If the gene of interest is expressed in the immobilised DNA sample, the radiolabelled probe will bind to it in a specific manner and this binding can be observed as an image on photographic film following autoradiography. This technique has become the standard method for locating specific sequences in cloned DNA and also for identifying sequences within digests of total eukaryotic DNA.

Polymerase chain reaction (PCR)

Since it was first described more than 15 years ago, PCR has revolutionised almost every field of biological and clinical research and has rapidly become established as one of the most widely used molecular biological techniques available. The technique is a rapid, inexpensive and simple method for the exponential amplification of very small amounts of DNA into much larger quantities. Over the past few years, PCR has become a routine method for amplifying specific sequences of DNA either in a cloned cDNA fragment or in a total DNA preparation and is used routinely in the diagnosis of a variety of genetic disorders. In medicine, for example, the PCR has had a major impact on diagnosis and screening of genetic diseases, including cancer, and has been used for the rapid detection of fastidious or slow-growing microorganisms and viruses (e.g. mycobacteria and HIV).

One advantage of PCR over other methods of DNA purification and separation is that the reaction can be carried out on total DNA that has not had to be fragmented with restriction enzymes. Restriction enzymes are endonucleases, isolated primarily from prokaryotes, that recognise specific sequences within double-stranded DNA and are used to 'cut' DNA into different sized fragments. There are a number of known restriction enzymes, each of which recognises a different sequence, and different stretches of DNA will produce different fragmentation patterns when cut with these enzymes since each sequence is unique. The different fragments can then be separated and visualised by agarose gel electrophoresis. Once a DNA fragment of interest has been amplified it is then separated on an agarose gel and subjected to Southern blotting as described above.

Analysis of RNA

Preparation and purification of mRNA

Unlike DNA, which is a relatively stable molecule, mRNA is rapidly degraded after death and has a very short half-life (minutes) once extracted from cells or tissues. One of the major reasons for this is contamination by RNases, a ubiquitous series of heat-stable enzymes that rapidly degrade RNA. These enzymes are present in blood, all tissues, most bacteria and moulds that are present in the environment and even on the fingertips of investigators. Therefore, any analysis of RNA needs to be carried out under very clean conditions and, at the absolute minimum, all operators should wear gloves. Since mRNA represents only 2–3% of all RNA species in a cell, some additional purification is required prior to analysis. One common method for the preparation of total RNA involves rapid homogenisation of fresh or rapidly frozen material in guanidinium thiocyanate, which inactivates RNases, followed by extraction with phenol/chloroform and precipitation of the extracted RNA with ethanol as described for DNA above. The RNA pellet is then extracted with high salt which solubilises double-stranded nucleic acids (the remaining traces of DNA and small RNAs) but not single-stranded rRNA or mRNA. The yield of total RNA by this method is in the region of 1 μg of total RNA per mg of fresh tissue, although this does depend upon the cell/tissue type under investigation. If the gene of interest is not expressed at particularly high levels it may be necessary to purify this preparation further to enrich for mRNA species. There are many commercial kits now available that make the preparation of mRNA relatively simple. Most are based on the principle that mRNA has a poly(A) tail (see above) and that, in the presence of salt, hydrogen bonds will form readily between synthetic homopolymers of either uridine [poly(U)] or thymidine [oligo(dT)], i.e. those bases that base pair specifically with A. When the salt is removed, the hydrogen bonds dissociate, thereby enabling the bound mRNA to be separated from the synthetic oligonucleotide. When oligo(dT) is immobilised on a solid support and mixed with total RNA, the poly(A) tail of the mRNA component will hybridise to the oligo(dT) in the presence of high salt whilst the rRNA is washed away. Rewashing the oligo(dT)–mRNA hybrid with water then releases an enriched mRNA preparation that can be precipitated with ethanol and the pellet resuspended in water prior to analysis.

Detection of specific RNA sequences

As with the detection of DNA, a number of different techniques are available for the detection of mRNA levels within a sample. These techniques include Northern blotting and reverse transcription PCR.

Northern blotting

This is a technique similar to Southern blotting, described above. Briefly, it separates an RNA sample according to size in a denaturing agarose gel followed by transfer and immobilisation of the denatured RNA onto a nitrocellulose or nylon filter. The filter is then used in a hybridisation assay with a radiolabelled cDNA probe that is specific for a selected gene. Quantitation of mRNA expression is carried out by autoradiography followed by densitometry of the resultant photographic signal(s).

Reverse transcription PCR (RT-PCR)

PCR can be used quantitatively to measure the levels of specific mRNAs in different cell populations or tissues or in the same tissue at different developmental stages by a technique called RT-PCR. In this reaction the mRNA first is reverse transcribed into complementary DNA (cDNA), which is then subjected to conventional PCR amplification. The amount of mRNA of interest is compared with the amount of amplified mRNA from a control gene (which produces a different-sized band by electrophoresis) in the same reaction (Figure 1.4). This method is particularly useful when analysing low-abundance mRNAs or when limiting amounts of material are available. However, Northern blotting remains the preferred technique for quantitating levels of expression of a particular mRNA species if sufficient starting material is available (~10–30 μg of total RNA or 2–5 μg of mRNA).

Analysis of proteins

Preparation and purification of proteins

Proteins can be isolated from cells or tissues by a number of procedures. Initial disruption of the cells is achieved either by osmotic shock, ultrasonic vibration, grinding or lysis in a detergent-containing buffer. It is important, however, to include a range of protease inhibitors in any buffers since, once the cell is disrupted, a number of proteases will be released into the milieu that could break down a number of labile proteins that normally would be separated from these degradative enzymes. These procedures dissociate most cellular membranes, including plasma membranes and those of the endoplasmic reticulum. This is then followed by fractionation into the various subcellular components of the

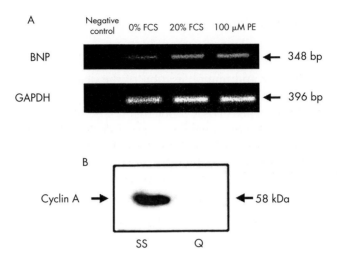

Figure 1.4   Examples of (A) reverse transcription polymerase chain reaction (RT-PCR) and (B) immunoblot analyses to determine mRNA and protein expressions, respectively. (A) Detection of brain natriuretic peptide (BNP) and glyceraldehyde-3-phosphate dehydrogenase (GAPDH) mRNA expressions in neonatal cardiac myocytes treated with media containing 0% fetal calf serum (FCS), 20% FCS or 100 μM phenylephrine (PE) for 48 hours. Total RNA extraction was carried out from 0% FCS, 20% FCS and 100 μM PE-treated myocytes and cDNA preparations carried out using 5 μg of total RNA. Semi-quantitative RT-PCR was performed using gene-specific primers and agarose gel (1%) electrophoresis was used to separate amplified products. Gels were stained with ethidium bromide and products visualised under ultraviolet light. (B) Detection of cyclin A expression in serum-stimulated (SS) and quiescent (Q) NIH 3T3 fibroblasts. Cell lysates (20 μg) were separated by 12% SDS-PAGE and the separated proteins transferred to a nitrocellulose membrane. The membrane then was incubated with rabbit anti-cyclin A antibody (Santa Cruz, USA) and primary antibody binding detected with a goat anti-rabbit secondary antibody cross-linked to horseradish peroxidase. Detection of specific binding was determined by enhanced chemiluminescence.

cell, which can be achieved either by filtration, chromatography and/or centrifugation. These latter steps enable separation of contaminating nucleic acids, mitochondria and lysosomes from the protein preparation. Further purification of some proteins that are heat stable (approximately 5% of all cellular proteins) can be achieved by boiling the protein extract for approximately 5 minutes followed by centrifugation that will pellet the heat-labile proteins in the sample. Once the protein extract has been purified in this manner it can then be analysed for the presence of specific proteins by one of the methods described below.

Detection of specific proteins

A variety of detection methods are available for determining the presence of specific proteins in an extract, most of which rely upon the interaction of the protein with a specific antibody. Whilst it is possible to visualise certain proteins on a polyacrylamide gel by staining the separated proteins with Coomassie blue or silver stain, these approaches do not provide direct evidence for the presence of a specific protein; an antibody that recognises a specific amino acid sequence in the desired protein would be required to demonstrate the presence of that protein.

Polyacrylamide gel electrophoresis and immunoblotting (Western blotting)

This method is one of the most commonly used analytical techniques for demonstrating the presence of a particular protein in a sample preparation. The method relies on the fact that proteins usually have a net positive or negative charge that reflects the mixture of charged amino acids that they contain. If an electric field is applied to a solution containing a protein molecule, the protein will migrate at a rate that depends upon its net charge and on its size and shape (electrophoresis). A modified version of this separation, called sodium dodecylsulfate-polyacrylamide gel electrophoresis (SDS-PAGE), was developed in the mid-1960s. SDS-PAGE uses a highly cross-linked gel of polyacrylamide as an inert matrix through which the proteins migrate, and the detergent SDS. SDS is negatively charged and large numbers of SDS molecules are bound by each protein molecule; this tends to overcome the intrinsic charge of the protein, ensuring that each protein migrates towards the positive electrode when a current is applied. Proteins of the same size then tend to behave similarly and larger molecules are retarded much more than smaller ones since the polyacrylamide acts as a molecular sieve. As a result, a complex mixture of proteins is fractionated into a series of discrete protein bands arranged in order of their molecular weight (Figure 1.4).

SDS-PAGE is a very powerful procedure for analysing and separating proteins and can be used to analyse all types of proteins, including those that are water-insoluble. The method is capable of separating around 50 different proteins from a complex mixture, although other techniques are available (e.g. two-dimensional (2D) electrophoresis) that are capable of separating more than 1000 proteins on a single gel. Recent advances in proteomics now enable 2D electrophoresis to be automated such that the range of proteins expressed in one extract (e.g. the control) can be compared with the expression profile of proteins expressed in another extract (e.g. following drug treatment). Those proteins that differ in their expressions between the two groups can then be identified with the help of a computer program, the protein is excised from the gel, purified and characterised further (e.g. by mass spectrometry).

In the immunoblotting procedure, a protein mixture is separated into proteins of different sizes by SDS-PAGE. The resolved proteins are then transferred to a nitrocellulose filter and incubated with an antibody that specifically recognises the protein of interest. A secondary antibody, which recognises the first antibody and is either attached to an enzyme (e.g. horseradish peroxidase) or is labelled with a radioactive isotope (e.g. ^{125}I), is then incubated with the filter. In the case of enzyme-linked antibodies, a colour reaction develops specifically in the region of the protein of interest when the substrate for the enzyme is subsequently incubated with the filter. This can be visualised either directly or as an image on photographic film (in the case of radiolabelled secondary antibodies, this image is visualised directly without the need for a substrate) (Figure 1.4). The levels of protein expression can then be determined by densitometry.

Immunoprecipitation

In this technique, the protein of interest is precipitated from a mixture of proteins by first incubating with an antibody that is specific for the protein of interest (primary antibody). A secondary antibody is then added to the mix that recognises an immunoglobulin component of the primary antibody. This secondary antibody is covalently linked to sepharose or agarose beads, making it possible to isolate the protein of interest by centrifugation as a complex comprising the protein of interest, the primary antibody and the secondary antibody attached to sepharose beads. The immunoprecipitate can then be separated by SDS-PAGE, which releases the isolated protein from the complex. The isolated protein can then be identified either with the same primary antibody by Western blotting or the nitrocellulose filter could be incubated with an antibody directed against another protein to see whether the first protein exists as a complex with another protein *in vivo*.

Immunohistochemistry

This technique enables the investigator to determine the expression and localisation of a particular protein in a tissue section. A thin section (a few micrometres thick) of the tissue of interest is prepared and incubated with the primary antibody. Following detection of the primary antibody with an appropriate fluorescent-labelled secondary antibody, the expression and localisation of the protein of interest can be observed by fluorescence microscopy.

Use of DNA as a drug – an introduction to gene therapy

A number of human diseases are known to be genetic in origin (e.g. Huntington's chorea and cystic fibrosis) and virtually all disease, except for some trauma, has a hereditary component (SoRelle, 2000). Thus, the opportunity to treat such disorders by replacing the defective gene(s) with a normal healthy gene (gene therapy) offers a novel therapeutic approach for patients who suffer from such diseases. The sequencing of the human genome (see Chapter 3) will permit the relatively simple identification of genes associated with a particular disease and also pinpoint exactly where on the three billion base pair DNA strand the gene is located. Once we have this information, new diagnostic tests can be developed that will enable individuals to be tested for those diseases to which they are prone and then given an indication of their risk of developing that disease. Such genetic profiling also will enable physicians to predict which drugs will and will not work for a particular patient. Indeed, this new field of medicine, called pharmacogenetics, will enable a doctor to tailor therapy to an individual's requirements. Despite these ideals, there still is a long way to go before such technology can become routine. Also, the possibility of using DNA as a drug for the treatment of genetic diseases is still very much in its infancy. One reason for this is that, unlike monogenetic disorders such as severe combined immune deficiency (SCID), which is caused by a mutation in the adenosine deaminase (ADA) gene (see Chapter 4), very few diseases are caused by a single gene mutation; most are caused by the mutation of multiple genetic components. For example, cancer usually involves multiple genetic lesions within the same cell and it is unlikely that the nature of every one of these oncogenic mutations are yet known. Indeed, as the number of diseases that are known to have at least some genetic component increases, so the definition of gene therapy has become much broader. Now, gene therapy routinely is evoked to encompass the use of DNA as a drug to alleviate the symptoms of a disease, even if the therapeutic genes are not strictly 'corrective' (in the sense of restoring a function known to be mutated in the affected cells). Hence, the delivery of cytotoxic genes to kill cancer cells (rather than to correct the oncogenic mutations within them) also is accepted as gene therapy. Thus, in its broadest terms, gene therapy represents 'an opportunity for the treatment of genetic disorders in adults and children by genetic modification of human body cells' (Report of the UK Health Minister's Gene Therapy Advisory Committee, 1995).

Although gene therapy is a simple concept, in practice it poses a number of complications. For instance, the correct gene must be inserted into the correct cells and expressed in those cells at the correct time. Also, gene expression normally should be maintained for long periods (for the lifespan of the patient in the case of inherited diseases) in order to minimise the number of times a patient requires treatment. Overcoming such problems for each disease is a formidable task and, despite the early promise of this form of treatment, this probably accounts for the limited clinical success that has been achieved to date with gene therapy.

All of the gene therapy trials currently approved for use in human patients target somatic cells that will live only as long as the patient. This ensures that the genetic treatment will affect only one generation and will not alter the genetic makeup of any offspring of the patient, assuming there is no inadvertent spread of the therapeutic gene(s) to the gametes. This is known as somatic gene therapy, and its purpose is to alleviate disease in the treated individual, and in that individual alone. In contrast, it also is possible to target directly the gametes (sperm and ova) in order to modify the genetic profile, not of the current, but of the subsequent generation of unborn 'patients'. Gene transfer at an early stage of embryonic development also might have similar effects by achieving gene transfer to both somatic and germ line cells. This is germ line gene therapy. The attraction of germ line gene therapy for the treatment of disease is that, at least in theory, permanent genetic cures might be achieved by delivering a functional copy of a mutated gene to every cell of the resulting progeny. However, there is extensive apprehension about the development of germ line gene therapy research programmes. The ability to alter the genetic profile of subsequent generations rightly invokes many spectres. Apart from the inability to predict the long-term sequelae of altering the germ line by delivery of exogenous genetic material at the scientific level, there are many ethical issues raised by the prospect of treating 'patients' whose consent it is impossible to obtain. In addition, although it currently is not possible to manipulate genetically traits such as 'intelligence' or 'beauty', there is a perceived fear of such technology being abused in eugenic-type breeding programmes in the future. As a result, the major ethical and regulatory bodies of gene therapy both in the US and in Europe have placed a moratorium on the consideration of any germ line gene therapy treatments of human patients because of 'insufficient knowledge to evaluate the risks to future generations'. However, it is important that such issues be addressed at a regulatory level sooner rather than later. A refusal to consider applications for germ line trials in patients will in no way prevent continued research into the direct genetic modification of the germ line and the relevant ethical and regulatory dilemmas will simply be deferred, rather than solved, by procrastination.

Despite the obvious advantages that might be gained from replacing a defective gene with a normal DNA sequence, a number of ethical, social and commercial issues surround the technology. For instance, one problem with this type of work is that the outcome of an error in technology might not be observed for many years, and recent concern from a number of countries has highlighted the need for restraint in matters associated with xenotransplantation (see Chapter 10). Furthermore, it is feared that unpredictable and perhaps irreversible side effects might occur in treated individuals. The social implications of such technology include the possibility that patients might suffer from depression as a result of being 'genetically altered' or might not be accepted by society in the way that they were before treatment. The unknown long-term consequences of the gene therapy also could play a significant role in the general well-being of the patient. Although genetic profiling, in which an individual has their genome analysed for potential mutations, has advantages for selecting suitable drug treatments and would permit such treatment to begin earlier, it does have certain downsides. One obvious caveat of this technology that has commercial implications is the fact that insurance companies and other such institutions also would want to access the available information prior to them granting life insurance policies etc. Quite clearly, a person shown to have a predisposition to a genetic disease could be severely penalised because of a mutation in their DNA, even though they might never develop the disease.

Probably the biggest setback for gene therapy occurred recently in the autumn of 1999 when Jesse Gelsinger, an 18-year-old high-school graduate from Arizona, died as a result of a gene therapy experiment. Gelsinger developed a fever and blood clots throughout his body within hours of treatment to correct partial ornithine transcarbamylase (OTC) deficiency, a rare metabolic disease that can cause a dangerous build-up of ammonia in the body. He died four days later (Lehrman, 1999). Although the exact reasons for the failure of the gene therapy remain unclear, researchers are investigating the adenovirus vector used to deliver the OTC gene to the liver. Although Gelsinger was the 18th and final patient in the phase I experiment, he was only the second person to receive a dose of 3.8×10^{13} virus particles, believed to be the highest so far with an adenovirus (Lehrman, 1999). As a direct consequence of this incident, the University of Pennsylvania Institute for Human Gene Therapy in the USA had its clinical trials programme terminated, since the Institute had failed to inform the US Food and Drug Administration of adverse effects experienced by other patients treated before Gelsinger. However, the researchers involved in the OTC trial were commended for their openness and for their prompt and full disclosure of the circumstances surrounding Gelsinger's case. Despite this attempt to preserve public confidence in gene therapy, six unreported deaths were documented by the *Washington Post* on 3rd November 1999 that had occurred in trials conducted at the Cornell Medical Center in Manhattan and at the Tufts University in Boston (Anon, 1999). In these cases, the two research team leaders, who are competing fiercely in a race to use gene therapy to grow new cardiac blood vessels for commercial exploitation, defended their decisions not to notify the National Institutes of Health, despite federal guidelines requiring such reporting. They both argued that these deaths were not due to the gene therapy but to the patients' underlying illnesses. Irrespective of the cause of death, these cases highlight the need to proceed with caution when using new technologies and for regulatory bodies to monitor closely, and report on, the progress of such trials.

Conclusions and summary

This chapter has described the basic concepts of DNA and RNA structure, transcription and translation and the procedures for purifying and identifying specific sequences or proteins in a nucleic acid or protein preparation. In addition, it has introduced the concept of using DNA as a drug to treat certain genetic diseases (gene therapy). Clearly a number of benefits exist for patients who could be treated by this route; however, a number of potential problems also can occur. Therefore, as is the case with any therapy the benefit-to-risk ratio must be assessed before a patient embarks on such a treatment programme. Subsequent chapters now will overview the different methods used for introducing DNA into target cells and tissues and address the use of gene therapy in the treatment of specific human diseases.

References

Anon (1999) The increasing opacity of gene therapy. *Nature* 402: 107.

Lehrman S (1999) Virus treatment questioned after gene therapy death. *Nature* 401: 517–518.

Report of the United Kingdom Health Minister's Gene Therapy Advisory Committee (1995) Guidance on making proposals to conduct gene therapy research on human subjects. *Hum Gene Ther* 6: 335–346.

SoRelle R (2000) Who owns your DNA? Who will own it? *Circulation* 101: e67–e68.

Watson J D, Crick F H C (1953) Molecular structure of nucleic acids: a structure for deoxyribose nucleic acid. *Nature* 171: 737–738.

Further reading

Alberts A, Bray D, Lewis J, *et al.*, eds (1994) *Molecular Biology of the Cell*, 3rd edn. New York: Garland Publishing.

Brooks G, ed. (1998) *Biotechnology in Healthcare: An Introduction to Biopharmaceuticals*. London: Pharmaceutical Press.

Kendrew J, ed. (1994) *The Encyclopedia of Molecular Biology*. Oxford: Blackwell Science.

Sambrook J, Fritsch E F, Maniatis T (1989) *Molecular Cloning. A Laboratory Manual*, 2nd edn. Cold Spring Harbor, NY: Cold Spring Harbor Laboratory Press.

Watson J D, Tooze J, Kurtz D T, eds (1983) *Recombinant DNA. A Short Course*. New York: Scientific American Books.

2

Methods for delivering DNA to target tissues and cells

Katrina A Bicknell and Gavin Brooks

In recent years, many diseases have been shown, at least in part, to have a genetic component to their aetiology. In some cases, the causal component of a particular disease state results from a mutation in the DNA encoding a single gene. For example, a mutation in the cystic fibrosis transmembrane conductance regulator (CFTR) gene predisposes an individual to cystic fibrosis (Riordan *et al.*, 1989). However, the majority of genetic diseases arise from mutations in more than one gene (Brooks and Vile, 1998). Thus, an important first step in establishing a therapy for a particular genetic disease that involves manipulation of the disrupted or affected gene(s) is the identification of the genetic component of that disease. Fortunately, this task will be made easier for the gene therapist with the completion of the sequencing of the human genome (see Chapter 3). Equally, there are other important considerations that must be addressed to establish the therapeutic potential of gene therapy in the treatment of any disease. Thus, the therapeutic DNA might be required to restore the activity of a gene that has been abolished or altered, to control the expression of a gene that has become deregulated and/or to block the function of an affected gene. All of these scenarios require the introduction of genetic material into affected cells to restore the original function of the mutated gene. The introduction of the therapeutic genetic material only into affected cells also might be necessary (e.g. in the treatment of cancers). Where available, the use of tissue- or cell-specific promoters to control the expression of the therapeutic DNA would ensure the expression of the introduced DNA only in the target cells and not in normal, neighbouring cells. Considerations such as specific characteristics of the targeted cells, the required duration of the gene therapy and/or the preferred route of administration of the therapeutic gene (Figure 2.1) might have an important influence on the therapeutic approach employed.

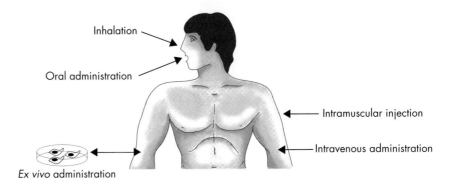

Figure 2.1 Possible routes for administration of therapeutic genetic material. The route of administration employed for the delivery of the therapeutic gene is dependent upon a number of factors, including the type of delivery system used and the cells targeted by the therapy. Potential routes of administration of therapeutic DNA include inhalation (e.g. via an aerosol), oral administration, intramuscular injection, intravenous injection or *ex vivo* administration, where target cells are removed from the patient, transduced in cell culture and then genetically altered cells are returned to the patient.

This chapter describes the various delivery systems that can be used to introduce genetic material into targeted cells, with a special emphasis on delivery methods that are suitable for human gene therapy approaches. The systems discussed include both viral and non-viral methods of DNA delivery.

Viral vectors for DNA delivery

Viral vectors for DNA delivery provide a powerful means for delivering therapeutic genes to targeted cells following *in vivo* or *ex vivo* administration. However, before viruses can be used to deliver therapeutic genetic material, they first must be modified to prevent the uncontrolled replication of the engineered viral vector and the potential for reversion of the therapeutic virus into an actively pathogenic form. In addition, viral genes that cause, or are involved in, the pathogenic host response also must be deleted or inactivated. The deletion of non-essential viral genes and of those involved in the replication and pathogenesis of the virus allows for the inclusion of non-viral genetic material in the viral genome.

The viral DNA-delivery vectors described in this section include both RNA and DNA viruses. The choice of viral vector in a gene therapy approach depends largely on the type of cell to be targeted by the therapy and also on the desired duration of expression of the therapeutic gene. The various properties of these vectors will be described in the following section.

Retroviral delivery vectors

Retroviruses have long been recognised as a powerful means of delivering foreign genes to target cells since they are relatively simple to construct as a vector-delivery system (Figure 2.2). Retroviruses are enveloped, single-stranded RNA viruses that enter target cells by a receptor-mediated endocytotic process (Figure 2.3). Once inside a host cell, the viral RNA is converted into DNA and is integrated into the genetic material of that cell. Since the retroviral DNA is incorporated into the genome of the host cell, the gene(s) encoded by this DNA will be maintained for the life of the host cell and upon division of the host cell, retroviral-encoded DNA will be inherited by the resulting daughter cells. Thus, the integration of the retroviral-encoded DNA into the host genome has the potential to permit the enduring expression of a therapeutic gene in a targeted cell.

As with all DNA-delivery systems, the use of retroviral vectors has both advantages and disadvantages (Table 2.1). Advantages of the system include the ability of retroviral vectors to integrate the therapeutic gene into the genetic material of targeted cells with high efficiency. Also, the introduced gene remains functional for the duration of the life of the cell and is inherited by any daughter cells. Additionally, retroviral vectors have been widely used and studied, therefore, as a delivery system they are well characterised and relatively safe. To ensure safety, the viral genes involved in the replication and pathogenesis of the retrovirus are removed in the viral vector and this reduces the risk of reactivation of the virulent form of the virus when expressed in target cells. One disadvantage, however, is that the retroviral-encoded therapeutic DNA can only enter the nucleus and be integrated into the genetic material of the host cell when the nuclear membrane of the infected cell is disrupted in the process of cell division (Roe *et al.*, 1993; Lewis and Emerman, 1994). Additionally, the size of the therapeutic DNA encoded by retroviral vectors is restricted to approximately 8 kb in size (Shin *et al.*, 2000) and this limits the use of such vectors for large genes, such as

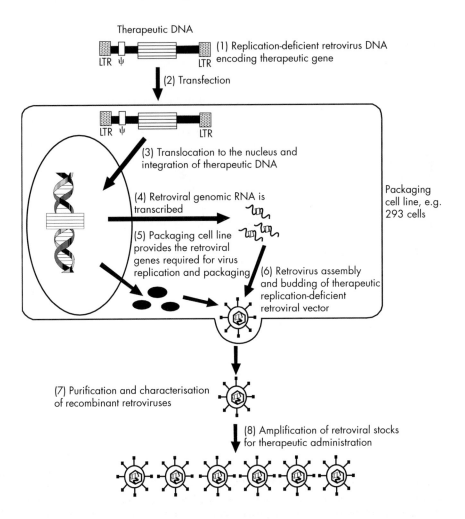

Figure 2.2 Retroviral vector construction for gene delivery. The therapeutic DNA is first cloned into the retroviral vector. Although replication-deficient, the retroviral vector must possess the sequences needed for retroviral integration and packaging, such as the long terminal repeats (LTRs) and the packaging sequence (ψ). A packaging cell line expressing retroviral genes necessary for replication and viral packaging then is transfected with the retroviral vector DNA. The transfected DNA is transported to the nucleus of the transfected cell and the retroviral vector DNA integrates into the genome of the transfected cell. The packaging cell line provides the retroviral genes necessary for viral replication, assembly and packaging and thus infective recombinant retroviral particles are released from transfected cells. The released recombinant retroviral particles must be purified and characterised to ensure they contain the therapeutic DNA and that they remain replication-deficient. Once characterised, the therapeutic retroviral vector must be amplified to produce stocks of sufficient titre for therapeutic administration.

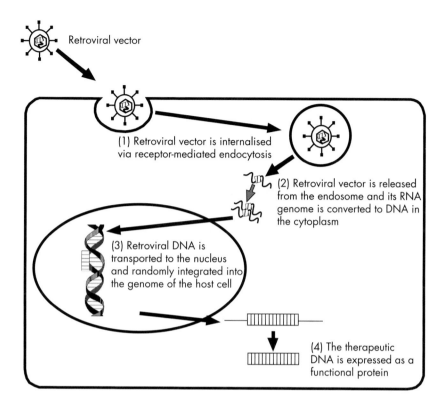

Figure 2.3   Retroviral-mediated gene delivery. The retroviral vector encoding the therapeutic gene binds to specific cell surface receptors and enters the cell by endocytosis. The viral vector then is released from the endosome and its RNA genome is converted to DNA before being transported into the nucleus of the cell. Once inside the nucleus, retroviral DNA is integrated randomly into the genome of the infected cell. The integrated retroviral and/or therapeutic DNA then is transcribed and translated into a functional protein using the transcriptional and translational machinery of the host cell. As the recombinant retroviral vector is integrated into the genome of the infected cell the expression of the therapeutic DNA is stable and is passed on to resultant progeny.

dystrophin (14 kb cDNA) (Koenig *et al.*, 1987), that cannot be delivered via this route. Although integration of the therapeutic gene into the genome of the host cell has been described previously as an advantage (see above), it should be noted that integration of the viral-encoded gene occurs randomly. Thus, disruption of essential host cell genes might have devastating effects and can result in tumorigenesis or loss of function of another essential gene.

Table 2.1 Advantages and disadvantages of viral-based gene delivery systems for gene therapy

Viral-based vectors	Advantages	Disadvantages
Retrovirus	Well characterised system Efficient gene transfer Long-term expression of stably integrated therapeutic gene possible	Safety issues Difficult to produce high-titre virus stocks Limited insert size (8 kb) Random integration of therapeutic gene Only some retrovirus-based vectors, e.g. lentiviruses can transduce non-dividing cells
Adenovirus	Enters dividing and non-dividing cells Not integrated into host genome Allows transient expression of therapeutic DNA	May stimulate severe host immune response Limited insert size (8 kb) Transient expression of therapeutic DNA limits therapeutic applications
Adeno-associated virus	Integrates into genome of host at a specific site Does not stimulate an immune response	Difficult to produce viral stocks

The first-generation retroviral vectors were largely derived from oncoretroviruses, such as the *Moloney murine leukaemia virus* (MoMLV), and were unable to transfer genes into non-dividing cells (Roe *et al.*, 1993; Lewis and Emerman, 1994). This limited the potential for their application as a delivery system in gene therapy since certain cell types that are targeted for such therapeutic approaches are non-dividing cells (e.g. cardiomyocytes and neurons). The utilisation of the lentivirus family of retroviruses, however, has overcome this shortcoming (Lewis and Emerman, 1994; Naldini *et al.*, 1996). Lentiviruses, which include *Human immunodeficiency virus type 1* (HIV-1), *Bovine immunodeficiency virus* (BIV), *Feline immunodeficiency virus* (FIV) and *Simian immunodeficiency virus* (SIV), are able to transfer genes to non-dividing cells (Lewis and Emerman, 1994; Naldini *et al.*, 1996). Obviously, safety concerns arise when HIV-based retroviral vectors are considered for gene therapy approaches since although the viral genes that encode the viral pathogenesis and replicative capacity of the HIV-based viral vector are inactivated or deleted, the risk of re-activation of the pathogenic virus must be considered carefully.

Retroviral vectors used in gene therapy are replication deficient, such that they are unable to replicate in the host cell and can infect only one cell (Mann *et al.*, 1983; Cone and Mulligan, 1984). This characteristic, although essential for the safety of viral vectors in gene therapy, imposes restrictions on the amounts of virus that can safely be administered (Kim *et al.*, 1998; Sheridan *et al.*, 2000). Figure 2.2 illustrates the experimental procedures used to produce retroviral vectors for use in gene therapy. Generation of the retroviral vector first involves insertion of the therapeutic gene into the replication-deficient retroviral genome. Since retroviral vectors are unable to replicate, the retroviral vector genome encoding the gene of interest must then be packaged into a viral envelope. Propagation and packaging of the viral vector requires the transfection of the viral vector into a packaging cell line, which provides the viral packaging machinery required for the production of infectious replication-deficient viral particles for *in vivo* or *ex vivo* administration (Mann *et al.*, 1983; Cone and Mulligan, 1984; Kim *et al.*, 1998; Sheridan *et al.*, 2000). Retroviral-mediated delivery of therapeutic DNA has been widely used in clinical gene therapy protocols, including the treatment of cancers, such as melanoma (Fujii *et al.*, 2000) and ovarian cancer (Tait *et al.*, 1999) (see Chapter 5), adenosine deaminase deficiency–severe combined immune deficiency (ADA–SCID) (Bordignon *et al.*, 1995; Onodera *et al.*, 1998) (see Chapter 4) and Gaucher's disease (Dunbar *et al.*, 1998).

Adenoviral and adeno-associated viral (AAV) delivery vectors

Adenoviruses are non-enveloped, double-stranded DNA viruses that normally elicit mild respiratory tract infections in humans upon infection. One of the major advantages of using adenoviral vectors for delivery of therapeutic DNA is that both dividing and non-dividing cells can be infected readily and most cells are susceptible to infection. Construction of these vectors (Figure 2.4) is slightly easier than for retroviruses (Figure 2.2), and various kits are now available from a range of manufacturers that simplify the procedure still further. During adenovirus infection, adenovirus particles enter host cells by receptor-mediated endocytosis and once inside the cytoplasm of the cell, the adenoviral DNA enters the host nucleus where viral reproduction occurs (Figure 2.5). In contrast to retroviral infection, adenoviral DNA is not integrated into the genome of the host cell; instead, adenoviral DNA remains separate (episomal) and the nuclear machinery of the host is re-organised

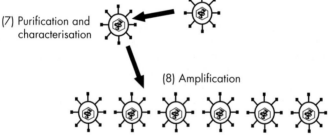

Figure 2.4   Adenoviral vector construction for gene delivery. (1) The therapeutic DNA must first be cloned into an adenoviral shuttle vector. (2) The adenoviral shuttle vector and replication-deficient adenoviral DNA are then co-transfected into a packaging cell line (e.g. 293 cells) that provides the adenoviral sequences required for viral replication and packaging. (3) Once inside the cell, the process of homologous recombination allows DNA to be swapped between the adenoviral DNA and the shuttle vector, thus generating recombinant adenoviruses that encode the therapeutic

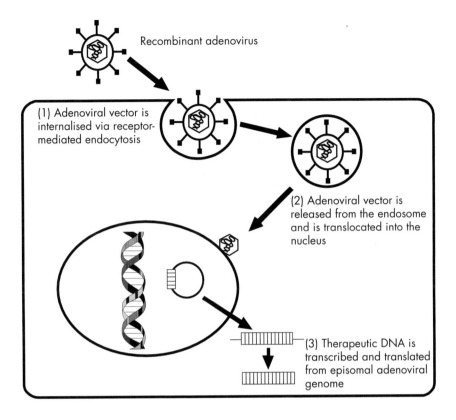

Recombinant adenovirus

(1) Adenoviral vector is internalised via receptor-mediated endocytosis

(2) Adenoviral vector is released from the endosome and is translocated into the nucleus

(3) Therapeutic DNA is transcribed and translated from episomal adenoviral genome

Figure 2.5   Adenoviral-mediated gene delivery. The recombinant adenoviral vector enters the cell by receptor-mediated endocytosis. In the endosome the viral particle is released from this internal cellular compartment and the adenoviral capsid is translocated into the nucleus. Once inside the nucleus, the therapeutic DNA is transcribed from the episomal recombinant adenoviral genome and, if necessary, the therapeutic RNA is translated. As the recombinant adenoviral vector is replication-deficient, the genome of the adenovirus is not replicated or packaged and therefore the infection is unable to spread to surrounding cells.

gene. (4) Generated adenoviruses are translocated to the nucleus, where they are then replicated and packaged (5) using proteins provided by the packaging cell line. (6) They are then released from the infected cells. (7) The recombinant adenoviruses are then purified and characterised to ensure that they have remained replication-deficient and that they express the appropriate therapeutic DNA. (8) Once characterised, the therapeutic recombinant adenovirus is amplified to generate high-titre stocks required for *in vivo* administration.

and employed by the infecting virus to facilitate viral replication. As is the case with retroviral vectors, the therapeutic gene replaces genes involved in the replication and pathogenesis of the adenovirus when adenoviral vectors are constructed. Therefore, nuclear transcription of the therapeutic gene in the host cell is initiated in place of adenoviral replication.

The fact that adenoviruses do not integrate their genetic material into the genome of the host cell has both advantages and disadvantages for gene therapy approaches (Table 2.1). For instance, the failure of the adenoviral vector to integrate ensures that no essential genes present in the genetic material of the host cell are disrupted by random integration of viral DNA into the genome. Additionally, the temporary expression of a therapeutic gene might be desirable in the treatment of acute disease states. For example, adenoviruses have been used to deliver therapeutic DNA to patients suffering from metastatic breast, ovarian and melanoma cancers (Stewart *et al.*, 1999; Alvarez *et al.*, 2000a,b). Treatment of chronic disorders, such as cystic fibrosis, however, require repeated administration of adenoviral therapy that could cause complications due to the innate immune response that these vectors induce (Byrnes *et al.*, 1995; Yang *et al.*, 1996a,b; van Ginkel *et al.*, 1997). Indeed, the severe immune response of the host contributes to the limited survival of the adenoviral DNA in targeted cells and results in a transient expression of the therapeutic gene since the adenoviral DNA is lost over time (Yang *et al.*, 1996a,b; Byrnes *et al.*, 1996; van Ginkel *et al.*, 1997; Michou *et al.*, 1997). However, it might be possible to extend the retention time of viral DNA in targeted cells by parallel immunosuppressant treatment and/or further manipulation of the viral genes involved in stabilising the viral DNA in the host cell.

A further advantage of using adenoviral vectors for gene therapy is that they are able to accommodate large foreign genetic sequences in their viral genome. First-generation adenoviral vectors were able to accommodate the introduction of therapeutic genes over 7 kb long (but rarely larger) into targeted cells (Bett *et al.*, 1993). However, the generation of gutless adenoviral vectors, which lack all viral genes, has facilitated adenoviral delivery of up to 30 kb of a therapeutic DNA sequence (Clemens *et al.*, 1996; Kochanek *et al.*, 1996; Parks and Graham, 1997; Morsy *et al.*, 1998) with decreased toxicity (Schiedner *et al.*, 1998). Classically, the therapeutic gene of interest could not be inserted directly into the adenoviral genome. Figure 2.4 describes the construction of an adenovirus expressing a therapeutic gene for use in gene therapy. First, the therapeutic gene must be inserted into a shuttle vector, which contains adenoviral sequences on either side of the inserted gene. This shuttle vector and a replication-deficient adenoviral genome DNA then are introduced or co-transfected into a packaging cell line [e.g. 293 cells (Graham *et al.*, 1977)], which expresses genes that allow the production of infective viral particles. Once inside the cell, the viral sequences on either side of the therapeutic gene in the shuttle vector allow the transfer of the therapeutic gene into the adenoviral genome. This event is called homologous recombination. The adenoviral genome expressing the therapeutic DNA then is packaged into virus particles or virions. These particles then are amplified to generate large numbers of viral particles for *in vivo* or *ex vivo* administration. Because the generation of replication-competent recombinant adenoviruses is a concern when using traditional methods for generating therapeutic adenoviruses, methods have been developed more recently that reduce the chance of this occurring (He *et al.*, 1998; Richards *et al.*, 2000).

One of the main concerns in using adenoviral vectors for the delivery of therapeutic genes in the clinic is the potential for patients to develop an immune response to the adenoviral vector, viral proteins or infected cells (Byrnes *et al.*, 1995; Yang *et al.*, 1996a,b; van Ginkel *et al.*, 1997). A pre-existing immune response to adenoviral infection could block adenoviral-driven gene therapy treatment completely or might result in an adverse reaction to the treatment, thereby threatening the life of the patient. Strategies for the development of adenoviral vectors that are less likely to stimulate an immune response currently are underway (Schiedner *et al.*, 1998; Morsy *et al.*, 1998). These second-generation vectors either have more viral genes deleted or inactivated or are devoid of viral genes altogether (the so called 'gutless' adenoviral vectors) (Clemens *et al.*, 1996; Kochanek *et al.*, 1996; Parks and Graham, 1997; Schiedner *et al.*, 1998; Morsy *et al.*, 1998).

The use of adeno-associated viral (AAV) vectors provides an alternative to adenoviral vectors for gene therapy and a means for long-term gene expression with a reduced risk of adverse reactions upon administration of the vector (Fisher *et al.*, 1997; Jooss *et al.*, 1998). AAV viruses are linear, single-stranded DNA parvoviruses that are not associated with any disease in humans (Rose *et al.*, 1969). Unlike the adenovirus DNA, the AAV genome is able to insert itself into the genetic material of the infected cell at a specific location. In humans, the site of AAV viral DNA integration is on chromosome 19 (Kotin *et al.*, 1990; Samulski *et al.*, 1991). In common with adenoviruses, AAVs can infect both dividing and non-dividing cells. The AAV life cycle involves two distinct stages: initially, the AAV enters the cell by receptor-mediated endocytosis and is transported to the nucleus. In the nucleus of the host cell the single-stranded viral DNA is synthesised to form a double-stranded viral DNA fragment, which then is integrated into the genome of the host cell. The integrated virus then remains latent in the infected host cell until subsequent infection of the cell with another virus, such as an adenovirus, that provides the sequences required for viral replication and packaging.

In the engineering of AAV vectors, most of the AAV genome can be replaced with the therapeutic gene (Samulski *et al.*, 1989), which significantly reduces potential adverse responses of the host to viral infection. However, the size of the therapeutic gene is limited to approximately 5 kb (Dong *et al.*, 1996; Hermonat *et al.*, 1997), potentially restricting the use of AAV vectors in gene therapy compared to adenoviral vectors. To propagate the recombinant AAV vector, a cell line must be infected with two DNA plasmids encoding AAV viral sequences. The first contains the therapeutic gene of interest and viral sequences necessary for DNA integration. The second plasmid encodes all other AAV sequences except those necessary for integration. With the AAV DNA integrated into the genetic material of the cell line, infection with a helper virus, such as an adenovirus, provides the necessary replicative and/or packaging capacity for AAV virus particles to be generated (Samulski *et al.*, 1989). The need to utilise a helper virus in the production of AAV vectors increases the safety concerns regarding the use of AAVs. Contamination of the AAV vector with replication-competent adenovirus or herpes simplex virus is difficult to eliminate with current methods available for AAV propagation. Although the AAV genome is relatively small and relatively simple, much less is known about the specific AAV sequences that are involved in infection and replication. Current research into the replication of AAVs might provide a means for generating AAV particles on a large scale without the use of helper viruses, thereby improving the safety of AAV vector use in human gene therapy.

Other viral methods of DNA delivery

Retroviral- and adenoviral-based vectors provide well-characterised and highly efficient methods for DNA delivery into cells for gene therapy purposes. Both methods of gene delivery have advantages and disadvantages that affect their applications in gene therapy approaches (Table 2.1). In view of their potential limitations, research into alternative viral vectors continues. For example, herpes simplex virus (HSV) vectors provide an alternative to previously described vectors. HSV is a large and relatively complex enveloped, double-stranded DNA virus that has the capacity to encode large therapeutic genes and, like AAV, can remain latent in infected cells providing the potential for long-term expression of the therapeutic gene (Carpenter and Stevens, 1996). Although able to infect many cell types, HSV vectors currently are limited in their use by vector toxicity (Lowenstein *et al.*, 1994).

An alternative method of DNA delivery involves the use of ultraviolet light (UV)-inactivated *Hemagglutinating virus of Japan* (HVJ), which has been complexed with liposomes (a non-viral method for DNA delivery discussed below) and the therapeutic DNA. The inactivated HVJ virus promotes fusion of the liposome–DNA complex with the cellular membrane of the target cells and delivers the liposome–DNA complex directly into the cell (Tomita *et al.*, 1994). This method has been used successfully to deliver therapeutic DNA *in vitro*, *ex vivo* and *in vivo* (Tomita *et al.*, 1994; Yoshida *et al.*, 1999; Kawauchi *et al.*, 2000; Morishita *et al.*, 2000). For example, this method has been used to deliver E2F oligonucleotide decoys into cardiac allografts to inhibit intimal thickening (Kawauchi *et al.*, 2000) and to reduce blood glucose levels in a diabetic animal model via delivery of the insulin gene by systemic administration (Morishita *et al.*, 2000).

The development of hybrid viral delivery systems allows the desirable features of each delivery system to be utilised whilst overcoming the problems associated with the negative features of individual delivery systems. Examples of chimaeric delivery systems that have been investigated in this way include recombinant adenoviruses expressing retroviral sequences that permit the stable integration of the therapeutic DNA without the disadvantages associated with retroviral-mediated delivery (Feng *et al.*, 1997; Caplen *et al.*, 1999) and adenovirus/AAV hybrid vectors that are simple to propagate and integrate stably into the genome of infected host cells (Ueno *et al.*, 2000).

Non-viral methods for DNA delivery

Although viral-based vectors are highly efficient at delivering DNA into cells, concern about their safety has led to the development of a number of non-viral vectors as a more suitable alternative. Non-viral methods of DNA delivery into cells have been used for the delivery of DNA *in vitro* in the laboratory for many decades. However, many of these approaches, such as the chemical methods of DNA delivery [e.g. calcium phosphate (Graham and Eb, 1973) or 2-(diethylamino)ether (DEAE)-dextran-mediated DNA delivery (Vaheri and Pagano, 1965)], cannot readily be employed for *in vivo* use mainly because of problems associated with low delivery efficiency and high cytotoxicity. Despite these limitations, non-viral delivery systems do offer many advantages over viral-based technologies and, therefore, the improvement and development of non-viral DNA-delivery technology has been the focus of intense research. Non-viral methods of DNA delivery are simple to use and the synthetic components of these systems, such as cationic lipids or polymers, can be produced in large quantities with relative ease. Perhaps the most desired feature of non-viral vectors is their safety for use *in vivo* as a specific host immune response to the vector is not encountered. Additionally, non-viral mechanisms of DNA delivery do not disrupt the genetic material of the targeted host cell and provide short-term expression of the therapeutic gene, a feature suitable for the treatment of acute conditions, such as the inhibition of vascular smooth muscle cell proliferation following balloon angioplasty (see Chapter 6). Improvements in the efficiency and longevity of non-viral DNA delivery will make these vectors a competitive choice over viral-based systems in the future. The following section overviews the non-viral delivery systems currently available for gene delivery.

Naked DNA

The direct transfer of naked DNA (i.e. a therapeutic gene sequence incorporated into a plasmid vector) that encodes a potentially therapeutic gene or DNA sequence is one of the simplest modes of DNA delivery. Naked DNA can be administered via two possible routes, either by *ex vivo* delivery or by *in vivo* delivery. The *ex vivo* method of naked DNA delivery provides a precise, but time-consuming, method for transfer of therapeutic DNA to target cells. In this procedure, target cells are removed from the patient and are grown in cell culture under sterile laboratory conditions. The therapeutic naked DNA then is introduced into these cultured cells, using a method such as microinjection, and expression of the introduced gene is confirmed before the transfected cells are re-implanted into the patient. Although this methodology has been used successfully for the introduction of DNA into endothelial and smooth muscle cells (Nakamura *et al.*, 1998; Mann *et al.*, 1999a), its reliance on the culture of harvested cells renders it unsuitable for many cell types.

In vivo delivery of naked DNA is by far the simplest method for the administration of therapeutic genetic material to a patient. This method of gene delivery was first described in 1990 when it was demonstrated that direct injection of DNA into skeletal muscle was sufficient for the successful introduction and expression of exogenous DNA encoding reporter genes such as chloramphenicol acetyltransferase, luciferase and β-galactosidase into myoblasts (Wolff *et al.*, 1990). The exact mechanism by which cells take up the naked DNA is poorly understood but it has been demonstrated that the genetic material may be introduced in a variety of ways, including intramuscular injection, inhalation and intravascular delivery (Wolff *et al.*, 1990). Efficiency of the delivery of naked DNA can be improved when administered in a pressure-mediated fashion, for example, by controlled non-distending pressure in cardiovascular tissue (Mann *et al.*, 1999a) or by hydrodynamic force in intravenous injection (Liu *et al.*, 1999). Compared with the *ex vivo* delivery of DNA, the *in vivo* method of gene transfer results in less precise delivery of DNA to the target cells and exogenous DNA might be subject to degradation by serum nucleases. Several modifications of this method have been described that increase the efficiency of uptake of naked DNA into target cells, including the particle bombardment or 'gene gun' approach (Yang *et al.*, 1990) and electroporation techniques (Rols *et al.*, 1998) described briefly below.

Particle bombardment technology has provided a convenient and rapid method for delivery of DNA directly into targeted cells (Figure 2.6). Briefly, tungsten or gold microparticles are coated with the therapeutic DNA and propelled at high velocity, commonly using a pulse of helium gas, directly into the target cell. This technology enables the localised delivery of DNA readily into skin or muscle (Fynan *et al.*, 1993) and, therefore, has applications as a method for delivery of DNA vaccines.

Another technique for delivery of naked DNA directly into target cells is electroporation (Wong and Neumann, 1982; Neumann *et al.*, 1982; Rols *et al.*, 1998). The use of high-voltage electrical pulses to temporarily permeabilise cell membranes and deliver DNA into cells is efficient and widely used in *in vitro* applications. Unfortunately, a large percentage of cells die following this technique, thus limiting its application *in vivo*, although cell death and damage to surrounding tissues have been minimised for *in vivo* applications through the use of low-voltage, high-frequency electrical pulses (Rols *et al.*, 1998). The successful delivery of DNA by electroporation *in vivo* has been reported in tissues such as skin and muscle (Rols *et al.*, 1998; Rizzuto *et al.*, 1999).

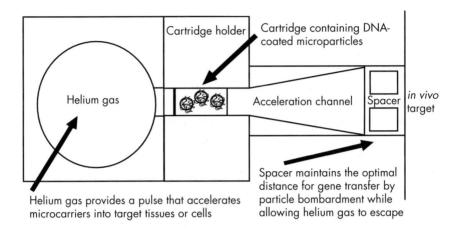

Figure 2.6   Delivery of DNA using particle bombardment or 'gene gun' technology. Initially, gold or tungsten microparticles are coated with the therapeutic DNA. These microcarriers then are loaded into a cartridge and subsequently into the cartridge holder of the gene gun. Helium gas then provides a pulse that accelerates the DNA-coated microcarriers through the acceleration channel of the gene gun and into the target tissue or cells. The spacer of the gene gun maintains the optimal distance required for gene transfer using this technology whilst minimising damage to the target. The spacer also permits escape of the helium gas.

Cationic lipids and polymers

The direct transfer of DNA into target cells is not feasible in many cases. In such instances, a delivery vehicle, such as cationic lipids or cationic polymers, must be used to facilitate efficient entry of the DNA into cells.

The use of cationic lipids to transfer DNA into cells was first described as an *in vitro* method of DNA delivery (Felgner *et al.*, 1987) and subsequently this technology has been widely adopted and shown to be suitable for the transfection of many different cell types. Cationic liposomes also have been used in clinical trials to deliver therapeutic DNA; for example, the liposomal-mediated delivery of the CFTR gene to the nasal epithelium in patients with cystic fibrosis (Caplen *et al.*, 1995; Hyde *et al.*, 2000; Noone *et al.*, 2000) and for the treatment of patients with melanoma (Nabel *et al.*, 1993, 1996). The cationic lipids in use currently are a mixture of neutrally and positively charged molecules. When the DNA and cationic lipids are mixed, DNA molecules condense and the positively charged lipid molecules bind to negatively charged phosphate groups on the DNA, which in turn form a lipid/DNA complex (Figure 2.7). Cells that come into contact with the DNA complexes take them up via a process of non-specific endocytosis. Once inside the cell, the cationic lipid binds to specific cellular membranes and the transported DNA is released into the cytoplasm of the cell. The therapeutic DNA then must be transported into the nucleus of the cell where the therapeutic gene can be expressed (Figure 2.7).

There are major barriers that must be overcome to improve the efficiency of cationic lipids as DNA-delivery vehicles. First, formation of the DNA/lipid complex can be a variable process and variation in such complexes might influence the efficiency of DNA delivery. Secondly, the efficiency by which the lipid/DNA complex is taken up by targeted cells must be improved.

Synthetic polymers, such as protective interactive non-condensing polymers (PINC), poly(L-lysine), cationic polymers or dendrimers, offer an alternative to cationic lipids as a vehicle for DNA delivery into target cells (Boussif *et al.*, 1995; Wadhwa *et al.*, 1995; Kukowska-Latallo *et al.*, 1996; Tang and Szoka, 1997; Mumper *et al.*, 1998). Cationic polymers are able to condense DNA efficiently and deliver the complex efficiently into a variety of cell types. Delivery of the DNA/polymer complex occurs in a similar fashion to that described above for cationic lipid/DNA complexes. Controlled chemical synthesis of the cationic polymers, however, ensures that the size and shape of the dendrimers is consistent and defined, thereby improving the reproducibility of DNA delivery. The use of cationic polymers also might permit the controlled expression of potentially therapeutic genes in gene therapy approaches. Thus, encapsulation of a DNA molecule or even a therapeutic viral vector within a biodegradable polymer has been demonstrated to permit the controlled release of the DNA in a targeted cell over a period of weeks or months (Naughton *et al.*, 1992; Singh *et al.*, 2000). Using such a system to deliver naked DNA has the advantage of providing a means of controlling the long-term expression of an introduced therapeutic gene whilst employing a non-viral DNA-delivery system.

The inclusion of proteins or peptides in the DNA complex that are recognised by receptors on targeted cells has led to an improvement in the efficiency of DNA uptake in several instances (Jenkins *et al.*, 2000). In addition, the use of such proteins could improve the targeting of DNA delivery to specific cells and the exclusion of other neighbouring cells. Indeed, there are reports of improved efficiency of DNA delivery by cationic lipid via the coupling of specific receptor ligands or peptides to

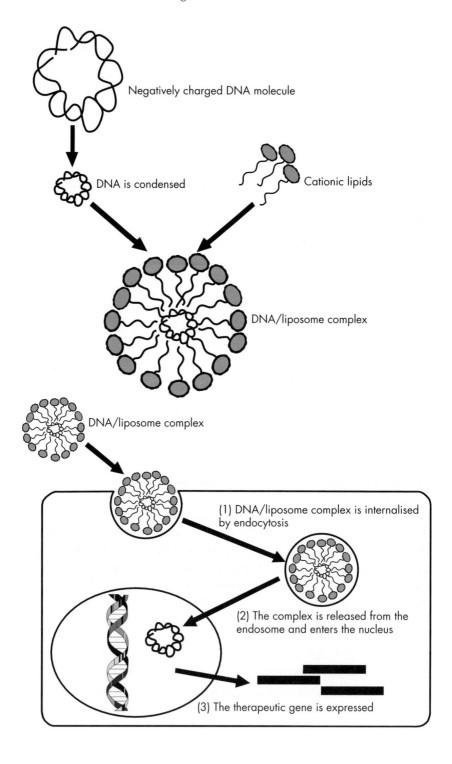

Negatively charged DNA molecule

DNA is condensed

Cationic lipids

DNA/liposome complex

DNA/liposome complex

(1) DNA/liposome complex is internalised by endocytosis

(2) The complex is released from the endosome and enters the nucleus

(3) The therapeutic gene is expressed

DNA/liposome complexes (Ellison *et al.*, 1996; Simoes *et al.*, 1998; Shinmura *et al.*, 2000). One such example is the recently reported receptor-mediated integrin-targeting DNA-delivery system that is capable of delivering very large DNA constructs of up to 110 kb both *in vitro* (Compton *et al.*, 2000) and *in vivo* (Jenkins *et al.*, 2000).

Other non-viral delivery methods

Another method of gene delivery suitable for gene therapy applications arose from the discovery of the family of transcription factors called the homeodomain proteins, which are able to translocate across the plasma membranes of living cells. This unusual property has formed the basis of the development of the penetratin family of polypeptides. These synthetic peptides retain the ability to translocate efficiently across the plasma membrane of living cells and are capable of carrying therapeutic oligonucleotides or peptides into the cytoplasm and nucleus of target cells (Derossi *et al.*, 1994). The mechanism of cellular internalisation by penetratin is not fully understood. It is not cell type-specific, receptor-mediated nor concentration-dependent but is thought to result from interaction of the peptide with membrane lipids (Derossi *et al.*, 1996; Thoren *et al.*, 2000). The efficient and rapid internalisation of penetratin and its cargo by all cell types at low concentrations, and with low cellular toxicity, are properties that make this non-viral DNA-delivery approach very attractive. Despite these desired characteristics, the penetratin system does have disadvantages, including the fact that when penetratin binds double-stranded DNA its translocation properties are lost (Derossi *et al.*, 1998). Thus, therapeutic DNA delivered via this system must be in the form of a single-stranded oligonucleotide. The size of the therapeutic DNA that can be delivered by penetratin is also limited to approximately 55 nucleotides (Derossi *et al.*, 1998). The route of administration of penetratin and its cargo also must be carefully considered since internalisation of penetratin is highly efficient and the penetratin–DNA complex will translocate rapidly into cells at the point of administration only.

Figure 2.7 Liposome-mediated DNA delivery. Negatively charged DNA is first condensed and then mixed with the cationic lipid mixture. The complexes of DNA and liposomes that form are then administered to the target tissue or cells, where the complexes are taken up by endocytosis. Once inside the cell, the complexes are released from the endosomes and enter the target cell nucleus, where the therapeutic DNA is transcribed and translated to express the therapeutic gene product.

Penetratin is not the only polypeptide that is internalised by living cells. Other proteins that have demonstrated similar internalisation properties include the TAT transcription factor of HIV (Vives *et al.*, 1997) and VP22 of the *Herpes simplex virus* (Elliott and O'Hare, 1997). High transfer efficiency and the low toxicity levels associated with gene-delivery systems that utilise translocating peptides make them attractive candidates for use in gene therapy.

Targeting the delivery of therapeutic DNA

The ability to deliver therapeutic DNA specifically to target cells and not to normal, surrounding cells is a desirable attribute in any DNA-delivery system and might be an important consideration in the design of gene therapy protocols. A number of approaches can be taken to target the delivery of the therapeutic DNA and these vary depending upon the delivery system employed. For instance, cell type-specific viral-mediated DNA delivery can be achieved via the manipulation of the natural tropism of viruses (Douglas *et al.*, 1996). The viral vectors employed for DNA delivery, like the viruses upon which they are based, enter host cells using a receptor-mediated mechanism. Altering the viral proteins involved in the recognition of these receptors on the host cell and engineering them to recognise alternative receptors found only on the targeted cell type would enable therapeutic viral-based DNA-delivery systems to target specific cells. Another method that can be used to ensure that a therapeutic gene only is expressed in a specific population of cells exploits the transcriptional control mechanisms present in all cells (Shering *et al.*, 1997). Transcriptional control of therapeutic gene expression can be achieved in gene therapy protocols that use either viral- or non-viral-based delivery systems. Placing expression of the therapeutic gene under the control of a cell type-specific promoter will ensure that, although the therapeutic DNA may be delivered to many different cell types, the gene can be expressed only in cells possessing the specific transcriptional machinery that allows expression from that promoter. One example of such a promoter is the myosin light chain-2v promoter that is present only in cardiac myocytes (Chen *et al.*, 1998). Thus, therapeutic genes placed under the transcriptional control of this promoter will be expressed only in cardiac myocytes, thereby enabling genes to be specifically targeted to heart muscle cells. The specific targeting of DNA delivery in various gene therapy protocols will be discussed in more detail in the following chapters.

Summary and conclusions

Currently there are a number of methods for transferring therapeutic DNA sequences into cells and tissues that are based on both viral and non-viral systems. No one system is ideal and all confer both advantages and disadvantages that might limit their clinical use (summarised in Table 2.2). When choosing a DNA-delivery system for a gene therapy protocol, careful consideration must be given to the required safety, route of administration, duration and level of therapeutic gene expression. Highly efficient DNA transfer, made possible by the development of viral-based DNA-delivery vectors, is reflected in their prevalence in a variety of gene therapy protocols and clinical trials. However, viral vectors are not suitable for all gene therapy procedures. In these circumstances, and despite providing a lower efficiency of gene delivery, non-viral DNA-delivery systems offer a number of advantages and a number of applications for human gene therapy, e.g. in the delivery of E2F decoy oligonucleotides to vascular tissue (Mann *et al.*, 1999b). The major advantage of non-viral DNA systems is the relatively low level of risk that is associated with their use. However, the efficiency and safety of all DNA-delivery systems, both viral- and non-viral-based systems, constantly is being refined. Hopefully, such modifications will lead to substantial improvements in the success of future gene therapy trials.

Table 2.2 Comparison of viral- and non-viral-based gene delivery systems

Property	Viral delivery	Non-viral delivery
Efficiency	Highly efficient gene delivery Potential for long-term gene expression (retroviral delivery)	Low efficiency of gene transfer
Size of therapeutic DNA	Limited by size that can be accommodated by viral genome and packaging of viral particles	Largely unlimited
Safety issues	Some viral vectors stimulate severe immune responses in the patient Concern regarding use of viral vectors based on HIV	Low toxicity to host
Longevity of expression	Transient (adenoviral-based systems) or long-term (retroviral- or AAV-based systems) expression	Transient expression

References

Alvarez R D, Barnes M N, Gomez-Navarro J, *et al.* (2000a) A cancer gene therapy approach utilizing an anti-erbB-2 single-chain antibody-encoding adenovirus (AD21): a phase I trial. *Clin Cancer Res* 6: 3081–3087.

Alvarez R D, Gomez-Navarro J, Wang M, *et al.* (2000b) Adenoviral-mediated suicide gene therapy for ovarian cancer. *Mol Ther* 2: 524–530.

Bett A J, Prevec L, Graham F L (1993) Packaging capacity and stability of human adenovirus type 5 vectors. *J Virol* 67: 5911–5921.

Bordignon C, Notarangelo L D, Nobili N, *et al.* (1995) Gene therapy in peripheral blood lymphocytes and bone marrow for ADA-immunodeficient patients. *Science* 270: 470–475.

Boussif O, Lezoualc'h F, Zanta M A, *et al.* (1995) A versatile vector for gene and oligonucleotide transfer into cells in culture and *in vivo*: polyethylenimine. *Proc Natl Acad Sci USA* 92: 7297–7301.

Brooks G, Vile R (1998) Gene therapy for the treatment of disease. In: Brooks G, ed. *Biotechnology in Healthcare. An Introduction to Biopharmaceuticals.* London: Pharmaceutical Press, 83–116.

Byrnes A P, Rusby J E, Wood M J, *et al.* (1995) Adenovirus gene transfer causes inflammation in the brain. *Neuroscience* 66: 1015–1024.

Byrnes A P, MacLaren R E, Charlton H M (1996) Immunological instability of persistent adenovirus vectors in the brain: peripheral exposure to vector leads to renewed inflammation, reduced gene expression, and demyelination. *J Neurosci* 16: 3045–3055.

Caplen N J, Alton E W, Middleton P G, *et al.* (1995) Liposome-mediated CFTR gene transfer to the nasal epithelium of patients with cystic fibrosis. *Nat Med* 1: 39–46.

Caplen N J, Higginbotham J N, Scheel J R, *et al.* (1999) Adeno-retroviral chimeric viruses as *in vivo* transducing agents. *Gene Ther* 6: 454–459.

Carpenter D E, Stevens J G (1996) Long-term expression of a foreign gene from a unique position in the latent herpes simplex virus genome. *Hum Gene Ther* 7: 1447–1454.

Chen J, Kubalak S W, Chien K R (1998) Ventricular muscle-restricted targeting of the RXRalpha gene reveals a non-cell-autonomous requirement in cardiac chamber morphogenesis. *Development* 125: 1943–1949.

Clemens P R, Kochanek S, Sunada Y, *et al.* (1996) In vivo muscle gene transfer of full-length dystrophin with an adenoviral vector that lacks all viral genes. *Gene Ther* 3: 965–972.

Compton S H, Mecklenbeck S, Mejia J E, *et al.* (2000) Stable integration of large (>100 kb) PAC constructs in HaCaT keratinocytes using an integrin-targeting peptide delivery system. *Gene Ther* 7: 1600–1605.

Cone R D, Mulligan R C (1984) High-efficiency gene transfer into mammalian cells: generation of helper-free recombinant retrovirus with broad mammalian host range. *Proc Natl Acad Sci USA* 81: 6349–6353.

Derossi D, Joliot A H, Chassaing G, *et al.* (1994) The third helix of the Antennapedia homeodomain translocates through biological membranes. *J Biol Chem* 269: 10444–10450.

Derossi D, Calvet S, Trembleau A, *et al.* (1996) Cell internalization of the third helix of the Antennapedia homeodomain is receptor-independent. *J Biol Chem* 271: 18188–18193.

Derossi D, Chassaing G, Prochiantz A (1998) Trojan peptides: the penetratin system for intracellular delivery. *Trends Cell Biol* 8: 84–87.

Dong J Y, Fan P D, Frizzell R A (1996) Quantitative analysis of the packaging capacity of recombinant adeno-associated virus. *Hum Gene Ther* 7: 2101–2112.

Douglas J T, Rogers B E, Rosenfeld M E, *et al.* (1996) Targeted gene delivery by tropism-modified adenoviral vectors. *Nature Biotechnol* 14: 1574–1578.

Dunbar C E, Kohn D B, Schiffmann R, *et al.* (1998) Retroviral transfer of the glucocerebrosidase gene into CD34+ cells from patients with Gaucher disease: *in vivo* detection of transduced cells without myeloablation. *Hum Gene Ther* 9: 2629–2640.

Elliott G, O'Hare P (1997) Intercellular trafficking and protein delivery by a herpesvirus structural protein. *Cell* 88: 223–233.

Ellison K E, Bishopric N H, Webster K A, *et al.* (1996) Fusigenic liposome-mediated DNA transfer into cardiac myocytes. *J Mol Cell Cardiol* 28: 1385–1399.

Felgner P L, Gadek T R, Holm M, *et al.* (1987) Lipofection: a highly efficient, lipid-mediated DNA-transfection procedure. *Proc Natl Acad Sci USA* 84: 7413–7417.

Feng M, Jackson W H, Jr, Goldman C K, *et al.* (1997) Stable *in vivo* gene transduction via a novel adenoviral/retroviral chimeric vector. *Nat Biotechnol* 15: 866–870.

Fisher K J, Jooss K, Alston J, *et al.* (1997) Recombinant adeno-associated virus for muscle directed gene therapy. *Nat Med* 3: 306–312.

Fujii S, Huang S, Fong T C, *et al.* (2000) Induction of melanoma-associated antigen systemic immunity upon intratumoral delivery of interferon-gamma retroviral vector in melanoma patients. *Cancer Gene Ther* 7: 1220–1230.

Fynan E F, Webster R G, Fuller D H, *et al.* (1993) DNA vaccines: protective immunizations by parenteral, mucosal, and gene-gun inoculations. *Proc Natl Acad Sci USA* 90: 11478–11482.

Graham F L, van der Eb A J (1973) A new technique for the assay of infectivity of human adenovirus 5 DNA. *Virology* 52: 456–467.

Graham F L, Smiley J, Russell W C, *et al.* (1977) Characteristics of a human cell line transformed by DNA from human adenovirus type 5. *J Gen Virol* 36: 59–74.

He T C, Zhou S, da Costa L T, *et al.* (1998) A simplified system for generating recombinant adenoviruses. *Proc Natl Acad Sci USA* 95: 2509–2514.

Hermonat P L, Quirk J G, Bishop B M, *et al.* (1997) The packaging capacity of adeno-associated virus (AAV) and the potential for wild-type-plus AAV gene therapy vectors. *FEBS Lett* 407: 78–84.

Hyde S C, Southern K W, Gileadi U, *et al.* (2000) Repeat administration of DNA/liposomes to the nasal epithelium of patients with cystic fibrosis. *Gene Ther* 7: 1156–1165.

Jenkins R G, Herrick S E, Meng Q H, *et al.* (2000) An integrin-targeted non-viral vector for pulmonary gene therapy. *Gene Ther* 7: 393–400.

Jooss K, Yang Y, Fisher K J, *et al.* (1998) Transduction of dendritic cells by DNA viral vectors directs the immune response to transgene products in muscle fibers. *J Virol* 72: 4212–4223.

Kawauchi M, Suzuki J, Morishita R, *et al.* (2000) Gene therapy for attenuating cardiac allograft arteriopathy using *ex vivo* E2F decoy transfection by HVJ-AVE-liposome method in mice and nonhuman primates. *Circ Res* 87: 1063–1068.

Kim S H, Yu S S, Park J S, *et al.* (1998) Construction of retroviral vectors with improved safety, gene expression, and versatility. *J Virol* 72: 994–1004.

Kochanek S, Clemens P R, Mitani K, *et al.* (1996) A new adenoviral vector: replacement of all viral coding sequences with 28 kb of DNA independently expressing both full-length dystrophin and beta-galactosidase. *Proc Natl Acad Sci USA* 93: 5731–5736.

Koenig M, Hoffman E P, Bertelson C J, *et al.* (1987) Complete cloning of the Duchenne muscular dystrophy (DMD) cDNA and preliminary genomic organization of the DMD gene in normal and affected individuals. *Cell* 50: 509–517.

Kotin R M, Siniscalco M, Samulski R J, *et al.* (1990) Site-specific integration by adeno-associated virus. *Proc Natl Acad Sci USA* 87: 2211–2215.

Kukowska-Latallo J F, Bielinska A U, Johnson J, *et al.* (1996) Efficient transfer of genetic material into mammalian cells using Starburst polyamidoamine dendrimers. *Proc Natl Acad Sci USA* 93: 4897–4902.

Lewis P F, Emerman M (1994) Passage through mitosis is required for oncoretroviruses but not for the human immunodeficiency virus. *J Virol* 68: 510–516.

Liu F, Song Y, Liu D (1999) Hydrodynamics-based transfection in animals by systemic administration of plasmid DNA. *Gene Ther* 6: 1258–1266.

Lowenstein P R, Morrison E E, Bain D, *et al.* (1994) Use of recombinant vectors derived from herpes simplex virus 1 mutant tsK for short-term expression of transgenes encoding cytoplasmic and membrane anchored proteins in post-mitotic polarized cortical neurons and glial cells in vitro. *Neuroscience* 60: 1059–1077.

Mann M J, Gibbons G H, Hutchinson H, *et al.* (1999a) Pressure-mediated oligonucleotide transfection of rat and human cardiovascular tissues. *Proc Natl Acad Sci USA* 96: 6411–6416.

Mann M J, Whittemore A D, Donaldson M C, *et al.* (1999b) *Ex-vivo* gene therapy of human vascular bypass grafts with E2F decoy: the PREVENT single-centre, randomised, controlled trial. *Lancet* 354: 1493–1498.

Mann R, Mulligan R C, Baltimore D (1983) Construction of a retrovirus packaging mutant and its use to produce helper-free defective retrovirus. *Cell* 33: 153–159.

Michou A I, Santoro L, Christ M, *et al.* (1997) Adenovirus-mediated gene transfer: influence of transgene, mouse strain and type of immune response on persistence of transgene expression. *Gene Ther* 4: 473–482.

Morishita R, Gibbons G H, Kaneda Y, *et al.* (2000) Systemic administration of HVJ viral coat-liposome complex containing human insulin vector decreases glucose level in diabetic mouse: a model of gene therapy. *Biochem Biophys Res Commun* 273: 666–674.

Morsy M A, Gu M, Motzel S, *et al.* (1998) An adenoviral vector deleted for all viral coding sequences results in enhanced safety and extended expression of a leptin transgene. *Proc Natl Acad Sci USA* 95: 7866–7871.

Mumper R J, Wang J, Klakamp S L, *et al.* (1998) Protective interactive noncondensing (PINC) polymers for enhanced plasmid distribution and expression in rat skeletal muscle. *J Controlled Release* 52: 191–203.

Nabel G J, Nabel E G, Yang Z Y, *et al.* (1993) Direct gene transfer with DNA-liposome complexes in melanoma: expression, biologic activity, and lack of toxicity in humans. *Proc Natl Acad Sci USA* 90: 11307–11311.

Nabel G J, Gordon D, Bishop D K, *et al.* (1996) Immune response in human melanoma after transfer of an allogeneic class I major histocompatibility complex gene with DNA-liposome complexes. *Proc Natl Acad Sci USA* 93: 15388–15393.

Nakamura M, Davila-Zavala P, Tokuda H, *et al.* (1998) Uptake and gene expression of naked plasmid DNA in cultured brain microvessel endothelial cells. *Biochem Biophys Res Commun* 245: 235–239.

Naldini L, Blomer U, Gallay P, *et al.* (1996) *In vivo* gene delivery and stable transduction of nondividing cells by a lentiviral vector. *Science* 272: 263–267.

Naughton B A, Dai Y, Sibanda B, *et al.* (1992) Long-term expression of a retrovirally introduced beta-galactosidase gene in rodent cells implanted in vivo using biodegradable polymer meshes. *Somat Cell Mol Genet* 18: 451–462.

Neumann E, Schaefer-Ridder M, Wang Y, *et al.* (1982) Gene transfer into mouse lyoma cells by electroporation in high electric fields. *EMBO J* 1: 841–845.

Noone P G, Hohneker K W, Zhou Z, *et al.* (2000) Safety and biological efficacy of a lipid-CFTR complex for gene transfer in the nasal epithelium of adult patients with cystic fibrosis. *Mol Ther* 1: 105–114.

Onodera M, Ariga T, Kawamura N, *et al.* (1998) Successful peripheral T-lymphocyte-directed gene transfer for a patient with severe combined immune deficiency caused by adenosine deaminase deficiency. *Blood* 91: 30–36.

Parks R J, Graham F L (1997) A helper-dependent system for adenovirus vector production helps define a lower limit for efficient DNA packaging. *J Virol* 71: 3293–3298.

Richards C A, Brown C E, Cogswell J P, *et al.* (2000) The admid system: generation of recombinant adenoviruses by Tn7-mediated transposition in *E. coli*. *Biotechniques* 29: 146–154.

Riordan J R, Rommens J M, Kerem B, *et al.* (1989) Identification of the cystic fibrosis gene: cloning and characterization of complementary DNA. *Science* 245: 1066–1073.

Rizzuto G, Cappelletti M, Maione D, *et al.* (1999) Efficient and regulated erythropoietin production by naked DNA injection and muscle electroporation. *Proc Natl Acad Sci USA* 96: 6417–6422.

Roe T, Reynolds T C, Yu G, *et al.* (1993) Integration of murine leukemia virus DNA depends on mitosis. *EMBO J* 12: 2099–2108.

Rols M P, Delteil C, Golzio M, *et al.* (1998) *In vivo* electrically mediated protein and gene transfer in murine melanoma. *Nat Biotechnol* 16: 168–171.

Rose J A, Berns K I, Hoggan M D, *et al.* (1969) Evidence for a single-stranded adenovirus-associated virus genome: formation of a DNA density hybrid on release of viral DNA. *Proc Natl Acad Sci USA* 64: 863–869.

Samulski R J, Chang L S, Shenk T (1989) Helper-free stocks of recombinant adeno-associated viruses: normal integration does not require viral gene expression. *J Virol* 63: 3822–3828.

Samulski R J, Zhu X, Xiao X, *et al.* (1991) Targeted integration of adeno-associated virus (AAV) into human chromosome 19. *EMBO J* 10: 3941–3950.

Schiedner G, Morral N, Parks R J, *et al.* (1998) Genomic DNA transfer with a high-capacity adenovirus vector results in improved *in vivo* gene expression and decreased toxicity. *Nat Genet* 18: 180–183.

Sheridan P L, Bodner M, Lynn A, *et al.* (2000) Generation of retroviral packaging and producer cell lines for large-scale vector production and clinical application: improved safety and high titer. *Mol Ther* 2: 262–275.

Shering A F, Bain D, Stewart K, *et al.* (1997) Cell type-specific expression in brain cell cultures from a short human cytomegalovirus major immediate early promoter depends on whether it is inserted into herpesvirus or adenovirus vectors. *J Gen Virol* 78: 445–459.

Shin N H, Hartigan-O'Connor D, Pfeiffer J K, *et al.* (2000) Replication of lengthened Moloney murine leukemia virus genomes is impaired at multiple stages. *J Virol* 74: 2694–2702.

Shinmura K, Morishita R, Aoki M, *et al.* (2000) Catheter-delivered *in vivo* gene transfer into rat myocardium using the fusigenic liposomal mediated method. *Jpn Heart J* 41: 633–647.

Simoes S, Slepushkin V, Gaspar R, *et al.* (1998) Gene delivery by negatively charged ternary complexes of DNA, cationic liposomes and transferrin or fusigenic peptides. *Gene Ther* 5: 955–964.

Singh M, Briones M, Ott G, *et al.* (2000) Cationic microparticles: a potent delivery system for DNA vaccines. *Proc Natl Acad Sci USA* 97: 811–816.

Stewart A K, Lassam N J, Quirt I C, *et al.* (1999) Adenovector-mediated gene delivery of interleukin-2 in metastatic breast cancer and melanoma: results of a phase 1 clinical trial. *Gene Ther* 6: 350–363.

Tait D L, Obermiller P S, Hatmaker A R, *et al.* (1999) Ovarian cancer BRCA1 gene therapy: phase I and II trial differences in immune response and vector stability. *Clin Cancer Res* 5: 1708–1714.

Tang M X, Szoka F C (1997) The influence of polymer structure on the interactions of cationic polymers with DNA and morphology of the resulting complexes. *Gene Ther* 4: 823–832.

Thoren P E, Persson D, Karlsson M, *et al.* (2000) The antennapedia peptide penetratin translocates across lipid bilayers – the first direct observation. *FEBS Lett* 482: 265–268.

Tomita N, Higaki J, Ogihara T, *et al.* (1994) A novel gene-transfer technique mediated by HVJ (Sendai virus), nuclear protein, and liposomes. *Cancer Detect Prev* 18: 485–491.

Ueno T, Matsumura H, Tanaka K, *et al.* (2000) Site-specific integration of a transgene mediated by a hybrid adenovirus/adeno-associated virus vector using the Cre/loxP-expression-switching system. *Biochem Biophys Res Commun* 273: 473–478.

Vaheri A, Pagano J S (1965) Infectious poliovirus RNA: a sensitive method of assay. *Virology* 27: 434–436.

van Ginkel F W, McGhee J R, Liu C, *et al.* (1997) Adenoviral gene delivery elicits distinct pulmonary-associated T helper cell responses to the vector and to its transgene. *J Immunol* 159: 685–693.

Vives E, Brodin P, Lebleu B (1997) A truncated HIV-1 Tat protein basic domain rapidly translocates through the plasma membrane and accumulates in the cell nucleus. *J Biol Chem* 272: 16010–16017.

Wadhwa M S, Knoell D L, Young A P, *et al.* (1995) Targeted gene delivery with a low molecular weight glycopeptide carrier. *Bioconjug Chem* 6: 283–291.

Wolff J A, Malone R W, Williams P, *et al.* (1990) Direct gene transfer into mouse muscle *in vivo. Science* 247: 1465–1468.

Wong T K, Neumann E (1982) Electric field mediated gene transfer. *Biochem Biophys Res Commun* 107: 584–587.

Yang N S, Burkholder J, Roberts B, *et al.* (1990) *In vivo* and *in vitro* gene transfer to mammalian somatic cells by particle bombardment. *Proc Natl Acad Sci USA* 87: 9568–9572.

Yang Y, Jooss K U, Su Q, *et al.* (1996a) Immune responses to viral antigens versus transgene product in the elimination of recombinant adenovirus-infected hepatocytes in vivo. *Gene Ther* 3: 137–144.

Yang Y, Su Q, Wilson J M (1996b) Role of viral antigens in destructive cellular immune responses to adenovirus vector-transduced cells in mouse lungs. *J Virol* 70: 7209–7212.

Yoshida M, Hayashi S, Sakuma-Mochizuki J, *et al.* (1999) Introduction of plasmid DNA and oligonucleotides into lung epithelial cells by the hemagglutinating virus of Japan (HVJ)-liposome method. *Somat Cell Mol Genet* 25: 49–57.

3

The Human Genome Project

Ian Dunham

The Human Genome Project is the global initiative to clone and sequence the DNA that makes up our genomes. It has its origin in the mid-1980s with the realisation that global approaches to mutation research and diseases like cancer which act at the level of our DNA would require a much better knowledge of how our genomes are constructed (Dulbecco, 1986; Cook-Deegan, 1989). Systematic study of genes and the genetic component of disease ultimately would require the full complement of human genes. Incredibly, in less than 15 years we are now at a position where the faith that motivated the early calls for the project has begun to be justified by, for instance, the beginnings of molecular classification of tumours (Golub *et al.*, 1999; Alizadeh *et al.*, 2000). At the same time we have seen the genome project announce the completion of the first working draft sequence of the genome (Macilwain, 2000) and it is now planned to complete the sequence by 2003.

In the field of gene therapy there is usually a wealth of information about the structure of the gene that is the target of intervention. However, information from the genome project has a number of roles to play. First, the genes that are to form the basis for future gene therapy may not yet have been identified. Indeed, at the current time this is quite likely since we still have an incomplete knowledge of many of the genes in the genome, and the genes which provide the genetic component for the common diseases such as cancer, heart disease, diabetes and schizophrenia are largely unidentified. Secondly, even when the protein-coding sequence and intron/exon organisation of the gene are established, there are likely to be important regulatory sequences that are also necessary for correct gene expression. Detailed information about the DNA sequence context of the gene will be required to elucidate the nature of these regulatory sequences. Finally, although a specific gene may be altered in a disease, it is possible that other genes, perhaps downstream of the aberrant gene product in critical pathways, or able to take over the mutant gene function, could be relevant targets for intervention

(Wakefield *et al.*, 2000). Therefore, while current work in gene therapy uses well-established genes for well-studied diseases, the genes that are now being discovered in the human genome may well be the subject of gene therapy protocols in the future.

The haploid human genome comprises three billion base pairs distributed over 22 autosomes and one of the pair of sex chromosomes. Over the years the genome has been charted at ever increasing levels of resolution, using a series of techniques starting with the whole chromosomes at the cytogenetic and somatic cell hybrid level, down to the DNA sequence itself (Figure 3.1). This chapter will examine the successively more detailed maps of our genome, and then look at the progress that is now being made in identifying human genes, and cataloguing the variation that exists between individuals.

Human genome maps

The cytogenetic map

Human chromosomes have characteristic banding patterns revealed by appropriate staining techniques, for instance treatment with Giemsa. The chromosomes are conventionally visualised as the G-banded karyotype with either 400 or 550 bands (Mitelman, 1995), although higher resolution banding is also possible. The technique of fluorescence *in situ* hybridisation (FISH) using fluorescently labelled genomic clones is a simple and effective means of mapping genes or other DNA segments to distinct locations on the cytogenetic map (Lichter *et al.*, 1991; Trask, 1991). Recently, the availability of large numbers of genomic DNA clones (see below) has provided ideal reagents to relate cytogenetic maps directly to DNA sequence (Leversha *et al.*, 1999; Kirsch *et al.*, 2000). Further information about validated clones for FISH can be found from the websites listed in Table 3.1. These resources are increasingly being used to investigate chromosomal deletions, duplications and translocations in disease both by FISH and comparative genome hybridisation using micorarrays (Pinkel *et al.*, 1998).

The genetic map

Genetic linkage mapping utilises the obligatory recombination events that occur in each meiosis to follow the fate of chromosomal DNA through

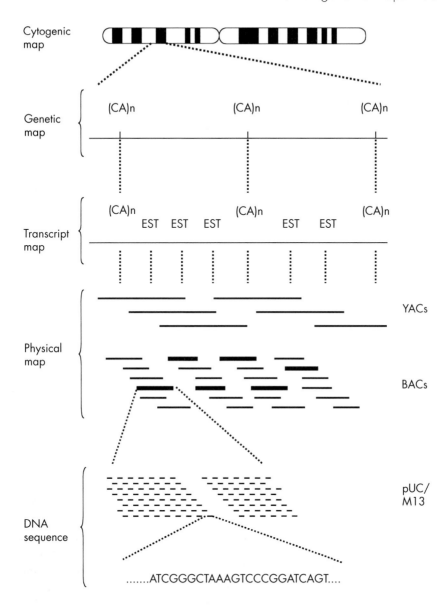

Figure 3.1 Increasing resolution maps of the human genome. Moving down through the maps as described in the text, the genome is progressively broken down into smaller segments, initially through long-range maps and then into clones.

the generations. Measuring the frequency at which the alleles of two markers are separated by recombination indicates the distance between the markers. Human genetic maps first used detectable enzymatic or

Table 3.1 Useful World Wide Web resources for the Human Genome Project. This list is not exhaustive and additional links can be found at these sites

Resource	URLs
General	
NCBI	http://www.ncbi.nlm.nih.gov/genome/guide/H_sapiens.html
NHGRI	http://www.nhgri.nih.gov/HGP/
Ethical, legal and social issues	http://www.ornl.gov/hgmis/elsi/elsi.html
The Sanger Centre	http://www.sanger.ac.uk/HGP/
Cytogenetic maps	
The Cancer Chromosome Aberration Project (CCAP)	http://www.ncbi.nlm.nih.gov/CCAP/
The Sanger Centre	http://www.sanger.ac.uk/HGP/Cytogenetics
University of Bari	http://www.biologia.uniba.it/rmc/
Genetic maps	
Généthon	http://www.genethon.fr/genethon_en.html
The Cooperative Human Linkage Center	http://lpg.nci.nih.gov/html-chlc/ChlcMaps.html
Center for Medical Genetics	http://www.marshmed.org/genetics/mainframe.htm
Transcript map	
Gene Map '99	http://www.ncbi.nlm.nih.gov/genemap99/
Physical maps	
BAC fingerprint database	http://genome.wustl.edu/gsc/human/human_database.shtml
Human genome sequence	
Ensembl	http://www.ensembl.org
NCBI	http://www.ncbi.nlm.nih.gov/genome/seq/
Ensembl Blast server	http://www.ensembl.org/Data/blast.html
NCBI Blast server	http://www.ncbi.nlm.nih.gov/genome/seq/page.cgi?F=HsBlast.html&&ORG=Hs
Genes	
UniGene	http://www.ncbi.nlm.nih.gov/UniGene/Hs.Home.html
Ensembl	http://www.ensembl.org
OMIM	http://www.ncbi.nlm.nih.gov/Omim/
The Genome Channel	http://compbio.ornl.gov/tools/channel/
SNPs	
The SNP consortium	http://snp.csml.org/
dbSNP	http://www.ncbi.nlm.nih.gov/SNP/

antigenic markers, for instance the ABO blood group antigens. In the 1980s polymorphic DNA sequences were detected by restriction enzyme digestion and Southern blotting, so-called restriction fragment length polymorphisms (RFLPs), and used to build the first generation of genome-wide genetic linkage maps (Donis-Keller *et al.*, 1987). However, for most of the 1990s the polymorphic marker of choice was the microsatellite. Microsatellites are short tracts of tandemly repeated di-, tri- or tetranucleotide sequences dispersed throughout the genome (most frequently runs of CA/GT), which differ remarkably in the number of repeats at a particular locus between different copies of the same chromosome (Weber and May, 1989). These length differences can be detected by polymerase chain reaction (PCR) amplification using unique sequence oligonucleotides flanking the microsatellite repeat. The different amplification products (alleles) are separated by acrylamide gel electrophoresis, and detected by silver staining, autoradiography or fluorescence. These methods were used to analyse the patterns of segregation of the alleles of many markers in a set of defined families collected by the Centre d'Etude Polymorphism Humain (CEPH), and a number of different genetic linkage maps were produced (Weissenbach *et al.*, 1992; Buetow *et al.*, 1994a,b; Murray *et al.*, 1994; Gyapay *et al.*, 1994; Dib *et al.*, 1996). The final Généthon map consisted of 5264 CA/GT microsatellite markers at an average density of 1.6 cM. A selected subset of these markers is available for genome linkage scans for genetic disease (Reed *et al.*, 1994).

   In recent years it has been realised that to achieve very high throughput, such as might be required for detection of the genetic factors involved in common multifactorial disease, markers suitable for automated typing are required. Single nucleotide polymorphisms (SNPs) (Figure 3.2) are stable biallelic single base substitution alleles found at high frequency across the human genome (about 1 per 1000 bp when two genomes are compared). These features make them highly suitable genetic markers for automated genotyping methods (Kwok and Gu, 1999). Recent efforts have resulted in a third-generation linkage map of the human genome based on SNPs (Wang *et al.*, 1998). Further extraction of these markers from the rich resource in our genomes will greatly increase the density available for linkage maps (see below).

The transcript (radiation hybrid) map

Radiation hybrid (RH) mapping is a method that enables placement of any PCR amplifiable marker on a map. When irradiated human cells are fused with hamster cells, a panel of hybrid cell lines can be produced that contains different collections of fragments of the human genome on a background of the hamster genome. If the hybrids are tested for the

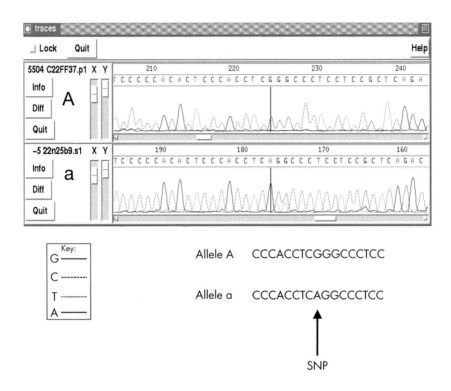

Figure 3.2   Single nucleotide polymorphisms (SNPs). DNA sequence traces taken from clones of the same genomic region but from different alleles are shown. A clear single base difference can be seen between the traces showing a G–A substitution between the alleles. In reality, multiple sequence reads would be required to definitively call this difference.

presence of any two PCR-based markers, the frequency at which the two markers will be present together in the same hybrid is a function of their proximity. The closer together they are, the more likely they are to be found in the same hybrid. With a sufficiently large panel of hybrids and sufficient markers it is possible to form a map of the markers (Walter *et al.*, 1994; Gyapay *et al.*, 1996; Stewart *et al.*, 1997).

The availability of automated DNA sequencers prompted extensive surveys of the mRNA transcript populations of human tissues. Short sequence reads from the ends of clones from cDNA libraries constructed by poly(A)- or random-primed reverse transcription of the cellular mRNA allowed sampling of the expressed transcripts (Figure 3.3). These sequences are called expressed sequence tags (ESTs) (Adams *et al.*, 1992). Large collections of ESTs have now been assembled (Adams *et al.*, 1995;

(A)

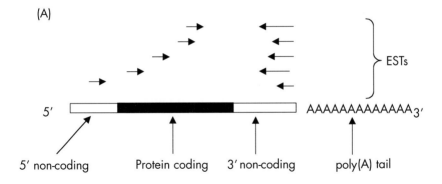

(B)

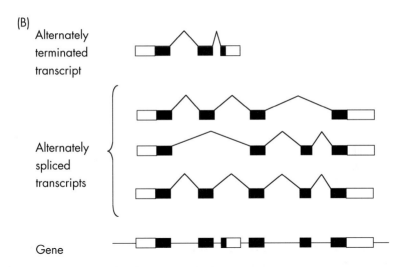

Figure 3.3 Expressed sequence tags (ESTs). (A) ESTs are short sequence reads from the ends of cDNA clones. The figure shows a generic mRNA transcript structure and the distribution of ESTs generated by sequencing different cDNA clones derived from this transcript. In the simplest case all the reads from the 3′ end of the clones will be overlapping, but since cDNA clones extend to different lengths at the 5′ ends, the 5′ reads may not overlap. (B) Further complexity is introduced by alternative splicing or termination. A generic gene is shown with boxes representing exons (protein-coding regions filled). A series of alternatively spliced transcript and an alternatively terminated transcript are also shown. EST sequencing from this set of transcripts would generate a series of ESTs which may not overlap or assemble into a single cluster.

Hillier *et al.*, 1996). There is redundant sampling of single transcript species in the EST collections, and individual ESTs may originate from different parts of a gene due to the method of cDNA priming, or the existence of alternative splicing and termination (Figure 3.3). Therefore attempts have been made to combine ESTs by sequence alignment to form clusters that might reconstitute the original cDNA sequence and hence represent at least an approximation to individual genes (Boguski and Schuler, 1995; Schuler *et al.*, 1996).

Combining RH mapping with PCR-based assays for the sequences represented in the EST clusters and microsatellites allows construction of a map of the transcripts (Schuler *et al.*, 1996). In 1998, the RH Mapping Consortium published a map of 30 000 transcript locations placed relative to a framework of well-ordered microsatellite markers (Deloukas *et al.*, 1998). Since then they have released a further version of the map (RH Mapping Consortium, 1999). The great benefit of this sort of map is that it allows location of candidate genes within the regions of linkage defined by genetic mapping using microsatellites, for instance from a whole genome linkage scan for a monogenic genetic disease.

The physical map

In order to have direct access to the DNA of the genome, maps must be assembled of human DNA segments cloned into suitable vectors. Initial efforts to generate physical maps of the human genome used libraries of human DNA cloned into yeast artificial chromosomes (YACs) (Burke *et al.*, 1987; Brownstein *et al.*, 1989). YACs are able to propagate segments of human DNA over a megabase (Mb) in size. Most of the human YAC maps used PCR-based markers to detect the presence of a specific locus within the YACs, so-called sequence tagged sites (STSs) (Olson *et al.*, 1989), although DNA–DNA hybridisation techniques were also used. Using sufficient STSs or hybridisation probes, contigs could be constructed covering large sections of the human genome. This approach resulted in two YAC-based maps of the whole genome (Chumakov *et al.*, 1995; Hudson *et al.*, 1995), as well as more detailed maps of a number of the human chromosomes (Chumakov *et al.*, 1992; Collins *et al.*, 1995; Doggett *et al.*, 1995; Gemmill *et al.*, 1995; Krauter *et al.*, 1995; Crollius *et al.*, 1996; Bouffard *et al.*, 1997).

Unfortunately, YACs have two serious disadvantages when used to clone human DNA, which meant they could not be used as the main substrate for sequencing of the genome. First, shotgun cloning and sequencing of the artificial chromosome separated from the yeast chromosomes was time consuming and inefficient. Second, and more importantly, cloning human DNA into YACs resulted in serious rearrangement of the DNA by deletion and production of chimaeras in which two regions that were physically unrelated in the genome were brought together in the same YAC (Green *et al.*, 1991). In order to provide maps that could be used efficiently for genomic sequencing, physical maps of the genome were constructed using libraries of DNA cloned in *E. coli*-based vectors, chiefly bacterial artificial chromosomes (BACs) (Shizuya *et al.*, 1992) and P1-derived artificial chromosomes (PACs) (Ioannou *et al.*, 1994). For effective production of sequence-ready maps in PACs and BACs a strategy was devised that combined the use of STS landmarks with restriction enzyme fingerprinting of the bacterial clones (Marra *et al.*, 1997; Gregory *et al.*, 1997) to form contigs which were anchored to the frameworks of the YAC and RH maps (Mungall *et al.*, 1997; Centre and Centre, 1998). The gaps between contigs were closed by directed chromosome walking using sequences from the ends of the BACs (Venter *et al.*, 1996) or probes isolated from the ends of contigs (see Dunham *et al.*, 1999a for techniques). Figure 3.4 illustrates part of a typical contig from human chromosome 9. At the current time a genome-wide map in bacterial clones covering at least 90% of the genome has been constructed from a whole BAC library fingerprinting approach integrated with STS landmarks, BAC end sequences, and FISH localisation of individual BACs (NHGRI, 2000). As with the YAC-based physical maps, particular attention has been paid to certain chromosomes to improve the detailed maps (Dunham *et al.*, 1999b; Hattori *et al.*, 2000; Han *et al.*, 2000). At the time of writing it has been estimated that 97% of the euchromatic (gene-containing) part of the genome has been covered in mapped bacterial clones. What remains to be done is to close the gaps between the remaining contigs by chromosome walking to complete coverage of the genome.

The human genome sequence

The strategy of the public domain International Human Genome Sequencing Consortium has been to use the restriction enzyme fingerprints in the BAC physical map of the genome to select clones that are representative of the genome (a minimum tiling path) (Centre and Centre, 1998). The individual BACs representing defined genomic

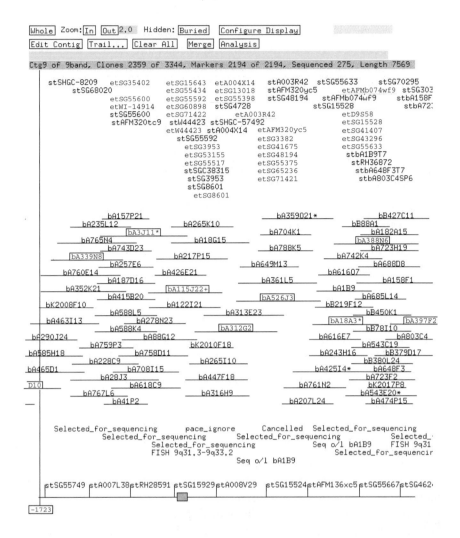

Figure 3.4   A bacterial artificial chromosome (BAC) contig from chromosome 9. A screenshot is shown of a bacterial clone contig from human chromosome 9 displayed in the contig-building program FPC (Soderlund *et al.*, 1997). The horizontal lines represent a series of BACs assembled into contigs using *Hind*III restriction enzyme fingerprinting data, combined with sequence tagged site (STS) content with the STSs shown above. The boxed BACs have been chosen as a minimal tiling path for genomic sequencing. The STSs in bold are mapped electronically using the genomic sequence.

regions are randomly subcloned into plasmid and/or M13 vectors and then the subclones sequenced using fluorescence-based dideoxy sequencing protocols and automated DNA sequencers (Centre and Centre, 1998) to achieve a defined coverage of the genomic DNA segment. The shotgun sequences are assembled by computer to produce contigs covering the BAC sequence. Two levels of coverage are defined (Figure 3.5). The lower level of coverage, which provides a slightly less accurate sequence, is called working or rough draft (Bouck et al., 1998; Collins et al., 1998) (see Working Draft, 2000). At this level each clone is shotgun sequenced to an average coverage so that each base of the sequence submitted should be covered four times by sequence reads, contributing high-quality information to that base. The quality of the base is defined by a quality score (Q), which is generated by the base-calling software, Phred (Ewing and Green, 1998; Ewing et al., 1998), so that the mean coverage of the working draft sequence should be at least four calls of $Q \geq 20$ per base. The second higher level of coverage is the completed or 'finished' sequence, in which more shotgun reads are added, but in addition directed sequencing is undertaken to resolve ambiguities and close any remaining gaps in the sequence (Centre and Centre, 1998; McMurray et al., 1998; Dunham et al., 1999b). The overall error rate of the finished sequence is less than one error in 10 000 bases (Felsenfeld et al., 1999), and may actually be considerably better (Dunham et al., 1999b). Importantly, each of the institutes involved in the public consortium releases its sequence data immediately to the public sequence databases upon the first assembly according to what has been called the Bermuda Statement (Bentley, 1996). The sequences are released every 24 hours and are continuously updated as more shotgun data are added.

On 25 June 2000 DNA sequence equivalent to 86.8% of the human genome (assumed to be 3.15 gigabases (Gb)) had been deposited into Genbank/EMBL/DDBJ (NCBI, 2000). Some of this sequence (21.1%) was in highly accurate finished form, and the remainder (65.7%) was working draft sequence. The weighted average size of a sequence contig in the working draft sequence is around 200 kb, but it is also the case that many BAC sequences consist of between 5 and 20 contigs per clone. This milestone was announced by the consortium, consisting of 16 institutions world-wide (NHGRI, 2000; Sanger, 2000). At the time of writing the sequence has not been published in a peer-reviewed journal (see Note added in proof, p. 65). At the same time, Celera Genomics announced that they had assembled a whole genome shotgun DNA sequence of the human genome to give 4.6 X coverage of 3.12 Gb (Celera, 2000). Again at the time of writing it seems that Celera Genomics assembled the sequence from sets of paired reads from 2-kb and 10-kb plasmids and some 50-kb clones. It is difficult to know the exact state of this assembly (see Note added in proof, p. 65).

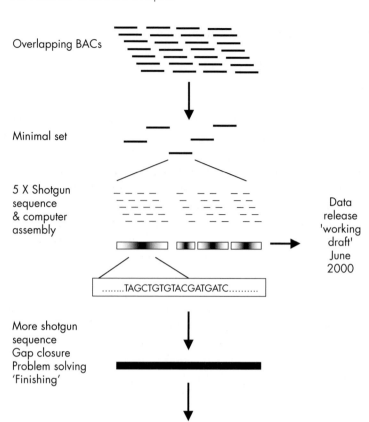

Overlapping BACs

Minimal set

5 X Shotgun
sequence
& computer
assembly

Data
release
'working
draft'
June
2000

.........TAGCTGTGTACGATGATC..........

More shotgun
sequence
Gap closure
Problem solving
'Finishing'

Data release and analysis
Complete product 2003

Figure 3.5 BAC-based genomic sequencing strategy. Sequence is generated by shotgun cloning and sequencing of BACs from the minimal tiling set as described in the text to form, successively, a working draft sequence and then a finished sequence. Shaded boxes indicate sequence contigs, with darker areas being higher quality sequence.

The working draft sequence must now be converted into the fully finished form across the entire genome. Currently it is predicted that this will happen by 2003. Already 21.1% of the sequence is in the highly accurate finished form, and the two smallest autosomes have been finished (Dunham *et al.*, 1999b; Hattori *et al.*, 2000). Chromosomes 20, 14 and 7 are progressing well (see NCBI, 2000, for progress updates). There is also the possibility that the public and private domain data could be combined in a freely accessible sequence, which would bring forward the finishing schedule.

Identifying genes and their structures

Identifying genes can be addressed at several levels. First, we wish to identify sequences that are likely to be part of a gene, to 'tag' that gene. Secondly, we would like to be able to identify all the exons that are part of a gene, and to annotate that structure. Ultimately we also wish to be able to define the tissues in which the gene is expressed and to define patterns of exon use through alternative splicing mechanisms. For the moment the first two structural levels are what has preoccupied the genome project, although increasingly microarray technology is beginning to look at the functional level as well.

As mentioned above, large collections of ESTs have now been assembled (Adams *et al.*, 1992, 1995; Hillier *et al.*, 1996) and clustering has been performed on these collections (Fields *et al.*, 1994; Schuler *et al.*, 1996). However, ESTs only sample part of the full-length message, and are imperfect representations of gene expression because of issues of redundancy, alternative splices and terminations (Figure 3.3B), as well as artefactual sequences which occur within cDNA libraries (Ewing and Green, 2000; Liang *et al.*, 2000). It also seems possible that even very large EST collections may not sample the majority of human genes (Ewing and Green, 2000; Liang *et al.*, 2000; Roest Crollius *et al.*, 2000). To address these issues there have been efforts to sequence full-length cDNA clones (Ohara *et al.*, 1997).

A second method for identifying genes is to use genomic sequence. There are two approaches that can be used for this. The first is to try to predict the presence of a gene by using software based on our current knowledge of gene features. A number of prediction packages have been developed for this approach (Burge and Karlin, 1997; Solovyev and Salamov, 1997; Claverie, 1997). However, calibration of these packages against genomic sequence with extensive experimental gene annotation suggests that although they are able to predict the presence of genes, at least partially, they are also prone to over-prediction and cannot be relied upon solely (Claverie, 1997; Dunham *et al.*, 1999b). The second approach is to use similarity searches to identify regions of genomic sequence with sequence similarity to known cDNAs, ESTs and protein sequences, and to use this information to delineate gene structures. It is also possible to use a combination of the prediction and similarity approaches either in a single software package (Kulp *et al.*, 1997) or as part of an overall annotation strategy. Both the completed sequences of chromosomes 21 and 22 used a combined annotation strategy. For chromosome 22, which is believed to be a relatively gene-dense chromosome, 545 genes and 134 pseudogenes were identified from the sequence (Dunham *et al.*, 1999b). Additionally it was speculated that a further 100 gene predictions which did not have support from similarity searching might also be real genes. In contrast, only 225 genes and 59 pseudogenes were identified from the chromosome 21 sequence. This was consistent with prior data that suggested that chromosome 21 was gene-poor. Taking the chromosome 22 and 21 data together would suggest that there might be less than 50 000 genes in the whole genome.

Identifying genes in the working draft sequence is still ongoing. However, the Ensembl database provides a first public analysis of the genes in the working draft sequence using a combined prediction and similarity matching approach (see Ensembl, 2000). The database provides tools for viewing genes identified within the sequence, and is being updated continuously. At the current time the Ensembl project have identified just under 40 000 confirmed genes in the sequence. There has been some debate about how many genes are likely to be found in the genome (Smaglik, 2000; Ewing and Green, 2000; Liang *et al.*, 2000; Roest Crollius *et al.*, 2000), but current estimates appear to be favouring a number below 50 000.

Human genome sequence variation and SNPs

One aim of the Human Genome Project is to provide a reference DNA sequence from which to detail sequence variation in human populations. This genotypic diversity is presumed to be the basis of heritable phenotypic differences such as drug response variation and susceptibility to disease. Hence, identification of sequence variation will provide the tools to enable discovery of the causative genetic factors (Collins *et al.*, 1997; Housman and Ledley, 1998). The major types of sequence variation in the genome are SNPs and small insertions or deletions of one or a few nucleotides. There have been a number of strategies used to identify SNPs in the human genome that have focused on candidate genes for common diseases (Nickerson *et al.*, 1998; Cambien *et al.*, 1999; Cargill *et al.*, 1999; Halushka *et al.*, 1999), genes with ESTs (Wang *et al.*, 1998; Buetow *et al.*, 1999; Garg *et al.*, 1999; Marth *et al.*, 1999; Picoult-Newberg *et al.*, 1999), or genomic sequence (Kwok *et al.*, 1996; Kawasaki *et al.*, 1997; Horton *et al.*, 1998; Lai *et al.*, 1998; Taillon-Miller *et al.*, 1998, 1999; Wang *et al.*, 1998). The gene-based approaches use either resequencing of the gene in a panel of individuals or electronic alignment of EST and cDNA sequences. For variations in genomic sequence the two main methods have been either to resequence the area of interest using PCR products (Kwok *et al.*, 1996; Lai *et al.*, 1998; Wang *et al.*, 1998), specially constructed shotgun libraries (Mullikin *et al.*, 2000; Altshuler *et al.*, 2000), or the overlapping sections of clones from the tiling paths of large-scale sequencing projects (Kawasaki *et al.*, 1997; Horton *et al.*, 1998; Taillon-Miller *et al.*, 1998). The SNPs identified by many of these projects are available through a public database, dbSNP (see Table 3.1).

A major effort to identify SNPs has been established by the SNP Consortium (SNP Consortium, 2000), an international partnership of pharmaceutical companies, genome sequencing centres and the Wellcome Trust. By April 2000 over 100 000 SNPs had been identified and mapped in the genome. With the benefit of the draft genome sequence, by the end of 2000 the consortium substantially surpassed its initial target of 300 000 genome-wide SNPs.

In combination we should soon have an SNP map of the genome with at least one SNP per 10 kb. This will be an extremely powerful resource for study of genetic disease.

Conclusion

The last decade has seen dramatic advances in our knowledge of the structure of the genome. We are now at the stage where genomic DNA sequence is available for most of the genome, and the resources of cytogenetic reagents, genetic markers and gene sequences can be integrated through the common metric of the DNA sequence. This should be an extremely powerful tool for designing reagents for gene therapy.

Note added in proof

In February 2001 the two initial assemblies of the human genome sequence were published, together with supporting papers on mapping, SNPs and other areas. See International Human Genome Consortium (2001) Initial sequencing and analysis of the human genome. *Nature* 409: 860–921. Venter, J C, *et al.* (2001) The sequence of the human genome. *Science* 291: 1304–1351.

Acknowledgements

The author wishes to thank all the members of the Sanger Centre past and present, and the other members of the International Human Genome Sequencing Consortium. Many thanks are also due to Luc Smink and Andy Mungall for their comments on the manuscript and for Sean Humphray for help with Figure 3.4. The author is supported by the Wellcome Trust.

References

Adams M D, Dubnick M, Kerlavage A R, *et al.* (1992) Sequence identification of 2,375 human brain genes. *Nature* 355: 632–634.

Adams M D, Kerlavage A R, Fleischmann R D, *et al.* (1995) Initial assessment of human gene diversity and expression patterns based upon 83 million nucleotides of cDNA sequence. *Nature* 377: 3–174.

Alizadeh A A, Eisen M B, Davis R E, *et al.* (2000) Distinct types of diffuse large B-cell lymphoma identified by gene expression profiling. *Nature* 403: 503–511.

Altshuler D, Pollara V J, Cowles C, *et al.* (2000) A human SNP map generated by reduced representation shotgun sequencing. *Nature* 407: 513–516.

Bentley D R (1996) Genomic sequence information should be released immediately and freely in the public domain. *Science* 274: 533–534.

Boguski M S, Schuler G D (1995) ESTablishing a human transcript map. *Nat Genet* 10: 369–371.

Bouck J, Miller W, Gorrell J H, *et al.* (1998) Analysis of the quality and utility of random shotgun sequencing at low redundancies. *Genome Res* 8: 1074–1084.

Bouffard G G, Idol J R, Braden V V, *et al.* (1997) A physical map of human chromosome 7: an integrated YAC contig map with average STS spacing of 79 kb. *Genome Res* 7: 673–692.

Brownstein B H, Silverman G A, Little R D, *et al.* (1989) Isolation of single-copy human genes from a library of yeast artificial chromosome clones. *Science* 244: 1348–1351.

Buetow K H, Edmonson M N, Cassidy, A B (1999) Reliable identification of large numbers of candidate SNPs from public EST data. *Nat Genet* 21: 323–325.

Buetow K H, Ludwigsen S, Scherpbier-Heddema T, *et al.* (1994a) Human genetic map. Genome maps V. Wall chart. *Science* 265: 2055–2070.

Buetow K H, Weber J L, Ludwigsen S, *et al.* (1994b) Integrated human genome-wide maps constructed using the CEPH reference panel. *Nat Genet* 6: 391–393.

Burge C, Karlin S (1997) Prediction of complete gene structures in human genomic DNA. *J Mol Biol* 268: 78–94.

Burke D T, Carle G F, Olson, M V (1987) Cloning of large segments of exogenous DNA into yeast by means of artificial chromosome vectors. *Science* 236: 806–812.

Cambien F, Poirier O, Nicaud V, *et al.* (1999) Sequence diversity in 36 candidate genes for cardiovascular disorders. *Am J Hum Genet* 65: 183–191.

Cargill M, Altshuler D, Ireland J, *et al.* (1999) Characterization of single-nucleotide polymorphisms in coding regions of human genes. *Nat Genet* 22: 231–238.

Celera (2000) http://www.celera.com/corporate/about/press_releases/celera062600_1.html

Centre T S, Centre G S (1998) Toward a complete human genome sequence. *Genome Res* 8: 1097–1108.

Chumakov I, Rigault P, Guillou S, *et al.* (1992) Continuum of overlapping clones spanning the entire human chromosome 21q. *Nature* 359: 380–387.

Chumakov I M, Rigault P, Le Gall I, *et al.* (1995) A YAC contig map of the human genome. *Nature* 377: 175–297.

Claverie J M (1997) Computational methods for the identification of genes in vertebrate genomic sequences. *Hum Mol Genet* 6: 1735–1744.

Collins F S, Guyer M S, Charkravarti A (1997) Variations on a theme: cataloging human DNA sequence variation. *Science* 278: 1580–1581.

Collins F S, Patrinos A, Jordan E, *et al.* (1998) New goals for the U.S. Human Genome Project: 1998–2003. *Science* 282: 682–689.

Collins J E, Cole C G, Smink L J, *et al.* (1995) A high-density YAC contig map of human chromosome 22. *Nature* 377: 367–379.

Cook-Deegan R M (1989) The Alta summit, December 1984. *Genomics* 5: 661–663.

Crollius H R, Ross M T, Grigoriev A, *et al.* (1996) An integrated YAC map of the human X chromosome. *Genome Res* 6: 943–955.

Deloukas P, Schuler G D, Gyapay G, *et al.* (1998) A physical map of 30,000 human genes. *Science* 282: 744–746.

Dib C, Faure S, Fizames C, *et al.* (1996) A comprehensive genetic map of the human genome based on 5,264 microsatellites. *Nature* 380: 152–154.

Doggett N A, Goodwin L A, Tesmer J G, *et al.* (1995) An integrated physical map of human chromosome 16. *Nature* 377: 335–365.

Donis-Keller H, Green P, Helms C, *et al.* (1987) A genetic linkage map of the human genome. *Cell* 51: 319–337.

Dulbecco R (1986) A turning point in cancer research: sequencing the human genome. *Science* 231: 1055–1056.

Dunham I, Dewar K, Kim U-J, Ross M T (1999a) In: Birren B, Green E D, Klapholz S, *et al.*, eds. *Genome Analysis: A Laboratory Manual Series*, Vol. 3: *Cloning Systems*. Cold Spring Harbor, NY: Cold Spring Harbor Laboratory Press, 1–86.

Dunham I, Hunt A R, Collins J E, *et al.* (1999b) The DNA sequence of human chromosome 22. *Nature* 402: 489–495.

Ensembl (2000) http://www.ensembl.org (accessed July 2000).

Ewing B, Green, P (1998) Base-calling of automated sequencer traces using phred. II. Error probabilities. *Genome Res* 8: 186–194.

Ewing B, Green, P (2000) Analysis of expressed sequence tags indicates 35,000 human genes. *Nat Genet* 25: 232–234.

Ewing B, Hillier L, Wendl M C, Green P (1998) Base-calling of automated sequencer traces using phred. I. Accuracy assessment. *Genome Res* 8: 175–185.

Felsenfeld A, Peterson J, Schloss J, Guyer M (1999) Assessing the quality of the DNA sequence from the Human Genome Project. *Genome Res* 9: 1–4.

Fields C, Adams M D, White O, Venter J C (1994) How many genes in the human genome? *Nat Genet* 7: 345–346.

Garg K, Green P, Nickerson, D A (1999) Identification of candidate coding region single nucleotide polymorphisms in 165 human genes using assembled expressed sequence tags. *Genome Res* 9: 1087–1092.

Gemmill R M, Chumakov I, Scott P, *et al.* (1995) A second-generation YAC contig map of human chromosome 3. *Nature* 377: 299–319.

Golub T R, Slonim D K, Tamayo P, *et al.* (1999) Molecular classification of cancer: class discovery and class prediction by gene expression monitoring. *Science* 286: 531–537.

Green E D, Riethman H C, Dutchik J E, Olson M V (1991) Detection and characterization of chimeric yeast artificial-chromosome clones. *Genomics* 11: 658–669.

Gregory S G, Howell G R, Bentley D R (1997) Genome mapping by fluorescent fingerprinting. *Genome Res* 7: 1162–1168.

Gyapay G, Morissette J, Vignal A, *et al.* (1994) The 1993–94 Genethon human genetic linkage map. *Nat Genet* 7: 246–339.

Gyapay G, Schmitt K, Fizames C, *et al.* (1996) A radiation hybrid map of the human genome. *Hum Mol Genet* 5: 339–346.

Halushka M K, Fan J B, Bentley K, *et al.* (1999) Patterns of single-nucleotide polymorphisms in candidate genes for blood-pressure homeostasis. *Nat Genet* 22: 239–247.

Han C S, Sutherland R D, Jewett P B, *et al.* (2000) Construction of a BAC contig map of chromosome 16q by two-dimensional overgo hybridization. *Genome Res* 10: 714–721.

Hattori M, Fujiyama A, Taylor T D, *et al.* (2000) The DNA sequence of human chromosome 21. The chromosome 21 mapping and sequencing consortium. *Nature* 405: 311–319.

Hillier L D, Lennon G, Becker M, *et al.* (1996) Generation and analysis of 280,000 human expressed sequence tags. *Genome Res* 6: 807–828.

Horton R, Niblett D, Milne S, *et al.* (1998) Large-scale sequence comparisons reveal unusually high levels of variation in the HLA-DQB1 locus in the class II region of the human MHC. *J Mol Biol* 282: 71–97.

Housman D, Ledley F D (1998) Why pharmacogenomics? Why now? *Nat Biotechnol* 16: 492–493.

Hudson T J, Stein L D, Gerety S S, *et al.* (1995) An STS-based map of the human genome. *Science* 270: 1945–1954.

Ioannou P A, Amemiya C T, Garnes J, *et al.* (1994) A new bacteriophage P1-derived vector for the propagation of large human DNA fragments. *Nat Genet* 6: 84–89.

Kawasaki K, Minoshima S, Nakato E, *et al.* (1997) One-megabase sequence analysis of the human immunoglobulin lambda gene locus. *Genome Res* 7: 250–261.

Kirsch I R, Green E D, Yonescu R, *et al.* (2000) A systematic, high-resolution linkage of the cytogenetic and physical maps of the human genome. *Nat Genet* 24: 339–340.

Krauter K, Montgomery K, Yoon S J, *et al.* (1995) A second-generation YAC contig map of human chromosome 12. *Nature* 377: 321–333.

Kulp D, Haussler D, Reese M G, Eeckman, F H (1997) Integrating database homology in a probabilistic gene structure model. *Pac Symp Biocomput* 232–244.

Kwok P Y, Deng Q, Zakeri H, Taylor S L, Nickerson, D A (1996) Increasing the information content of STS-based genome maps: identifying polymorphisms in mapped STSs. *Genomics* 31: 123–126.

Kwok, P Y, Gu Z (1999) Single nucleotide polymorphism libraries: why and how are we building them? *Mol Med Today* 5: 538–543.

Lai E, Riley J, Purvis I, Roses, A (1998) A 4-Mb high-density single nucleotide polymorphism-based map around human APOE. *Genomics* 54: 31–38.

Leversha M A, Dunham I, Carter N P (1999) A molecular cytogenetic clone resource for chromosome 22. *Chromosome Res* 7: 571–573.

Liang F, Holt I, Pertea G, *et al.* (2000) Gene index analysis of the human genome estimates approximately 120,000 genes. *Nat Genet* 25: 239–240.

Lichter P, Boyle A L, Cremer T, Ward, D C (1991) Analysis of genes and chromosomes by nonisotopic *in situ* hybridization. *Genet Anal Tech Appl* 8: 24–35.

Macilwain, C (2000) World leaders heap praise on human genome landmark. *Nature* 405: 983–984.

Marra M A, Kucaba T A, Dietrich N L, *et al.* (1997) High throughput fingerprint analysis of large-insert clones. *Genome Res* 7: 1072–1084.

Marth G T, Korf I, Yandell M D, *et al.* (1999) A general approach to single-nucleotide polymorphism discovery. *Nat Genet* 23: 452–456.

McMurray A A, Sulston J E, Quail, M A (1998) Short-insert libraries as a method of problem solving in genome sequencing. *Genome Res* 8: 562–566.

Mitelman F, ed. (1995) *ISCN (1995): An International System for Cytogenetic Nomenclature.* Basel: S. Karger.

Mullikin J C, Hunt S E, Cole C G, *et al.* (2000) A SNP map of human chromosome 22. *Nature* 407: 516–520.

Mungall A J, Humphray S J, Ranby S A, *et al.* (1997) From long range mapping to sequence-ready contigs on human chromosome 6. *DNA Seq* 8: 151–154.

Murray J C, Buetow K H, Weber J L, *et al.* (1994) A comprehensive human linkage map with centimorgan density. Cooperative Human Linkage Center (CHLC). *Science* 265: 2049–2054.

NCBI (2000) http: //www.ncbi.nlm.nih.gov/genome/seq/ (accessed May 2000).

NHGRI (2000) http: //www.nhgri.nih.gov/NEWS/sequencing_consortium.html#press (accessed May 2000).

Nickerson D A, Taylor S L, Weiss K M, *et al.* (1998) DNA sequence diversity in a 9.7-kb region of the human lipoprotein lipase gene. *Nat Genet* 19: 233–240.

Ohara O, Nagase T, Ishikawa K, *et al.* (1997) Construction and characterization of human brain cDNA libraries suitable for analysis of cDNA clones encoding relatively large proteins. *DNA Res* 4: 53–59.

Olson M, Hood L, Cantor C, Botstein D (1989) A common language for physical mapping of the human genome. *Science* 245: 1434–1435.

Picoult-Newberg L, Ideker T E, Pohl M G, *et al.* (1999) Mining SNPs from EST databases. *Genome Res* 9: 167–174.

Pinkel D, Segraves R, Sudar D, *et al.* (1998) High resolution analysis of DNA copy number variation using comparative genomic hybridization to microarrays. *Nat Genet* 20: 207–211.

Reed P W, Davies J L, Copeman J B, *et al.* (1994) Chromosome-specific microsatellite sets for fluorescence-based, semi-automated genome mapping. *Nat Genet* 7: 390–395.

RH Mapping Consortium (1999) http: //www.ncbi.nlm.nih.gov/genemap99/ (accessed June 2000).

Roest Crollius H, Jaillon O, Bernot A, *et al.* (2000) Estimate of human gene number provided by genome-wide analysis using *Tetraodon nigroviridis* DNA sequence. *Nat Genet* 25: 235–238.

Sanger (2000) http: //www.sanger.ac.uk/Info/Press/000626.shtml (accessed July 2000).

Schuler G D, Boguski M S, Stewart E A, *et al.* (1996) A gene map of the human genome. *Science* 274: 540–546.

Shizuya H, Birren B, Kim U J, *et al.* (1992) Cloning and stable maintenance of 300-kilobase-pair fragments of human DNA in *Escherichia coli* using an F-factor-based vector. *Proc Natl Acad Sci USA* 89: 8794–8797.

Smaglik P (2000) Researchers take a gamble on the human genome. *Nature* 405: 264.

SNP Consortium (2000) http: //snp.cshl.org/ (accessed June 2000).

Soderlund C, Longden I, Mott, R (1997) FPC: a system for building contigs from restriction fingerprinted clones. *Comput Appl Biosci* 13: 523–535.

Solovyev V, Salamov A (1997) The Gene-Finder computer tools for analysis of human and model organisms genome sequences. *Proc Int Conf Intell Syst Mol Biol* 5: 294–302.

Stewart E A, McKusick K B, Aggarwal A, *et al.* (1997) An STS-based radiation hybrid map of the human genome. *Genome Res* 7: 422–433.

Taillon-Miller P, Gu Z, Li Q, *et al.* (1998) Overlapping genomic sequences: a treasure trove of single-nucleotide polymorphisms. *Genome Res* 8: 748–754.

Taillon-Miller P, Piernot E E, Kwok, P Y (1999) Efficient approach to unique single-nucleotide polymorphism discovery. *Genome Res* 9: 499–505.

Trask B J (1991) Fluorescence *in situ* hybridization: applications in cytogenetics and gene mapping. *Trends Genet* 7: 149–154.

Venter J C, Smith H O, Hood L (1996) A new strategy for genome sequencing. *Nature* 381: 364–366.

Wakefield P M, Tinsley J M, Wood M J, *et al.* (2000) Prevention of the dystrophic phenotype in dystrophin/utrophin-deficient muscle following adenovirus-mediated transfer of a utrophin minigene. *Gene Ther* 7: 201–204.

Walter M A, Spillett D J, Thomas P, *et al.* (1994) A method for constructing radiation hybrid maps of whole genomes. *Nat Genet* 7: 22–28.

Wang D G, Fan J B, Siao C J, *et al.* (1998) Large-scale identification, mapping, and genotyping of single-nucleotide polymorphisms in the human genome. *Science* 280: 1077–1082.

Weber J L, May P E (1989) Abundant class of human DNA polymorphisms which can be typed using the polymerase chain reaction. *Am J Hum Genet* 44: 388–396.

Weissenbach J, Gyapay G, Dib C, *et al.* (1992) A second-generation linkage map of the human genome. *Nature* 359: 794–801.

Working Draft (2000) http: //www.nhgri.nih.gov/Grant_info/Funding/Statements/ RFA/quality_standard.html (accessed June 2000).

4

Gene therapy for single gene disorders

Christine Kinnon and Adrian J Thrasher

In many respects, the application of gene therapy to the treatment of single gene disorders appears to be a straightforward prospect. In general terms, it requires the introduction of a single gene into a specified cell type. There are estimated to be over 4000 human diseases caused by single gene defects, and it should, in theory, be possible to treat many of these by this kind of therapy. Clearly, the defective gene must first be identified and cloned, and with the completion of the Human Genome Project this should not prove to be the rate-limiting step. However, the prospect in many cases is not as straightforward as it seems. The most pertinent problems that can arise with this type of therapy are associated with obtaining sufficiently high levels of gene delivery and maintaining appropriate levels of gene expression without repeated intervention.

In many cases, successful attempts have been made to correct cells from patients with diseases caused by single gene defects in an *in vitro* situation. There has also been substantial success reported in treating appropriate animal models. On the basis of such attempts clinical trials have been initiated for a variety of diseases, although these have met with little success. Recently, however, there has been a report of a successful clinical trial of gene therapy for X-linked severe combined immunodeficiency (SCID). In this chapter we will concentrate on describing the application of clinical trials of gene therapy for SCID.

Cystic fibrosis

The largest of the clinical trials of gene therapy have involved transfer of the cystic fibrosis transmembrane conductance regulator (CFTR) gene in cystic fibrosis, and over 100 patients have received such therapy to date (reviewed in Crystal, 1995; Zeitlin, 2000). The CFTR gene was identified in 1989. It encodes an epithelial chloride ion channel which, when defective, affects the secretion of mucus in the lungs and digestive tract. The normal CFTR protein is expected to exert a dominant function over the mutant CFTR, which makes it a good candidate disorder for treatment by gene therapy. Since the target epithelial cells are terminally differentiated and relatively short-lived, there is no necessity for integration of the transgene, which means that gene delivery can be achieved using non-integrating vectors. Although both adenoviral vectors and liposomes have been shown to work effectively in *in vitro* gene therapy studies for cystic fibrosis, clinical studies delivering DNA to the nasal, and more recently lung, epithelia have shown only weak and short-lived correction (see, for example, Alton *et al.*, 1999; Harvey *et al.*, 1999). There is an added complication in that repeated administration of adenoviral vectors have reduced effectiveness and can cause adverse reactions in some patients (Harvey *et al.*, 1999).

Severe combined immunodeficiencies (SCIDs)

Without doubt the greatest clinical experience with gene therapy is in use of murine retroviral vectors for the treatment of SCID, particularly for patients with adenosine deaminase deficiency (ADA) (Blaese *et al.*, 1995; Bordignon *et al.*, 1995; Kohn *et al.*, 1995; Hoogerbrugge *et al.*, 1996), though more recently success has been reported for patients with X-linked SCID (Cavazzana-Calvo *et al.*, 2000).

SCIDs are a group of inherited disorders characterised by a profound reduction or absence of T-lymphocyte function (reviewed in Fischer, 2000). The resulting deficits in both cell-mediated and humoral immune responses invariably lead to premature mortality in the absence of haematopoietic stem cell transplantation. Since the first successful HLA-matched bone marrow transplants (BMT) were performed in two primary immunodeficiency disorders over 30 years ago, transplantation technology has advanced considerably. The cure rate for SCID using matched sibling donors is now over 95% and one recent study reported 100% cure (Buckley *et al.*, 1999). However, for only 30% of patients does such a donor exist, and for T cell-depleted haplo-identical parental grafts, the success rate falls to 60%. Complications can relate to toxicity arising from any conditioning regimen, the presence of mature T cells in the marrow graft, pre-existing infection and delayed reconstitution of immune function post transplant (Fischer *et al.*, 1990; Buckley *et al.*, 1999; Fischer, 1999). *In utero* transplantation of haplo-identical cells has been attempted to pre-empt the development of clinical disease, and to utilise the proliferative and possibly tolerogenic fetal environment to facilitate engraftment (Flake *et al.*, 1996; Wengler *et al.*, 1996). The efficacy and safety of this approach awaits comparison with conventional transplantation, and remains limited to those families with previously affected children.

X-linked severe combined immunodeficiency

The X-linked form of SCID (X-SCID) is often distinguishable from other forms by its characteristic pattern of inheritance and the observation that affected boys have no T cells or natural killer (NK) cells and often have apparently normal levels of B cells (T–NK–B+ SCID), although these are intrinsically abnormal. X-SCID accounts for about 50–60% of all cases of SCID and is caused by defects in the interleukin 2 receptor (IL-2R) γ-chain gene (reviewed in Fischer, 2000). The γc (common gamma) chain is expressed constitutively in haematolymphoid cells and is a component of several other cytokine receptors, including IL-4R, IL-7R, IL-9R and IL-15R. It is postulated that in each of the affected receptors the unique chain recognises the specific cytokine, and thus confers the signalling specificity, while γc transduces the signal via its cytoplasmic domain. The early blocks in T- and NK-cell development are thought to be caused by the failure of the IL-7 and IL-15 receptors, respectively, to transmit survival and proliferative signals. Defects in IL-2 and IL-4 signalling may contribute to the intrinsic B-cell defects.

Adenosine deaminase and purine nucleoside phosphorylase deficiencies

SCID can arise as a result of deficiencies in certain enzymes involved in purine metabolism. As many as 25% of all cases of SCID may be caused by defects in adenosine deaminase (ADA), while a few cases (about 4%) are caused by defects in purine nucleoside phosphorylase (PNP).

ADA deficiency in humans results primarily in immunological dysfunction with T and B lymphopenia (reviewed in Hershfield and Mitchell, 1995). The highest enzymatic activity of ADA is found in immature thymocytes, and deficiency results in impaired intrathymic differentiation. Accumulation of deoxyadenosine in T cells is accompanied by preferential conversion to the toxic compound deoxyadenosine triphosphate (dATP), and the build up of other toxic metabolites. Despite ubiquitous constitutive expression of ADA, lymphocytes are particularly susceptible to toxicity from accumulating metabolites, possibly because of predominant inhibition of T cell-specific molecules during intrathymic differentiation (Benveniste *et al.*, 1995).

Other autosomal recessive SCIDs

There are now many forms of SCID described which are individually quite rare, usually only a few families or individuals are affected. These are caused by the inheritance of defective autosomal genes. Many of these genes are involved in T-cell development, signalling or proliferation (reviewed in Fischer, 2000).

Jak-3 defects

The Jak-3 kinase is known to associate with γc chain-containing cytokine receptors and Jak-3 mutations have been identified in a small number of SCID patients with immunophenotypes equivalent to X-SCID, including blocked NK-cell differentiation.

Recombination activating genes (RAG1 and RAG2) defects

As many as half of T–B– SCID patients may be affected by mutations in the RAG1 and/or RAG2 genes. These proteins are involved in the process of VDJ rearrangement, which is essential for production of functional immunoglobulin and T-cell receptor (TCR) proteins.

ZAP 70 defects

Mutations in ZAP 70, a TCR-associated protein tyrosine kinase that is associated with the ζ chains of the TCR–CD3 complex, produce a distinctive form of SCID characterised by absence of CD8+ and abundance of CD4+ peripheral T cells (CD4+CD8–B+ SCID).

TCR–CD3 abnormalities

Rarely, defective expression and function of the TCR–CD3 complex of T cells can occur as a result of mutations in the γ or ε genes of the CD3 complex, resulting in a variable phenotype disease.

Somatic gene therapy for SCID

Although rare, primary immunodeficiencies are in many ways ideally
suited to the application of this technology, and have become model conditions on which to design and test gene therapy protocols. Rapid progress
in understanding the molecular basis for some of these disorders, including ADA-SCID, X-SCID, Jak-3 kinase deficiency and ZAP 70 deficiency,
has facilitated the development of therapeutic strategies based on genetic
manipulation of autologous cells (Osborne *et al.*, 1990; Ferrari *et al.*,
1991; Candotti *et al.*, 1996; Hacein-Bey *et al.*, 1996; Taylor *et al.*, 1996;
Bunting *et al.*, 1998; Cavazzana-Calvo *et al.*, 2000; Soudais *et al.*, 2000).

Treatment for ADA-SCID

Enzyme replacement therapy with bovine ADA conjugated to poly-
ethylene glycol (PEG-ADA), has resulted in significant improvement in
lymphocyte cell numbers and function in many ADA-SCID patients, but
the response is variable, and may be transient (Hershfield, 1995). This
probably reflects the main site of PEG-ADA activity which is extracellular, and which only partially complements the cellular deficiency. Complete absence of ADA results in lethality before 2 years of age. However,
retention of only 1–5% of activity often leads to attenuated disease, and
individuals with as little as 10% activity have been found to be immunologically normal, while levels of ADA 50 times above normal have also
been associated with normal immunity. These considerations have
important implications for the design of gene therapy vectors, but
suggest that relatively simple expression systems may be efficacious for
this condition. Furthermore, spontaneous reversion to normal of inherited mutations *in vivo* (resulting in somatic mosaicism) has recently been
demonstrated in two patients with attenuated disease (one with ADA-
SCID and another with X-SCID) suggesting that corrected cells have a
distinct growth and differentiation advantage over mutants (Hirschhorn
et al., 1996; Stephan *et al.*, 1996).

Retroviral vectors for gene therapy of ADA-SCID

A variety of techniques have been developed for transferring genetic
material into human cells, each with its associated advantages and disadvantages (Table 4.1). The most commonly used vectors tend to be

Table 4.1   Gene transfer methods

Vector	Capacity	In vitro transduction efficiency	In vitro integration efficiency	Strengths	Weaknesses
Retroviruses (MoMLV)	<8 kb	High	High (only in dividing cells)	Stable	Moderately efficient
Lentiviruses (HIV)	<8 kb	High	High	Stable, efficient	Safety concerns
Adenovirus	<35 kb	High	Low	Efficient	Transient, immuno-genic, safety concerns
Adeno-associated virus	4 kb	High	High	Stable	Inefficient for PHSC
Physical methods (including liposomes and electro-poration)	Potentially unlimited	Low	Low	Non-viral	Inefficient, transient

virus-based, because of the relatively high efficiencies of transduction that can be obtained. Where stable integration of transferred sequences is required, then retroviruses have most often been the vectors of choice. The murine oncoretrovirus *Moloney murine leukemia virus* (MoMLV) has formed the backbone of the retroviral vectors that have so far been used in clinical trials for SCID. The single-stranded RNA genome is reverse transcribed to double-stranded DNA which integrates into the chromosome of the target cell during cell division, where it becomes a stable genetic element passed on to all subsequent progeny cells. Thus, although stability can be achieved it is dependent on the process of cell division. Furthermore, integration is at random sites in the target cell genome which could potentially lead to unpredictable gene expression or insertional mutagenesis. Another potential problem is the generation of replication-competent recombinant viruses, though the risks are min-imised. Gene transfer to human cells has been optimised using the murine amphotropic retrovirus envelope protein, though the receptor expression on human cells may be limited (Orlic *et al.*, 1996). Future clinical trials may benefit from more effective gene transfer mediated by alternative envelope proteins, including the gibbon ape leukemia virus (GALV) protein (Demaison *et al.*, 2000) and the feline endogenous viral envelope (RD114) protein (Porter *et al.*, 1996).

T lymphocyte gene therapy for ADA-SCID

The ability of HLA-matched genotypically identical stem cell transplants for severe ADA deficiency to selectively reconstitute the lymphoid compartment in the absence of cytoablative conditioning suggested that biochemical correction of autologous T cells by somatic gene transfer could provide a similar therapeutic outcome. This was supported by preclinical studies which demonstrated a survival advantage of transduced ADA-SCID T cells in immunodeficient mice (Ferrari *et al.*, 1991).

The first ever approved clinical trial of gene therapy began in 1990 at the National Institutes of Health (NIH), and involved repeated *ex vivo* transduction of autologous peripheral blood T cells with a MoMLV-based retroviral vector expressing human ADA, followed by expansion and reinfusion into two patients (Blaese *et al.*, 1995). Although both patients had attenuated disease, at the time of enrolment both were lymphopenic, anergic and had depressed immune reactivity to specific antigens despite receiving optimal PEG-ADA enzyme replacement therapy. Within five to six months of gene therapy, the lymphocyte count in one patient had risen into the normal range, and remained stable for at least 2 years after the last infusion of transduced cells. Levels of ADA in blood lymphocytes stabilised at roughly half that found in heterozygote carriers, and was associated with return of delayed-type hypersensitivity (DTH) skin test reactivity, cytolytic responses and antibody production. The second patient also responded with an initial increase in peripheral T lymphocyte numbers to levels in the high normal range, although these fell over time to levels just above those at enrolment. In contrast to the first patient, ADA levels remained very low, correlating with low gene transfer efficiency (<10% as efficient as the other patient). Some return of immune reactivity was demonstrated, but could have arisen as a result of infusion of an expanded T-cell population, and was variable anyway prior to enrolment.

This trial demonstrates the potential efficacy of gene transfer to autologous T cells for therapy of ADA-SCID, and at the present time is suggestive of clinical benefit. The outcome is confused by the concurrent administration of exogenous PEG-ADA, which to a variable extent complements the cellular immunodeficiency. Discontinuation of this treatment would seem to be the obvious test for efficacy of gene transfer, but normalisation of T lymphocyte ADA levels alone may also be insufficient to correct the immunodeficiency fully, and may necessitate continued therapy. One concern with T lymphocyte gene therapy is the potential for insertional mutagenesis arising from multiple integration events during the transduction procedure. At present there is no evidence to suggest that this has occurred. Interestingly, attempts to utilise cytokine-mobilised peripheral blood progenitor cells from ADA-SCID patients for gene transfer have been limited by poor yield (Sekhsaria et al., 1996).

Stem cell gene therapy for ADA-SCID

The optimal target cell for curative gene therapy of many haematopoietic disorders is the pluripotent haematopoietic stem cell (PHSC). Much interest has therefore been directed towards attempts to achieve this goal. The first attempt in a clinical setting to transduce bone marrow cells from a patient with ADA deficiency was conducted by Bordignon and colleagues in Milan, and was combined with re-infusion of genetically modified peripheral blood lymphocytes (Bordignon et al., 1995). In this study, two retroviral vectors, distinguishable by molecular techniques, were used to transfer an ADA minigene into either bone marrow or lymphocytes from two patients with attenuated ADA-SCID who had become immunologically refractory to exogenous enzyme replacement. Administration of genetically modified cells resulted in normalisation of lymphocyte counts, antigen-specific immune responses, and mitogen and antigen-specific proliferation. The T-cell repertoire (V_β) was also shown to normalise progressively. Significantly, one year after discontinuation of gene therapy, peripheral T cells derived from the transduced lymphocyte population were gradually replaced by T cells derived from bone marrow, suggesting a proliferative advantage. Both children enrolled in this trial continued to receive enzyme replacement therapy, although relative dosages were decreasing. Withdrawal of PEG-ADA should reveal the true efficacy of gene transfer, and may enhance the proliferative advantage of corrected cells.

In a separate study, CD34+ cells obtained from the bone marrow of three children with ADA deficiency were used as targets for transduction by a retroviral vector encoding the human ADA cDNA (Hoogerbrugge et al., 1996). Mononuclear cells and granulocytes retaining the vector genome were detectable by PCR in the peripheral circulation for up to three months after gene transfer, and in one patient, in the bone marrow at six months. Detection of the vector genome after this period of time was not possible. One patient did not receive enzyme replacement until three months after infusion in an attempt to maximise proliferative advantage, although it is likely that because gene transfer efficiency was very low, this was not a sufficient time period for genetically corrected clones to reveal themselves.

Limiting factors for stem cell gene therapy

The inefficiency of retroviral transduction of the human PHSC population has been highlighted. The requirement for the current generation of retroviral vectors to transduce actively dividing cells may be a limiting factor because PHSCs are relatively quiescent. It was thought that cells harvested from umbilical cord blood might be better targets for retrovirus-mediated gene transfer, and they were therefore used in a clinical trial for ADA-SCID. In this study, three prenatally diagnosed infants received infusions of transduced cord blood CD34+ cells shortly after birth and were commenced on enzyme replacement therapy. Eighteen months after transplantation the proportion of lymphocytes retaining the transgene and levels of ADA activity in unselected cells was extremely low (Kohn *et al.*, 1995). It was expected that gradual withdrawal of PEG-ADA might facilitate the proliferation of gene-corrected cells, however this does not appear to be the case, cessation of PEG-ADA treatment in one patient 4 years after gene therapy treatment led to a decline in immune function. This suggests that although there is evidence for long-term engraftment of transduced stem cells and accumulation of peripheral T cells containing the transgene, there is still a need for improved efficiency of gene transfer and expression before clinical benefit can be achieved for this disease (Kohn *et al.*, 1998).

Clinical gene therapy for X-SCID

The most exciting results in this field have recently been reported from a clinical trial of gene therapy in two infants with X-SCID (Cavazzana-Calvo *et al.*, 2000). Following successful preclinical studies for X-SCID (Candotti *et al.*, 1996; Hacein-Bey *et al.*, 1996; Taylor *et al.*, 1996; Soudais *et al.*, 2000), CD34+ bone marrow cells were harvested from two X-SCID patients aged 11 months and 8 months, and preactivated and infected daily for 3 days with retroviral γc vector-containing super-natant. Following this, the CD34+ cells were infused into the patients without prior chemoablation. Two weeks after infusion, peripheral blood cells were found to be positive for the γc transgene by PCR. T-cell counts increased between one and two months and continued to rise over the next eight months. The children were able to leave protective iso-lation three months after treatment. After a ten-month period, γc trans-gene expression and function in the appropriate cell types, and antigen-specific responses in the normal range, could be observed. It can be concluded that gene therapy has provided full correction of the disease phenotype and that these children are 'cured' of their disease. Similar results have now been obtained for two additional children.

The improved success of this clinical trial over those previously conducted for ADA-SCID is attributable to several factors. First, X-SCID is not the same disease as ADA-SCID, and the children were not on enzyme replacement therapy prior to or during the gene transfer. This substantiates the idea that gene transfer confers a selective advantage for the transduced cells in this disease. Secondly, since the relatively poor results obtained in the clinical trials for ADA-SCID were reported there has been a substantial improvement in methodology, with use of opti-mised cytokine cocktails and a fibronectin fragment for gene transfer to CD34+ cells. The application of these improved protocols to the treat-ment of ADA-SCID patients may well prove to be efficacious in future clinical trials.

Alternative vector systems

Lentiviral vectors

Despite these encouraging results it is still vital to develop improved vectors for the transduction of PHSC, since there will not be a selective advantage for transduced stem cells in other diseases. It has also been known for some time that prolonged exposure of human PHSCs to growth factors and cytokine cocktails for efficient transduction using murine retroviruses is detrimental to their repopulating activity. It has been suggested that one way around this is to use lentivirus-based vectors. The pre-integration complex of human immunodeficiency virus (HIV)-based lentiviral vectors incorporates localisation signals able to mediate active transport through the nucleopores of an intact nuclear membrane during cell interphase, thereby removing the requirement for cell division (Naldini, 1998). In order to maximise safety, the current generation of replication-defective HIV-based lentiviral vectors are generated by transient transfection of a producer cell line with three plasmids; one expresses the core proteins and enzymes essential for viral replication, reverse transcription and integration, the second encodes the envelope protein, usually vesicular stomatitis virus G protein (VSV-G), and the third contains essential sequences for optimal packaging, reverse transcription and integration of the transgene (reviewed in Trono, 2000). The generation of self-inactivating (SIN) vectors further reduces the risk of vector mobilisation and recombination, while exogenous gene expression is controlled by an internal heterologous promoter. Such pseudotyped lentiviral vector systems have been used to transduce human CD34+ haematopoietic progenitors and stem cells *in vitro* in the absence of cytokine stimulation with limited evaluation *in vivo* (see, for example, Miyoshi *et al.*, 1999: reviewed in Trono, 2000). In our experience, however, the efficiency of gene transfer to CD34+ cells using lentiviral vectors is significantly enhanced by exposure of cells to cytokines, although the time required, 24 hours, is significantly less than that required for gene transfer using murine retroviruses (Demaison *et al.*, personal communication). It is possible that after only 24 hours in culture the original engraftment phenotype is preserved. The development of enhanced lentiviral vectors has clear advantages for the experimental manipulation of haematopoietic stem cells, and also other non-dividing cell types such as neurons (Naldini *et al.*, 1996) and retinal cells (Miyoshi *et al.*, 1997), and should be useful for future application in clinical trials of gene therapy.

Adeno-associated viral vectors

Adeno-associated virus (AAV) is a non-pathogenic human parvovirus which has attracted considerable interest as a gene transfer vector (reviewed in Russell and Kay, 1999; also see Chapter 2). Replication of this virus is usually dependent on co-infection with a helper virus. In the absence of helper virus (usually adenovirus) the wild-type AAV genome can integrate stably into the host cell genome by non-homologous recombination, usually in a tandem head-to-tail orientation. Analysis of flanking sequences from latently infected cells has shown that integration occurs at multiple sites within a single specific locus, AAVS1, in 60–70% of cases, which maps to human chromosome 19q13.3-qter. AAV vectors in which the *rep* gene is deleted probably integrate randomly, suggesting that *rep* gene products (Rep78 and Rep68) are important for this process.

Vectors based on AAV have been used successfully to transduce dividing cells *in vitro*, and non-dividing cells *in vivo* (see, for example, Ali *et al.*, 2000, reviewed in Russell and Kay, 1999). However, this system has proved to be unsuitable for targeting PHSCs on two counts. First, although AAV is capable of transducing non-dividing cells, the transduction efficiency is 200 times less than that of S-phase cells (Podsakoff *et al.*, 1994). Secondly, cell surface heparan sulfate proteoglycans, the primary receptor for AAV, are expressed at relatively low levels on human PHSCs, with marked donor variability, thus limiting the applicability of AAV-mediated transduction for this particular cell type (Summerford and Samulski, 1998). Most recently, AAV has successfully been used in a clinical trial of gene therapy for factor IX haemophilia (Kay *et al.*, 2000). Adults with severe haemophilia B were injected intramuscularly with factor IX-expressing AAV and the results showed evidence of gene expression even at low doses of vector, suggesting therapeutic benefit.

Conclusions

SCID remains one of the most attractive disorders for the application of somatic gene transfer technology. The clinical experience to date suggests a mood of cautious optimism. With more clinical trials planned for X-SCID and other SCIDs, including the Jak-3 and RAG deficiencies, in the near future, it is likely that further progress will ensue. Following on from this, the range of diseases that can be treated by PHSC gene therapy is likely to increase to include other primary immunodeficiencies, such as chronic granulomatous disease (CGD), haematological disorders, some forms of cancer and the inherited metabolic disorders. There is, however, a continuing need for the optimisation of gene transfer and expression mechanisms in the laboratory. Continuing development of improved gene transfer systems is necessary to ensure that somatic gene transfer can provide clinical benefit in the treatment of a variety of single gene disorders.

References

Ali R R, Sarra G-M, Stephens C, *et al.* 2000. Restoration of photoreceptor ultrastructure and function in retinal degeneration slow (*rds*) mice by gene therapy. *Nat Genet* 25: 306–310.

Alton E W, Stern M, Farley R, *et al.* (1999) Cationic lipid-mediated CFTR gene transfer to the lungs and nose of patients with cystic fibrosis: a double-blind placebo-controlled trial. *Lancet* 353: 947–954.

Benveniste P, Zhu W, Cohen A (1995) Interference with thymocyte differentiation by an inhibitor of S-adenosylhomocysteine hydrolase. *J Immunol* 155: 536–544.

Blaese R M, Culver K W, Miller A D, *et al.* (1995) T lymphocyte-directed gene therapy for ADA-SCID: initial trial results after 4 years. *Science* 270: 475–480.

Bordignon C, Notarangelo L D, Nobili N, *et al.* (1995) Gene therapy in peripheral blood lymphocytes and bone marrow for ADA-immunodeficient patients. *Science* 270: 470–475.

Buckley R H, Schiff S E, Schiff R I, *et al.* (1999) Hematopoietic stem-cell transplantation for the treatment of severe combined immunodeficiency. *N Engl J Med* 340: 508–516.

Bunting K D, Sangster M Y, Ihle J N, *et al.* (1998) Restoration of lymphocyte function in Janus kinase 3-deficient mice by retroviral-mediated gene transfer. *Nat Med* 4: 58–64

Candotti F, Oakes S A, Johnston J A, *et al.* (1996) In vitro correction of JAK3-deficient severe combined immunodeficiency by retroviral-mediated gene transduction. *J Exp Med* 183: 2687–2692.

Cavazzana-Calvo M, Hacein-Bey S, de Saint Basile G, *et al.* (2000) Gene therapy of human severe combined immunodeficiency (SCID)-X1 disease. *Science* 288: 669–672.

Crystal R G (1995) Transfer of genes to humans: early lessons and obstacles to success. *Science* 270: 404–410.

Demaison C, Brouns G, Blundell M P, *et al.* (2000) A defined window for efficient gene marking of severe combined immunodeficient-repopulating cells using a gibbon ape leukemia virus-pseudotyped retroviral vector. *Hum Gene Ther* 11: 91–100.

Ferrari G, Rossini S, Giavazzi R, *et al.* (1991) An in vivo model of somatic cell gene therapy for human severe combined immunodeficiency. *Science* 251: 1363–1366.

Fischer A (1999) Thirty years of bone marrow transplantation for severe combined immunodeficiency. *N Engl J Med* 340: 559–561.

Fischer A (2000) T-lymphocyte immunodeficiencies. In: Roifman C, ed. *Primary T-Cell Immunodeficiencies: Immunology and Allergy Clinics of North America.* Philadelphia: WB Saunders, 113–127.

Fischer A, Landais P, Friedrich W, *et al.* (1990) European experience of bone-marrow transplantation for severe combined immunodeficiency. *Lancet* 336: 850–854.

Flake A W, Roncarolo M G, Puck J M, *et al.* (1996) Treatment of X-linked severe combined immunodeficiency by in utero transplantation of paternal bone marrow. *N Engl J Med* 335: 1806–1810.

Hacein-Bey H, Cavazzana-Calvo M, Le Deist F, *et al.* (1996) Gamma-c gene transfer into SCID X1 patients' B-cell lines restores normal high-affinity interleukin-2 receptor expression and function. *Blood* 87: 3108–3116.

Harvey B G, Leopold P L, Hackett N R, *et al.* (1999) Airway epithelial CFTR mRNA expression in cystic fibrosis patients after repetitive administration of a recombinant adenovirus. *J Clin Invest* 104: 1245–1255.

Hershfield M S (1995) PEG-ADA: an alternative to haploidentical bone marrow transplantation and an adjunct to gene therapy for adenosine deaminase deficiency. *Hum Mutat* 5: 107–112.

Hershfield M S, Mitchell B S (1995) Immunodeficiency diseases caused by adenosine deaminase deficiency and purine nucleotide deficiency. In: Scriver C R, Beaudet A L, Sly W S, *et al.* eds. *The Metabolic and Molecular Basis of Inherited Disease*, 7th edn. New York: McGraw-Hill, 1725–1768.

Hirschhorn R, Yang D R, Puck J M, *et al.* (1996) Spontaneous in vivo reversion to normal of an inherited mutation in a patient with adenosine deaminase deficiency. *Nat Genet* 13: 290–295.

Hoogerbrugge P M, van Beusechem V W, Fischer A, *et al.* (1996) Bone marrow gene transfer in three patients with adenosine deaminase deficiency. *Gene Ther* 3: 179–183.

Kay M A, Manno C S, Ragni M V, *et al.* (2000) Evidence for gene transfer and expression of factor IX in haemophilia B patients treated with an AAV vector. *Nat Genet* 24: 257–261.

Kohn D B, Weinberg K, Nolta J A, *et al.* (1995) Engraftment of gene-modified umbilical cord blood cells in neonates with adenosine deaminase deficiency. *Nat Med* 1: 1017–1023.

Kohn D B, Hershfield M S, Carbonaro D, *et al.* (1998) T lymphocytes with a normal ADA gene accumulate after transplantation of transduced autologous umbilical cord blood CD34+ cells in ADA-deficient SCID neonates. *Nat Med* 4: 775–780.

Miyoshi H, Takahashi M, Gage F H, *et al.* (1997) Stable and efficient gene transfer into the retina using an HIV-based lentiviral vector. *Proc Natl Acad Sci USA* 94: 10319–10323.

Miyoshi H, Smith K A, Mosier D E, *et al.* (1999) Transduction of human CD34+ cells that mediate long-term engraftment of NOD/SCID mice by HIV vectors. *Science* 283: 682–686.

Naldini L (1998) Lentiviruses as gene transfer agents for delivery to non-dividing cells. *Curr Opin Biotechnol* 9: 457–463.

Naldini L, Blömer U, Gallay P, *et al.* (1996) In vivo gene delivery and stable transduction of nondividing cells by a lentiviral vector. *Science* 272: 263–267

Orlic D, Girard L J, Jordan C T, *et al.* (1996) The level of mRNA encoding the amphotropic retrovirus receptor in mouse and human hematopoietic stem cells is low and correlates with the efficiency of retrovirus transduction. *Proc Natl Acad Sci USA* 93: 11097–11102.

Osborne W R, Hock R A, Kaleko M *et al.* (1990) Long-term expression of human adenosine deaminase in mice after transplantation of bone marrow infected with amphotropic retroviral vectors. *Hum Gene Ther* 1: 31–41.

Podsakoff G, Wong K K Jr, Chatterjee S (1994) Efficient gene transfer into non-dividing cells by adeno-associated virus-based vectors. *J Virol* 68: 5656–5666.

Porter C D, Collins M K, Tailor C S, *et al.* (1996) Comparison of efficiency of infection of human gene therapy target cells via four different retroviral receptors. *Hum Gene Ther* 7: 913–919.

Russell D W, Kay M A (1999) Adeno-associated virus vectors and hematology. *Blood* 94: 864–874.

Sekhsaria S, Fleisher T A, Vowells S, *et al.* (1996) Granulocyte colony-stimulating factor recruitment of CD34+ progenitors to peripheral blood: impaired mobilization in chronic granulomatous disease and adenosine deaminase-deficient severe combined immunodeficiency disease patients. *Blood* 88: 1104–1112.

Soudais C, Shiho T, Sharara L I, *et al.* (2000) Stable and functional lymphoid reconstitution of common cytokine receptor chain deficient mice by retroviral-mediated gene transfer. *Blood* 95: 3071–3077.

Stephan V, Wahn V, Le Deist F, *et al.* (1996) Atypical X-linked severe combined immunodeficiency due to possible spontaneous reversion of the genetic defect in T cells. *N Engl J Med* 335: 1563–1567.

Summerford C, Samulski R J (1998) Membrane-associated heparan sulfate proteoglycan is a receptor for adeno-associated virus type 2 virions. *J Virol* 72: 1438–1445.

Taylor N, Uribe L, Smith S, *et al.* (1996) Correction of interleukin-2 receptor function in X-SCID lymphoblastoid cells by retrovirally mediated transfer of the gamma-c gene. *Blood* 87: 3103–3107.

Trono D (2000) Lentiviral vectors: turning a deadly foe into a therapeutic agent. *Gene Ther* 7: 20–23.

Wengler G S, Lanfranchi A, Frusca T, *et al.* (1996) In-utero transplantation of parental CD34 haematopoietic progenitor cells in a patient with X-linked severe combined immunodeficiency (SCIDXI). *Lancet* 348: 1484–1487.

Zeitlin P L (2000) Cystic fibrosis gene therapy trials and tribulations. *Mol Ther* 1: 5–6.

5

Gene therapy approaches for cancer

Iain McNeish and Michael J Seckl

Few areas of research have raised as much interest and introspection, not to mention false optimism, as gene therapy (Friedmann, 1989). Indeed, few subjects can have produced quite so many philosophical editorials (Verma, 1994; Leiden, 1995; Blau and Khavari, 1997). The possibility of using DNA as a therapeutic tool first became theoretically feasible with the isolation and cloning of the genes responsible for inherited monogenetic disorders such as cystic fibrosis (Riordan *et al.*, 1989; Rommens *et al.*, 1989), Lesch-Nyhan syndrome (Brennand *et al.*, 1983; Melton *et al.*, 1984) and adenosine deaminase (ADA)-deficient severe combined immune deficiency (SCID) (Orkin *et al.*, 1983). In theory, these disorders could be cured by the introduction and expression of a normal functional copy of the faulty gene in the appropriate tissue, but the practical requirements for such gene therapy are formidable. After the gene has been isolated, its regulatory sequences must also be identified to ensure that expression of the transgene occurs in the appropriate tissue and at the appropriate time. Then practical ways have to be found of delivering the gene to the requisite organ and, finally, once expression is achieved, it must continue indefinitely, to obviate the requirement for multiple and repeated treatments. Perhaps not surprisingly, initial clinical trials of gene therapy in cystic fibrosis (Knowles *et al.*, 1995) and ADA-deficient SCID (Blaese *et al.*, 1995) met with very limited success.

At a superficial level, cancer is an even less attractive candidate for gene therapy than either cystic fibrosis or ADA-deficient SCID: the progression from normal tissue to invasive malignancy may involve up to six or more separate genetic events (Bodmer, 1994), all of which, in theory, would have to be corrected to reverse the malignant phenotype. Similarly, it would also be necessary to restore normal gene function to 100% of the cells within a tumour population, which is impractical with current vector technology. However, novel gene therapy strategies for cancer have evolved that do not rely on gene complementation, and which thus circumvent some, but by no means all, of the difficulties listed above.

Cancer gene therapy strategies

Broadly, four separate pathways have developed, namely immuno-therapy, introduction of tumour suppressor genes/induction of apoptosis, enzyme prodrug therapy and inhibition of tumour angiogenesis.

Immunotherapy

Immunotherapy strategies were initially the most common approaches to cancer gene therapy in clinical trials (Roth and Cristiano, 1997). Their ultimate success will depend upon the recognition by T lymphocytes of a tumour-specific or tumour-associated antigen presented on the cell surface in association with class I and II major histocompatibility complex (MHC) proteins, having been processed into peptides between 8 and 12 amino acids long. It is evident that tumours do express antigens that can be recognised by the immune system, as witnessed by the isolation in several spontaneously arising tumours of immune cells with demonstrable reactivity against autologous tumour (Peoples *et al.*, 1995). There is an ever-expanding list of known or potential antigens expressed by tumours that could be exploited for therapeutic purposes. These include unique antigens expressed only by individual types of tumour (e.g. the bcr/abl protein produced by the Philadelphia chromosome translocation in chronic myeloid leukaemia); shared tumour-specific antigens expressed by a wide variety of tumours, but not normal adult cells (e.g. carcinoembryonic antigen in colorectal, pancreatic and other tumours); tissue-specific antigens expressed by both the tumour and the tissue from which it arose (e.g. tyrosinase in melanoma and melanocytes); and viral antigens in known virus-associated tumours (e.g. human papillomavirus E6 protein in cervical cancer) (Pardoll, 1998).

However, it has long been known that tumour cells are able to evade the immune system through several mechanisms, which are currently incompletely understood. Secretion of inhibitory factors such as transforming growth factor β (TGFβ) (Sulitzeanu, 1993), downregulation of MHC class I and II (Browning and Bodmer, 1992), disrupted antigen-presentation pathways (Restifo *et al.*, 1991), the absence of co-stimulatory signals (Gilligan *et al.*, 1998), emergence of antigenic loss variants (Wortzel *et al.*, 1983), impaired ability to transduce activation signals (Wang *et al.*, 1995) and the ability to induce T-cell apoptosis (Gimmi *et al.*, 1996) may all be involved.

There are three alternative but overlapping pathways by which immunotherapy may be attempted, namely the induction of cytokine or co-stimulatory molecule expression, genetic modification of lympho-cytes and tumour antigen vaccines. Much of the work in this area has employed malignant melanoma or renal cell carcinoma as model tumours as they represent two cancers to which host immune responses can be reliably demonstrated (Timmerman and Levy, 1998).

Induction of cytokine or co-stimulatory molecule expression

This strategy is the single most common approach to the gene therapy of malignant disease, accounting for over half of all clinical protocols up to the beginning of 1997 (Roth and Cristiano, 1997). Frequently employed cytokines include interleukin 2 (IL-2), interleukin 12 (IL-12) and granulocyte–macrophage colony-stimulating factor (GM-CSF). Many clinical protocols involve an *ex vivo* approach, with the excision of a single tumour nodule, viral transduction *in vitro*, followed by selec-tion for the transgene, irradiation of the modified cells and finally their re-implantation. The hope is that a generalised antitumour immune response will be elicited. In theory, the cytokines in question could be administered systemically, removing the need for viral modification. However, the level of systemic cytokine required to induce an anti-tumour response inevitably produces systemic toxicity. The *ex vivo* approach should permit the local production of high concentration cyto-kine within the microenvironment of the tumour, without significant systemic levels being produced.

IL-2 is secreted mainly by activated T helper (Th) cells and stimu-lates the proliferation and activation of a wide variety of cells, including cytotoxic T lymphocytes (CTLs), natural killer (NK) cells and lym-phokine-activated killer (LAK) cells, as well as acting in an autocrine fashion to aid expansion of antigen-specific Th cells. There are numerous reports that the induction of IL-2 expression by a wide variety of tumour cells leads to tumour rejection, mediated by CTLs and NK cells, but not Th cells, with variable reports of protective immunity induced (Cordier *et al.*, 1995; Toloza *et al.*, 1996). Interestingly, IL-2 secretion is effective in nude mice that lack T cells, implying that CTL function is not essen-tial (Bui *et al.*, 1997). It has also been noted that there is an optimal level of IL-2 expression, with levels in excess of this resulting in poorer anti-tumour effects (Schmidt *et al.*, 1995). The results of a few clinical trials have been published (e.g. Palmer *et al.*, 1999), in which it is possible to demonstrate the generation of tumour-specific CTL generation, but there have been few, if any, objective clinical responses. This is clearly disappointing but further work is still required before it will be possible to determine the role of these approaches in the treatment of cancer.

IL-12 is almost as widely employed as IL-2. It is expressed primarily by activated macrophages and its main function is the promotion of a Th1-like response via the secretion, by the relevant subclass of Th cells, of interferon γ (IFNγ), IL-2 and tumour necrosis factor α (TNFα) (Tahara and Lotze, 1995). This, in turn, promotes cell-mediated immunity. Again, it has been shown that induction of IL-12 secretion can result in regression of a wide variety of tumours, with the development of protective immunity against re-challenge (Brunda *et al.*, 1993). Unlike IL-2, it is important that functional CTLs are present, as they are the eventual effectors of IL-12 influence. There is also now evidence that part of the effect of IL-12 is mediated by impairment of tumour angiogenesis (Cavallo *et al.*, 1999).

It was first shown in 1993 that GM-CSF expression by irradiated B16 melanoma cells was capable of inducing long-lasting and specific antitumour immunity (Dranoff *et al.*, 1993), which was dependent upon both CD4+ and CD8+ cells as well as the irradiation of the melanoma cells prior to inoculation. GM-CSF has a wide variety of functions, including aiding NK cell-mediated rejection of tumours, the recruitment of professional antigen-presenting cells (APCs) and the enhancement of co-stimulatory molecule expression on the surface of APCs, and it is the ability to cause the maturation of APCs that is thought to underlie its efficacy in gene therapy. APCs will detect antigens released by the tumour (presumably by irradiation-induced damage in the case of the B16 melanoma cells), process them and present them in association with class I and II MHC to T cells in local lymph nodes, thereby eliminating the need for the tumour to present antigen directly itself.

A clinical trial of GM-CSF in renal cell carcinoma has been published (Simons *et al.*, 1997) as well as a further case report (Ellem *et al.*, 1997) and a published protocol (Dranoff *et al.*, 1997). In the renal cell carcinoma trial, 16 patients were re-injected with irradiated tumour cells transduced and expressing the cytokine, resulting in one partial response. In the case report, a patient with extensive metastatic melanoma was again treated with re-injected GM-CSF-expressing autologous irradiated tumour cells. There was short-lived partial regression of some deposits, but many lesions remained refractory.

There are many other reports of the use of a bewildering variety of cytokines, including both IFNα (Tuting *et al.*, 1997) and IFNγ (Abdel-Wahab *et al.*, 1997), IL-4 (Benedetti *et al.*, 1997), IL-6 (Mullen *et al.*,

1996) and IL-7 (Sharma *et al.*, 1996, 1997) in a wide variety of tumour models.

The recognition by T-cell receptors (TCR) of antigen/MHC complex alone is not sufficient to induce T-cell activation. Indeed, the binding of TCR to antigen/MHC in isolation can lead to a state of T-cell anergy (Figure 5.1). The function of co-stimulatory molecules, therefore, is to be recognised by T cells in association with the antigen/MHC complex and it is only this dual recognition that leads to T-cell activation. The most studied co-stimulatory molecule is B7.1 (CD80), which is recognised by CD28 on the surface of T cells in a manner that is neither MHC-restricted nor antigen-specific. B7.1 is usually expressed on APCs but not on tumour cells, such that a T-cell response to a tumour would require uptake of tumour antigen by APCs, which could then activate T cells. By inducing B7.1 expression on a tumour cell, one could render it into an effective APC. There is evidence from *in vitro* work that adeno-viral delivery of the B7.1 gene to human ovarian and cervical cancer cells increases the immunogenicity of those cells, as detected by mixed tumour/lymphocyte reactions (Gilligan *et al.*, 1998). There is also ample evidence from murine models that introduction of B7.1 into tumour cells causes their rejection in immunocompetent mice (Baskar *et al.*, 1993; Townsend and Allison, 1993). A phase I study of liposome-mediated

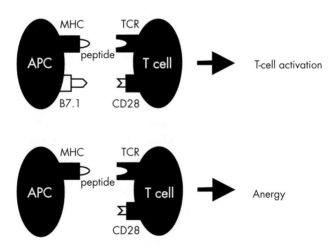

Figure 5.1   Recognition of peptide–MHC complex by the T cell in association with B7.1/CD28. In the presence of co-stimulation by B7.1, recognition of the peptide–MHC complex by the T-cell receptor leads to T-cell activation. However, if the co-stimulatory signal is absent, T-cell anergy is produced.

B7.1 delivery to colorectal metastases within the liver has been reported and, whilst there were no adverse effects, there were no objective clinical responses (Rubin *et al.*, 1997). There was, however, detection of B7.1 protein expression in 50% of the patients, all of whose tumours were B7.1 negative prior to treatment.

Given its role in aiding antigen presentation in order to activate CD8+ cells, it is not surprising that there are reports of combining B7.1 with GM-CSF or IL-12 (Chong *et al.*, 1998) and IL-2 (Salvadori *et al.*, 1995). In the former, expression of B7.1 with either GM-CSF or IL-12 resulted in failure to develop tumours and in protection against re-challenge in a colorectal carcinoma, but not a melanoma, model, implying that it may be necessary to choose specific combinations of cytokines and co-stimulatory molecules for specific tumour types.

Genetic modification of lymphocytes

The strategy here is to modify the lymphocytes, rather than the tumour cells, in order to induce an antitumour immune response. It was noted over a decade ago that the administration of tumour-infiltrating lymphocytes (TILs) with IL-2 could induce antitumour responses in models of melanoma and a subsequent clinical trial demonstrated impressive response rates of approximately 50% in patients with metastatic melanoma (Rosenberg *et al.*, 1988). However, this approach is hindered by the fact that TILs have to be isolated from each patient and expanded *ex vivo*. The subsequent discovery of an array of specific antigens expressed by tumours, especially melanomas, allowed the *in vitro* generation of highly specific TIL cultures by stimulating them with the appropriate peptide-pulsed (i.e. co-cultured *in vitro*) targets.

Currently extremely popular is the modification of dendritic cells (DCs). These bone marrow-derived cells function as extremely potent APCs and are capable of activating naïve T cells (Cella *et al.*, 1997). There is evidence from several groups that the expression of a model tumour antigen (β-gal) in DCs is capable of protecting mice from challenge with β-gal-expressing colon carcinoma cells (Song *et al.*, 1997) and even causes the regression of established pulmonary metastases (Specht *et al.*, 1997). Similarly, intratumoral injection of DCs modified with an adenovirus encoding CD40 ligand led to significant tumour regression in a murine model (Kikuchi *et al.*, 2000). However, one of the difficulties with DCs is that they are relatively hard to isolate and culture and they are extremely resistant to transduction (Schuler and Steinman, 1997).

Several phase I trials in which dendritic cells have been used have been published. In one of the first, 16 patients with advanced melanoma were immunised with peptide-loaded DCs pulsed with either HLA A1- or HLA A2-binding peptides from known melanoma antigens (12 patients) or crude autologous tumour lysates (4 patients). Also included was the highly immunogenic keyhole limpet haemocyanin (KLH) to aid recruitment of CD4+ T cells and promote the maturation of a CTL memory response. The results were impressive, with two complete responses and three partial responses, some lasting for 15 months (Nestle *et al.*, 1998). Interestingly, two of the responders were in the crude tumour lysate group, where the nature of the antigen being presented by the DCs was unknown. This potentially makes DC therapy even more powerful, as it may not be necessary to identify specific antigens from individual patients prior to commencing therapy. It appears that predictors of clinical response include skin test responses to recall antigens and cytokine secretion by T cells after non-specific stimulation (Lodge *et al.*, 2000).

Tumour antigen vaccines

The classification of immunotherapy strategies as discrete groups disguises the considerable overlap that exists between them: both the DC work and the re-introduction of GM-CSF-transduced tumour cells mentioned above could well be classified as vaccination strategies. The existence of multiple known or potential tumour antigens was discussed above and there have been attempts at tumour vaccination, at the crudest levels, by mixing tumour cell lysates with known immunogens such as the bacillus Calmette–Guérin (BCG) or by infecting tumour lysates with influenza virus (Pardoll, 1998). Recently, more sophisticated approaches have been undertaken, including successful clinical trials. In one trial, a modified peptide derived from the known melanoma antigen gp100 was administered subcutaneously with incomplete Freund's adjuvant (IFA), producing very high peptide-specific T-cell responses, although no objective clinical responses. However, if high-dose IL-2 was administered shortly after the vaccine, the frequency with which T-cell responses were detected fell dramatically, but objective clinical responses were seen in 42% of patients (including one complete response) with regression of distant tumour deposits (Rosenberg *et al.*, 1998). The implication is that the fall in detectable T-cell responses on co-administration of IL-2 resulted from T cells localising to the tumour nodules (Rosenberg *et al.*, 1998).

Introduction of tumour suppressor genes and induction of apoptosis

The multiple genetic events that occur in the progression from normal tissue to invasive malignancy are composed of gain-of-transforming function and loss-of-tumour-suppressor function mutations. There are some reports of attempts to inhibit the gain-of-transforming function mutations (Wagner, 1995), but the vast majority of work in this field involves the re-introduction of tumour suppressor function. The tumour suppressor genes that are known to be mutated in different cancers are many, but those that have been studied most frequently for gene therapy purposes are *p53*, *Rb* and the cyclin-dependent kinase inhibitors, such as *p16* and *p21*. All of these are involved in cell cycle control, with p53 having a pivotal role both in the control of the progression through the cell cycle and the induction of apoptotic cell death. In response to any potentially toxic stresses, such as hypoxia and DNA damage, p53 can prevent the passage of cells from G_0/G_1 into S phase by transactivating a number of proteins including p21. p21, in turn, can bind to the cyclin/cdk complexes and inhibit the phosphorylation of Rb. The phosphorylation status of Rb varies through the cell cycle under tight control. During G_1, Rb is un- or underphosphorylated, whilst from late G_1 through to the end of M phase, Rb is extensively phosphorylated and it is in the underphosphorylated form that *Rb* exerts its main growth inhibitory effect (Weinberg, 1995). Rb exists preferentially within the nuclear matrix, where it binds to the E2F family of transcriptional regulators. The binding of Rb to E2F causes the latter to change from a transcriptional activator to a repressor, whilst the phosphorylation of Rb causes these two proteins to dissociate, allowing E2F to activate a series of genes important for regulation (Hirama and Koeffler, 1995). Thus, anything that can affect the phosphorylation status of Rb can have a profound effect on cell cycle regulation.

p53 is also known to be the main downregulator of Bcl-2. Bcl-2 normally blocks apoptosis by heterodimerising with the pro-apoptotic protein Bax (Favrot *et al.*, 1998). Interestingly, p53 is also a strong inducer of Bax expression and thus can play an important role in promoting apoptosis in normal cells. However, in tumours with *p53* mutations this regulation of Bax and Bcl-2 is lost and apoptosis fails to occur (Yin *et al.*, 1997).

Restoration of wild-type p53 expression

Given its central role in both cell cycle control and induction of apoptosis and also the frequency with which it is mutated in human cancers

(Lane, 1995), it is not surprising that restoration of wild-type p53 function has been widely studied. There is extensive evidence *in vitro* that wild-type p53 expression can suppress the growth of a wide variety of tumour cell types (Favrot *et al.*, 1998), although pancreatic carcinoma seemed to be resistant to this effect (Kimura *et al.*, 1997). A similar pattern was also observed with induction of apoptosis in *in vivo* models of a number of tumours (Favrot *et al.*, 1998). The first clinical trial was reported in 1996 (Roth *et al.*, 1996). Nine patients with non-small cell lung cancer and known to have *p53* gene mutations were treated with up to five direct intratumoral injections of a recombinant retrovirus encoding wild-type human *p53*. The results were encouraging, in that three of seven evaluable patients had regression of the injected lesion, whilst two others had stable disease, although there was progression of non-injected lesions in all patients. Interestingly, although RT-PCR analysis failed to detect any evidence of wild-type *p53* expression, there was evidence of some gene transfer from PCR and *in situ* hybridisation analysis. The overall estimated gene transfer efficiency was low, although in some limited areas, there were up to 20% p53-positive cells. Given this low overall rate of gene transfer, the objective clinical responses seen imply that some form of 'bystander effect' must exist, confirming earlier *in vitro* observations (Cai *et al.*, 1993). How this bystander effect is mediated is not known, but the possibilities include the passage of effectors of apoptosis between cells, the establishment of an antitumour immune response or the inhibition of tumour angiogenesis. There has been a preliminary report of naked DNA-mediated *p53* transfer to patients with localised hepatocellular carcinoma, which shows evidence of partial responses in some patients (Habib, 1997), as well as an indication that expression of p53 may act as a radiosensitiser in glioma cells *in vitro* (Badie *et al.*, 1999).

Other tumour suppressor genes

Work on other tumour suppressor genes is less advanced than that on *p53* and has generally proven less fertile. Transfecting cells with *p21* leads to variable results, including cell cycle arrest, induction of apoptosis and differentiation (Sheikh *et al.*, 1995), although tumour regression has been seen following adenoviral delivery of the *p21* gene in renal cell carcinoma (Yang *et al.*, 1995) and cervical carcinoma (Tsao *et al.*, 1999) models. There has also been an attempt to compare the efficacy of various cyclin-dependent kinase inhibitors *in vitro* and *in vivo*. Although adenoviral delivery of the genes of several of the inhibitors was able to produce apoptosis *in vitro* and to prevent tumour development *in vivo*, only *p16^INK4A* was able to produce the regression of established tumours in a transgenic murine mammary adenocarcinoma model (Schreiber *et al.*, 1999).

There have also been encouraging reports that infection of Rb-null or Rb-positive cells with an adenoviral vector encoding either full-length *Rb* or an amino-terminal truncation caused inhibition of tumour growth, but without evidence of apoptosis or differentiation (Huang *et al.*, 1988; Xu *et al.*, 1996). One novel strategy has been to employ a selectively replicating adenovirus that carries a 24-bp deletion in the E1A region. This was able to cause lysis of glioma cells that were Rb-null, but not in Rb-positive fibroblasts nor in the glioma cells once Rb expression had been restored (Fueyo *et al.*, 2000).

Activation of apoptosis by caspases

More recently, attention has focused upon the pathways by which apoptosis is executed within cells and there has been a growing awareness of the importance of the caspase family of cysteine proteases in the induction and execution of apoptosis (reviewed in Nicholson, 1999). The execution caspases (caspases 3, 6 and 7) are produced as catalytically inert pre-pro-enzymes, with a large subunit, a small subunit and a pro-domain (Figure 5.2). The active enzyme is revealed only after the pro-domain has been removed and the two subunits have been cleaved, the latter occurring in response to an apoptotic stimulus.

Expression of pro-caspase 3 alone in tumour cells appears insufficient to induce apoptosis, but the addition of another stimulus, such as the simultaneous expression of Fas ligand (Shinoura *et al.*, 2000), or the addition of proteasome inhibitors (Tenev *et al.*, 2000) can induce extensive apoptosis of tumour cells *in vitro*. Similarly, the combination of caspase 3 and exposure to the cytotoxic drug etoposide produces apoptosis *in vitro* and a significant reduction in tumour volumes in a rodent hepatoma model (Yamabe *et al.*, 1999). Another strategy has been to reverse the orientation of the two subunits of caspase 3, which produces a constitutively active enzyme (Srinivasula *et al.*, 1998). Recently, a novel caspase activator known as Smac (Du *et al.*, 2000) or DIABLO (Verhagen *et al.*, 2000) has been identified, which may provide new pathways to be exploited in the induction of tumour cell apoptosis.

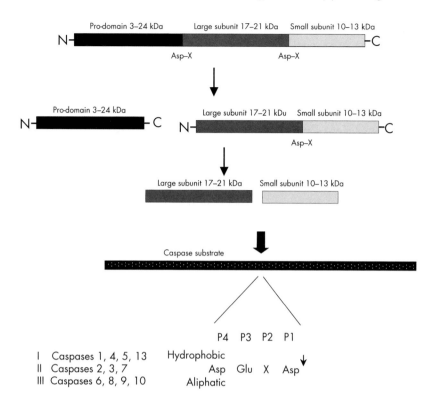

Figure 5.2 Caspase structure and proteolytic specificity. Caspases are released as pre-pro-enzymes, with a large subunit, a small subunit and a pro-domain, which is removed. The two active subunits are subsequently cleaved to reveal the active form of the enzyme in response to pro-apoptotic stimuli. Active caspase enzymes recognise specific tetrapeptides within target proteins and cleave them at the P1 Asp site. Based on their tetrapeptide preferences, the 11 human caspases can be divided into three families.

Virus-directed enzyme/prodrug therapy (VDEPT)

VDEPT (represented schematically in Figure 5.3) has two fundamental features. The first is the delivery to tumour cells, via a recombinant virus, of the gene encoding a non-human enzyme. The enzyme has been selected for its ability to convert a non-toxic prodrug into a cytotoxic species, which will then kill the cell in which it has been formed. The production of active drug by the tumour cells themselves should allow the generation of higher drug concentrations within the tumour microenvironment than could be achieved by systemic administration alone, and thus lead to a higher therapeutic index.

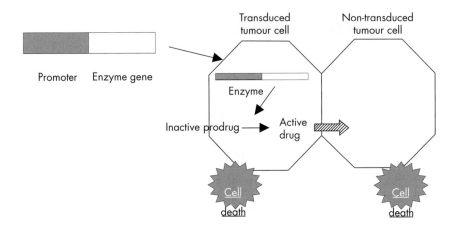

Figure 5.3 Virus-directed enzyme prodrug therapy with bystander killing of non-transduced cell. The gene encoding an enzyme is delivered to tumour cells. Expression of the enzyme within the tumour cell permits conversion of an inactive prodrug into its active species, thereby leading to cell death. Active drug is able to pass into neighbouring, non-transduced cells, killing them also – a phenomenon known as the 'bystander effect'.

The concept of VDEPT arose from studies in antibody-directed enzyme prodrug therapy (ADEPT) where the enzyme itself (rather than its gene) was delivered to tumour cells by means of an antibody directed against a tumour-specific antigen (Niculescu-Duvaz and Springer, 1997). The advantages of VDEPT over ADEPT include the fact that the enzyme is generated within the tumour cell itself, rather than being present in the interstitium, thus generating higher concentrations of the active species inside the cell and allowing ready access to any co-factors that may be required for enzyme activity. Also, the inherent immunogenicity of antibody–enzyme conjugates may preclude multiple administrations.

The second important feature of VDEPT is the so-called bystander effect. This describes the ability of active species generated in one cell to kill neighbouring, non-transduced cells, thereby eliminating the need to transduce every tumour cell, which is clearly impractical with current vector technology.

The ideal enzyme would consist of a single polypeptide species of reasonably low molecular weight and independent of post-translational modifications. Fundamentally, the catalytic activity or substrate specificity must be distinct from any human enzyme and so those in use derive predominantly from bacteria and viruses. The desirable parameters of potential enzyme prodrug combinations are a high differential toxicity of the active species relative to the prodrug, and a low K_m and a high K_{cat}, which will maximise production of the active species at any given concentration of prodrug and enzyme. The physicochemical properties of the prodrug and its cytotoxic species, such as lipophilicity, will influence tissue distribution, cellular uptake and bystander killing. The half-life of the activated cytotoxic agent will also affect its distribution and efficacy: a longer half-life should allow a more homogeneous distribution within a tumour, but this may be offset by a greater potential to diffuse into the vascular compartment, increasing the systemic concentration of the cytotoxic agent. Many different potential enzyme/prodrug combinations have been described, but the general principles can be illustrated by consideration of the following systems.

Thymidine kinase/ganciclovir

In 1986, Moolten described the successful *in vitro* and *in vivo* sensitisation of murine tumour cells to the then novel anti-herpes drug, ganciclovir (GCV), via expression of the herpes simplex virus 1 (HSV) thymidine kinase (*tk*) gene (Moolten, 1986). The HSV, but not mammalian, tk enzyme is capable of phosphorylating various nucleoside analogues, including ganciclovir and its relative acyclovir. Treatment of HSV tk-positive cells with ganciclovir leads to the formation of ganciclovir triphosphate (Figure 5.4), a potent antimetabolite that interrupts DNA synthesis by erroneous incorporation as a false nucleotide. Thus, in Moolten's original work, there was inhibition of growth of tk-positive cells following 3 days incubation with GCV at concentrations of 10^{-7} M, whereas tk-negative cells were not inhibited until concentrations of GCV reached 10^{-4} M.

Since the original description of the effectiveness of HSV *tk*/GCV, there have been many reports of its use in the treatment, both *in vitro* and *in vivo*, of multiple tumour types, including breast (Sacco *et al.*, 1995), glioma (Chen *et al.*, 1994), pancreatic (DiMaio *et al.*, 1994), mesothelioma (Sterman *et al.*, 1998) and colon (Chen *et al.*, 1995), with the *tk* gene delivered by retrovirus (Culver *et al.*, 1992), adenovirus (O'Malley *et al.*, 1995), naked DNA (Vile and Hart, 1993a) and liposomes (Fife *et al.*, 1998).

It was noticed in the original description of the effect of the HSV *tk*/GCV combination that the mixing of tk-positive and tk-negative cells at high density in a ratio of 1:9 resulted in almost complete eradication of the tk-negative cells upon treatment with GCV at a concentration of 4×10^{-6} M. In contrast, when the cells were plated at the

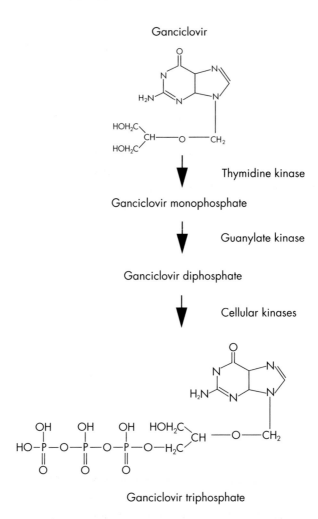

Figure 5.4   The activation of ganciclovir by herpes simplex virus thymidine kinase (HSV *tk*). Ganciclovir (GCV) is converted into its monophosphate by HSV *tk*. Guanylate kinase and other cellular kinases then add additional phosphate groups to create GCV triphosphate, the active species.

same ratio at low density, there was almost complete survival of the tk-negative cells, implying that direct cell-to-cell contact between the enzyme expressing and non-enzyme-expressing cells was capable of transferring sensitivity to GCV between cells, a process initially described as 'metabolic co-operation' (Moolten, 1986). It was subsequently shown in subcutaneous adenocarcinoma and fibrosarcoma models in mice that only 10% tk-positive cells were required for marked growth inhibition and that the normal tissue adjoining and overlying the tumours was unaffected by administration of GCV (Culver *et al.*, 1992). In the same study, the delivery of HSV *tk* gene via injection of retroviral producer cells into experimental rat glioma produced complete regression in 11 out of 14 animals on exposure to GCV. It has also been noted that a bystander effect can exist within the peritoneal cavity. Injecting tk-positive and tk-negative sarcoma cells at a ratio of 1:9 into the peritoneum of mice resulted in significant extension of survival following treatment with GCV, compared with those mice that received 100% tk-negative cells alone. If the ratio was 50:50, some of the mice survived long term (>70 days) (Freeman *et al.*, 1993). Interestingly, Freeman also noted that it was possible to prolong the survival of pre-existing tk-negative intraperitoneal tumours by injecting tk-positive tumour cells and GCV, without any attempt at gene transfer. However, other groups have shown that injecting tk-positive 3T3 fibroblasts into experimental gliomas in rats does not produce any bystander effect (Ram *et al.*, 1993).

Samejima and co-workers confirmed that cell-to-cell contact, or at least close proximity, was required for bystander killing in rodent fibroblasts expressing tk and that the process could be inhibited by co-administration of forskolin, the activator of adenylate cyclase. They also demonstrated that there was evidence of apoptosis in the cells killed by the bystander effect and suggested that phagocytosis by non-enzyme-expressing cells of apoptotic bodies released from dying cells could explain the mechanism of the bystander effect (Samejima and Merulo, 1995). However, it has become evident from more recent work that gap junctional activity is of fundamental importance to the bystander effect in the HSV *tk*/GCV enzyme/prodrug combination. It was demonstrated that the bystander effect seen in HeLa cells (Mesnil *et al.*, 1996) and SKHep J hepatocellular carcinoma cells (Elshami *et al.*, 1996), both of which have little gap junctional activity, increased dramatically when transfected with connexin 43 and connexins 43 and 32 respectively, which are major gap junctional proteins. This finding could explain why non-transduced normal tissue immediately adjacent to tumours, with little gap junctional connection with those tumour cells, was not affected by administration of GCV, whilst the tumour cells were rapidly eliminated.

There appears to be an additional mechanism that can give rise to a bystander effect *in vivo*. In a model of pulmonary metastases of the murine melanoma B16 line, it was noticed that the antitumour effect of HSV *tk*/GCV was markedly greater in immunocompetent mice than in immunodeficient mice. This effect was not due to the immunogenicity of tk itself and subsequent re-challenge of GCV-treated mice showed that some protection against wild-type tumour had been generated in the immunocompetent mice. This implies that the death of tumour cells following exposure to GCV results in the establishment of a systemic tumour-specific immunity (Vile *et al.*, 1994). These findings were con-firmed in murine colorectal carcinoma (Gagandeep *et al.*, 1996) and rat hepatoma (Kianmanesh *et al.*, 1997) models and have also been shown for the cytosine deaminase/5-fluorocytosine enzyme prodrug combi-nation (Mullen *et al.*, 1994) (see below). Vile and co-workers have suggested further that the protective immunity seen in the B16 murine melanoma model is due to a Th1-type response (Vile *et al.*, 1997), that the induction of heat shock protein 70 expression is a requirement for this immunity and that immunity is established after necrotic but not apoptotic cell death (Melcher *et al.*, 1998).

More recently, it has been suggested that there is an opposite, 'Good Samaritan' effect whereby the tk-positive cells are protected from the effects of the toxic metabolites of GCV via gap junctional activity, thereby allowing a more prolonged production of those toxic metabo-lites. The presumed mechanism is that the gap junctions allow rapid passage of the activated GCV away from the tk-positive cell, thereby sparing that cell (Wygoda *et al.*, 1997).

Although at least 20 clinical trials of HSV *tk*/GCV had been approved by the beginning of 1997 (Roth and Cristiano, 1997), only a very small number have been published. In the first (Izquierdo *et al.*, 1996), producer cells releasing *tk*-encoding retroviruses were implanted stereotactically into recurrent primary brain tumours in five patients, who then received 14 days of intravenous GCV at a dose of 5 mg/kg twice daily. One tumour in one patient showed a partial response, with progressive disease in all other injected tumours. The second trial proto-col was very similar (Ram *et al.*, 1997), with retroviral producer cells releasing *tk*-encoding virions injected into 19 tumours in 15 patients with recurrent primary and metastatic intracerebral tumours. Two tumours were resected 7 days after producer cell injection and *in situ* hybridisation revealed only very small clusters of *tk*-positive cells. Accordingly, in the remaining patients who were treated with GCV twice daily for 14 days, there was a complete response in only two nodules (both in the same patient), a partial response in three nodules with no response in the remainder and no responses in any uninjected lesion. All the nodules that responded were under 2 ml in volume prior to treat-ment. On a more positive note, there were no severe adverse events.

A similar, but larger scale multicentre trial has been published more recently (Shand *et al.*, 1999). Forty-eight patients with recurrent glioblastoma multiforme (GBM) were again injected with producer cells releasing *tk*-encoding retroviruses following resection of the recurrent tumour. GCV administration followed 14 days later at a dose of 5 mg/kg intravenously twice daily for another 14 days. Fourteen of 48 patients had demonstrable vector DNA in peripheral blood (as assessed by polymerase chain reaction), thought to be secondary to transduction of lymphocytes within the resected tumour bed, which then migrated into the peripheral circulation. Disappointingly, the median survival for the patients was only 8.6 months, which is no better than would be expected in a population of patients who had surgical resection of recurrent GBM without any other treatment. Ten patients had tk-positive residual tumours present at post mortem examination, indicating that, whilst there had been tumour cell transduction, subsequent GCV treatment had failed to kill them, either because GCV penetrated poorly into the CNS or because the cells were not in the correct phase of the cell cycle at the time of treatment.

In the first reported trial of this enzyme/prodrug combination in non-CNS tumours, an adenovirus encoding HSV *tk* was administered at doses of between 1×10^9 and 1×10^{12} plaque-forming units into the pleural cavity of 20 patients with pleural mesothelioma, followed by 14 days of GCV again at a dose of 5 mg/kg twice daily (Sterman *et al.*, 1998). Although no formal attempts were made to establish whether there were any clinical responses, there was evidence of gene transfer in 11 of 20 patients in a dose-related manner, again with minimal toxicity.

There has now been a reported phase I trial in recurrent localised prostate cancer (Herman *et al.*, 1999) in which an adenovirus encoding HSV *tk* was injected directly into the prostate of 18 men at doses of between 1×10^8 and 1×10^{11} infectious units. Twenty-four hours later, 14 days of intravenous GCV (dose as in previous trials) was commenced. Three patients had an objective response (fall in serum prostate-specific antigen of at least 50%), the longest lasting 12 months.

There were only two severe adverse reactions, both at the highest dose level. One was thrombocytopenia, which resolved after 5 days, and the other was hepatotoxicity, with transient elevation of bilirubin, transaminases and alkaline phosphatase. There has also been a report of severe hepatotoxicity in a rat colorectal carcinoma model following portal vein delivery of adenoviruses encoding the *tk* gene and GCV administration. This implies that activated GCV may be toxic to non-cycling hepatocytes, as this toxicity was not seen in rats that received the adenoviral *tk* without GCV nor in those rats that received a control adenovirus expressing β-galactosidase, followed by GCV (van der Eb *et al.*, 1998). Another potential safety concern was highlighted in a syngeneic rat glioma model (Dewey *et al.*, 1999). Following adenovirally delivered HSV *tk* and treatment with GCV, the brains of long-term (over three months) surviving rats demonstrated extensive inflammation, with microglial and T-lymphocyte infiltration, as well as widespread demyelination. There was also evidence of persistent tk expression three months after a single injection of 2×10^7 infectious units of the adenovirus, implying both that the duration of transgene expression after adenoviral delivery may be much longer *in vivo* than previously imagined and also that the administration of GCV in clinical trials of *tk*/GCV should, perhaps, continue for much longer than the 14 days that most trials currently utilise.

In light of the results of clinical trials and given the probable benefits of immune system involvement in bystander killing *in vivo*, there have been some attempts to increase the potency of the HSV *tk*/GCV system by combining it with immunotherapy. There are reports that IL-2 (Chen *et al.*, 1995), IL-4 (Benedetti *et al.*, 1997) and IL-7 (Sharma *et al.*, 1997) can combine successfully with *tk*/GCV to increase the elimination of colorectal metastases, gliomas and non-small cell lung cancer models, respectively. The significance of these results is that prodrug-mediated killing of one tumour nodule may allow elimination of distant nodules that do not express the prodrug-converting enzyme. There has also been a report of combined cytosine deaminase/5-fluorocytosine (*cd*/5-FC) and HSV *tk*/GCV gene therapy being more effective than either alone in eliminating murine mammary adenocarcinoma tumours (Uckert *et al.*, 1998). Others have attempted to improve the efficacy of *tk*/GCV by utilising the thymidine kinase gene of other herpesvirus species (Loubiere *et al.*, 1999). There is some evidence that equine herpesvirus *tk* mediates more rapid phosphorylation of GCV than that of HSV. Similarly, the thymidine kinase and phosphotransferase homologues of human herpesvirus 8 are both capable of phosphorylating GCV and may have potential for use in VDEPT (Cannon *et al.*, 1999). Other enhancements include the isolation of HSV *tk* mutants better able to phosphorylate GCV (Kokoris *et al.*, 1999), use of alternative prodrugs such as famciclovir and penciclovir that can also be activated by HSV *tk*, but which are orally active. This would facilitate a much longer duration of treatment than is currently possible with intravenous GCV, which would permit more cells to enter S phase and thereby become sensitive to the effects of the activated prodrug. Finally, there has been some elucidation of the pathways by which activated GCV induces apoptosis in transfected cells. These include the accumulation of p53, CD95/Fas and activation of both caspase 3 and caspase 8 (Beltinger *et al.*, 1999) and we have recently demonstrated that co-expression of pro-caspase 3 in ovarian carcinoma cells leads to greater cell death upon exposure to *tk*/GCV (McNeish *et al.*, 2000).

Cytosine deaminase/5-fluorocytosine

The second most commonly employed enzyme/prodrug combination utilises the cytosine deaminase (*cd*) gene, which deaminates the antifungal drug 5-fluorocytosine (5-FC) into 5-fluorouracil (5-FU) (Figure 5.5), the main chemotherapy drug used in the treatment of gastrointestinal malignancies for 30 years. 5-FU itself is converted into 5-fluorouridine 5'-triphosphate and 5-fluoro-2'-deoxyuridine 5'-monophosphate, which function as potent inhibitors of both DNA and RNA synthesis via inhibition of thymidylate synthase and erroneous incorporation as false bases. That there is some inhibition of RNA synthesis as well as DNA synthesis should also produce some toxicity to quiescent cells, although the toxicity of 5-FU still depends critically upon the length of S phase (Mirjolet *et al.*, 1998). Initial reports in transfected or retrovirally trans-duced murine fibroblast lines demonstrated effective killing of cd-positive cells on exposure to 5-FC at a concentration of 5–10 μg/ml, whilst the parental cd-negative cells were unaffected by concentrations in excess of 100 μg/ml. However, in cell-mixing experiments, there

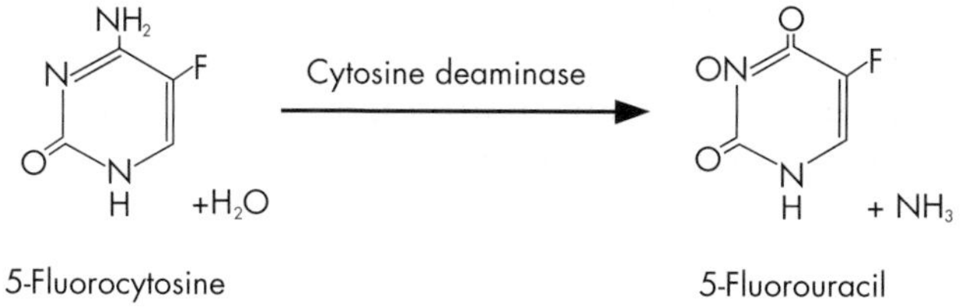

Figure 5.5   The conversion of 5-fluorocytosine (5-FC) into 5-fluorouracil (5-FU) by the action of cytosine deaminase. Cytosine deaminase catalyses the conversion of 5-FC into 5-FU in a step reaction. 5-FU itself is then converted into 5-fluorouridine 5'-triphosphate and 5-fluoro-2'-deoxyuridine 5'-monophosphate, which are both active compounds inhibiting DNA and RNA synthesis.

appeared to be selective killing of the cd-positive cells, with sparing of the cd-negative ones, implying no bystander effect (Mullen *et al.*, 1992). A group that had independently cloned the cd gene from *E. coli* (Austin and Huber, 1993) confirmed the sensitisation of cd-positive WiDR human colorectal carcinoma cells to 5-FC via its conversion to 5-FU (Huber *et al.*, 1993), but showed that there was marked bystander killing *in vitro* when 33% of cells were cd-positive and that this effect did not rely upon cell-to-cell contact. Also, there was a significant reduction in growth rates of mixed cd-positive and -negative subcutaneous WiDR xenografts in nude mice on treatment with 5-FC. It was possible to demonstrate this effect with only 2% cd-positive cells, implying a very powerful bystander effect *in vivo* with this enzyme/prodrug combination (Huber *et al.*, 1994). This same study also demonstrated that it was possible to generate a concentration of 5-FU of >400 μM within cd-positive tumours following systemic 5-FC administration. There is no apparent explanation for the discrepant results between the two groups in terms of bystander activity, although other groups have subsequently recorded bystander activity for *cd*/5-FC (Szary *et al.*, 1997; Shirakawa *et al.*, 1998). Equally, it has also been reported that *cd* gene delivery to normal liver can generate sufficient 5-FU to cause the regression of adjacent cd-negative colorectal metastases, without significant toxicity to those hepatocytes (Topf *et al.*, 1998), which implies both a powerful bystander effect and lack of toxicity of 5-FU to non-cycling cells.

Although the protocols of several clinical trials of *cd*/5-FC have been approved, only one trial has actually been completed (Pandha *et al.*, 1999), in which plasmid DNA encoding *cd* under the control of the c-*erb*B-2 proximal promoter was injected directly into cutaneous metastases of 12 women with recurrent breast cancer positive for c-*erb*B-2. Overexpression of c-*erb*B-2 is seen in approximately 20% of breast carcinomas and is associated with poor prognosis. There was evidence of cd expression in 11 of 12 tumour nodules injected and transgene expression was limited to c-*erb*B-2-positive cells, indicating that transcriptional targeting using this promoter is feasible in human patients. Only eight of the 12 patients received 5-FC (200 mg/kg per day as a 48-hour infusion) and there was evidence of some local tumour response in two of these eight patients. There were also two minor responses in patients who received the *cd* gene but no 5-FC, which may reflect an immune response to the injected plasmid DNA.

An attempt was made to compare the efficacy of *tk*/GCV and *cd*/5-FC in WiDR cells and it was demonstrated that, on exposure to GCV, there was no reduction in size of subcutaneous xenografts that contained

10% tk-positive cells, yet there was a marked antitumour effect in cd-positive tumours on exposure to 5-FC with only 4% of cells enzyme positive (Trinh *et al.*, 1995). However, the poor bystander effect for the tk tumours can be explained by the electron microscope finding that WiDR tumours do not express gap junctions.

As with HSV *tk*/GCV, there are now reports of combining *cd*/5-FC with immunotherapy. One recent report demonstrated that adenoviral GM-CSF and adenoviral *cd* gene transfer to melanomas in mice resulted in greater growth inhibition than with either *cd*/5-FC or GM-CSF alone and that the combination also resulted in greater protective immunity to re-challenge with parental cells (Cao *et al.*, 1998).

Nitroreductase/CB1954

The active species of both *tk*/GCV and *cd*/5-FC are antimetabolites, which means that they will be predominantly toxic to cells that are replicating their DNA. Even within a rapidly growing tumour nodule, the proportion of cells that will be actively dividing may be as low as 6% (Tubiana and Malaise, 1976). The large proportion of cells resting in G_0 has been proposed to be a major factor underlying resistance to GCV. In one study, tumours outgrew 30 days continuous GCV treatment, but remained sensitive on re-treatment, indicating that cells can remain in G_0 for long periods and that acquired resistance to the prodrug was not the cause of the original regrowth (Golumbek *et al.*, 1992). This potential shortcoming and the realisation that enzyme-catalysed activation of alkylating agents from non-toxic prodrugs could provide some advantages over antimetabolites have prompted the search for alternative enzyme prodrug combinations. One of the most promising of these involves the prodrug 5-(aziridin-1-yl)-2,4-dinitro-benzamide (CB1954).

CB1954 is a weak, monofunctional alkylating agent which originally provoked interest in the 1960s following the discovery that Walker rat carcinosarcoma cells were extremely sensitive to CB1954-mediated killing (Cobb *et al.*, 1969; Knox *et al.*, 1988b). The origin of the Walker cell sensitivity was later found to lie in the expression of DT diaphorase, an FAD-containing dehydrogenase that employs either NADH or NADPH as a co-factor. DT diaphorase catalyses the bioreduction of CB1954 to its 4-hydroxylamino derivative, which is then converted by thioesters such as acetyl co-enzyme A into a powerful bifunctional alkylating agent (Knox *et al.*, 1988a). The activated cytotoxic species is not phase-specific and can kill non-cycling cells (Bridgewater *et al.*, 1995).

Human DT diaphorase performs this reduction much less efficiently than the rat enzyme (Boland *et al.*, 1991), which probably explains the lack of efficacy of CB1954 in human subjects in an unpublished pilot clinical trial in the early 1970s. The molecular basis for this difference between human and rat DT diaphorase may lie at residue 104, which is a tyrosine in the rat enzyme and glycine in the human (Chen *et al.*, 1997). Cells that have the capacity to bioreduce CB1954 have been demonstrated to be 100 000 times more sensitive on a dose basis than those that do not (Roberts *et al.*, 1986). An *E. coli* nitroreductase (NTR) has been identified that is capable of reducing CB1954. It was shown to be a monomeric FMN-containing flavoprotein with a molecular mass of 24 kDa that also employed either NADH or NADPH as a co-factor. By comparison of amino acid sequences, it was also shown that this NTR had homology to the 'classical nitroreductase' of *Salmonella typhimurium* and a nitroreductase in *Enterobacter cloacae* (Anlezark *et al.*, 1992). It was further demonstrated that the *E. coli* NTR reduced CB1954 up to 60 times more rapidly than rat DT diaphorase (Knox *et al.*, 1992), although both the 4-hydroxylamino and the less toxic 2-hydroxylamino derivatives are generated in equal proportions (Figure 5.6).

NTR was selected for use in conjunction with CB1954, initially for antibody-directed enzyme prodrug therapy (Anlezark *et al.*, 1992) and, subsequently, for VDEPT once the gene encoding NTR, *nfnB*, had been identified and cloned from the B strain of *E. coli* (Michael *et al.*, 1994).

Several studies have confirmed the prediction that mammalian cells expressing NTR would be sensitised to CB1954 and have demonstrated the existence of a bystander effect with this system (Bridgewater *et al.*, 1995; Green *et al.*, 1997; Friedlos *et al.*, 1998), although one study has reported minimal bystander effect (Clark *et al.*, 1997). There have now been several *in vivo* studies. In the first, NTR was expressed selectively in secretory epithelial cells of the mammary gland from an ovine β-lactoglobin promoter (Clark *et al.*, 1997) and treatment with CB1954 resulted in ablation of the mammary epithelial tissue, with sparing of the adjacent myoepithelial cells, which were NTR negative, implying no bystander effect. However, in the second study (Drabek *et al.*, 1997), in which NTR was expressed in T cells under the control of elements from the human CD2 locus, CB1954 administration resulted in severe reduction in total cell numbers within the thymus with evidence of extensive apoptosis. There was also extensive cell reduction within the spleen, which contained a high number of non-T cells, implying a degree of bystander killing *in vivo*. This study also demonstrated that high doses

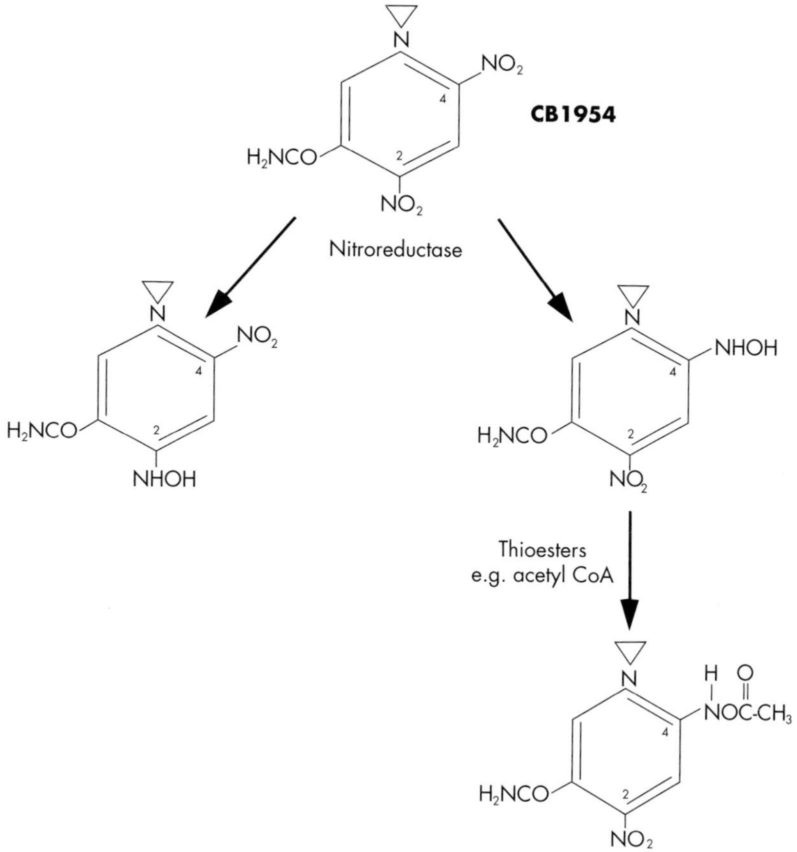

Figure 5.6 The activation of CB1954 by *E. coli* nitroreductase. CB1954 is converted into either its 2- or its 4-hydroxylamino derivative. Only the 4-hydroxylamino derivative is then converted by cellular thioesters into the active species, which is a highly potent bifunctional alkylating agent.

of CB1954 (50 mg/kg/day for 5 days) were also very toxic to BalbC and C3H/He mice and there have been some attempts to discover less toxic alternative prodrugs that can also be activated by NTR (Bailey and Hart, 1997; Friedlos *et al.*, 1997). More recently, it has been shown that human xenografts stably expressing NTR growing in nude mice can be eliminated after only two bolus doses of CB1954 (McNeish *et al.*, 1998) and that intraperitoneal injection of recombinant adenoviral particles encoding NTR, followed by two bolus doses of CB1954 leads to a significant increase in survival (Weedon *et al.*, 2000).

Others

There are many other potential enzyme/prodrug systems, some of which evolved from ADEPT strategies. Some of the more promising ones are listed in Table 5.1. Several of these novel combinations will generate toxic antimetabolite agents, which are likely to meet with the same potential hurdles as *tk*/GCV. The possible advantage that carboxypeptidase G2 (CPG2)-mediated activation of 4-[2-chloroethyl)(2-meslyoxyethyl) amino] benzoyl glutamic acid (CMDA) has over other combinations is that the active species produced by CPG2 requires no further modification by cellular enzymes. This contrasts with 5-FU and both activated CB1954 and GCV: clearly, if enzymes required for further drug modification become deficient in tumour cells, resistance to the activated drug could occur. Like activated CB1954, the active species of CMDA is an alkylating agent, toxic to non-cycling cells and less likely to induce resistance (Frei *et al.*, 1988). One potential disadvantage of CPG2 is that the enzyme in its natural configuration is secreted and removal of the signal peptide is required to prevent this. There is *in vitro* evidence that expression of this altered CPG2 is capable of sensitising a range of ovarian and colorectal carcinoma cells to CMDA and that a modest bystander effect exists (Marais *et al.*, 1996).

Cytochrome P450 isoenzyme 4B1 (CYP4B1) was first identified as an activator of the mould toxin 4-ipomeanol, following a mysterious cattle pulmonary illness. It has also been shown to activate 2-aminoanthracene, although the precise nature of both active species is unknown, but glioma cells stably expressing the rabbit isoform of the enzyme are sensitised both *in vitro* and *in vivo* to both prodrugs, with evidence of single-strand DNA breaks and an adequate bystander effect (Rainov *et al.*, 1998).

Another cytochrome P450 enzyme, the human isoenzyme 1A2 (CYP1A2), is capable of activating the analgesic drug paracetamol (acetaminophen), which is used world-wide as an analgesic drug, but can be hepatotoxic when taken in overdose. There are several pathways of paracetamol elimination, one of which involves CYP1A2, which oxidises the drug into the toxic metabolite N-acetylbenzoquinoneimine (NABQI). Normally, NABQI is detoxified by direct conjugation with reduced glutathione, but in overdose, however, the glutathione conjugation pathway is saturated, leading to excess NABQI and direct hepatic toxicity. An early report indicates that the expression of CYP1A2 in Chinese hamster V79 cells dramatically increases their sensitivity to acetaminophen-mediated toxicity (Thatcher *et al.*, 1999). There is evidence of bystander

Table 5.1   Other potential enzyme/prodrug combinations for use in VDEPT

Enzyme	Prodrug	Active species	Reference
Human thymidine phosphorylase	5'-Deoxy-5-fluorouridine	5-FU	Evrard et al., 1999
Varicella zoster virus (VZV) thymidine kinase	9-(β-D-Arabino-furanosyl)-6-methoxy-9H-purine (araM)	AraATP	Huber et al., 1991
E. coli purine nucleoside phosphorylase	9-(β-D-2-deoxy-erythropento-furanosyl)-6-methylpurine	6-Methylpurine	Sorscher et al., 1994; Hughes et al., 1995
Carboxypeptidase G2	4-[2-Chloroethyl) (2-meslyoxyethyl) amino] benzoyl glutamic acid (CMDA)	4-[2-Chloro-ethyl)(2-meslyoxyethyl) amino] benzoic acid	Marais et al., 1996
Rabbit cytochrome P450 isoenzyme 4B1	2-Aminoanthracene 4-Ipomeanol	Unknown Unknown	Rainov et al., 1998
Human cytochrome P450 isoenzyme 1A2	Acetaminophen (paracetamol)	N-Acetyl benzoquinone-imine (NABQI)	Thatcher et al., 1999
Human carboxyl-esterase	7-Ethyl-10 -[4-(1-piperidino)-1-piperidino] carbonyloxy camptothecin (CPT-11; irinotecan)	7-Ethyl-10-hydroxy-camptothecin (SN38)	Kojima et al., 1998
Linamarase	2-(β-D-glucopyra-nosyloxy)-2-methyl-propanenitrile (linamarin)	Cyanide	Cortés et al., 1998

killing of non-CYP1A2-expressing V79 cells at low concentrations of acetaminophen when mixed with only 5% of CYP1A2-positive cells. This effect is not cell-type specific, with evidence of killing of human ovarian carcinoma SKOV3 and colon carcinoma HCT116 cells when mixed with CYP1A2-expressing V79 cells.

The chemotherapeutic drug irinotecan, also known as CPT-11 (7-ethyl-10-[4-(1-piperidino)-1-piperidino] carbonyloxy-camptothecin), is active against lung, cervical, ovarian and colorectal carcinomas. As with 5-FU, it should strictly be classified as a prodrug as its piperidino side chain is cleaved by the enzyme carboxylesterase to reveal the active species, SN-38 (7-ethyl-10-hydroxy-camptothecin). Uniquely amongst the other active species mentioned above, SN-38 functions as an inhibitor of mammalian DNA topoisomerase I, an enzyme whose functions include releasing the torsional stress of supercoiled DNA. However, SN-38 is insoluble and is therefore impractical as a chemotherapeutic agent in its own right. Administration of irinotecan is frequently associated with severe, but unpredictable, toxicity, especially diarrhoea. This may be due to a genetically determined person-to-person variability in the expression of the activating carboxylesterase enzyme, resulting in highly variable levels of SN-38 production. Expression of high levels of carboxylesterase by tumour cells would permit much lower doses of irinotecan to be administered, with resultant reduction in toxicity. It has been shown that adenoviral delivery of the human carboxylesterase gene to A549 lung carcinoma cells increases both SN-38 production and sensitivity to irinotecan, and can produce growth delay in subcutaneous A549 xenografts in nude mice (Kojima *et al.*, 1998).

The enzyme–prodrug combination linamarase and 2-(β-D-glucopyranosyloxy)-2-methylpropanenitrile (linamarin) is of interest because the enzyme derives not from a virus or fungus, but from the cassava plant, *Manihot esculenta* Crantz. Linamarase is a β-glucosidase that hydrolyses linamarin into glucose and acetone cyanohydrin. The latter is unstable at pH greater than 6 and spontaneously degrades into acetone and hydrogen cyanide. The hydrolysis of linamarin does not take place in normal mammalian tissue and the prodrug is excreted unchanged in the urine. Expression of linamarase in range of human and rodent cells has been shown to increase both their sensitivity to linamarin and the production of cyanide.

The cyanide ion (CN^-) is freely diffusible and HCN is a gas, which would suggest that any bystander effect of this system would not rely upon gap junctional activity or cell-to-cell contact. There is *in vitro* evidence that a 50 : 50 mixture of linamarase-expressing and non-expressing murine ΨCRIP cells are completely eradicated on exposure to concentrations of linamarin that are non-toxic to the parental cells (Cortés *et al.*, 1998).

Given the toxicity of cyanide and the diffusible nature of the active species, there would be considerable concern that the use of this enzyme–prodrug combination *in vivo* would be associated with extensive toxicity. In a rat glioma model, direct infusion of linamarin into the brains of rats bearing linamarase-positive tumours resulted in complete tumour eradication with no discernible toxicity to the animals. However, there was no attempt to deliver the linamarin systemically, as there is evidence that bacteria present in normal gut flora of both rodents and humans contain β-glucosidases that are capable of releasing cyanide from linamarin. This problem would have to be overcome safely if this enzyme–prodrug combination were ever to reach clinical trials.

Inhibition of tumour angiogenesis

Angiogenesis describes the process by which primary tumours and metastases recruit a functional blood supply without which it is not possible for them to grow beyond a size of 2–3 mm^3 (Folkman, 1990). Independent of gene therapy, drugs designed selectively to damage tumour vasculature have been developed, and there have been promising early reports of their activity (Arap *et al.*, 1998). There are three gene therapy approaches to anti-angiogenic therapy. First, the suppression of angiogenic factors such as vascular endothelial growth factor (VEGF); secondly, the disruption of signalling pathways used by angiogenic factors; and thirdly, the delivery of genes for anti-angiogenic molecules. A related approach is to use the neo-vasculature as a means to target the expression of other toxic genes to tumours. Tumour targeting is discussed in detail below.

The delivery of VEGF antisense can lead to the regression of tumours *in vivo* (Saleh *et al.*, 1996). Tumours, perhaps inevitably, have alternative angiogenic factors that can be expressed in addition to VEGF, such as basic fibroblast growth factor (bFGF), suggesting that the isolated targeting to VEGF alone is unlikely to prove an adequate target (Lau and Bicknell, 1999). The strategy of targeting the downstream pathways used by factors such as VEGF has also shown some promise, utilising the native soluble FLT-1 truncated VEGF receptor (Goldman *et al.*, 1998) or soluble receptor for Tie2, an endothelium-specific receptor tyrosine kinase that is known to play a role in tumour angiogenesis (Lin *et al.*, 1998).

The list of known anti-angiogenic molecules is now lengthy, and includes angiostatin, endostatin, thrombospondin 1 and platelet factor 4. Recent reports have suggested that the adenoviral delivery of the endostatin gene can reduce the growth of breast and lung carcinoma xenograft models in mice (Sauter *et al.*, 2000). Similarly, retroviral delivery of the protease gene permits the cleavage of plasminogen to generate angiostatin within tumours and produces some slowing of lung carcinoma xenografts in nude mice (Matsuda *et al.*, 2000). Finally, there is some suggestion that part of the antitumour effect of other gene therapy strategies, such as overexpression of wild-type p53 and immunotherapy with IL-12, are mediated via an anti-angiogenesis (Ricciono *et al.*, 1998; Cavallo *et al.*, 1999).

Tumour targeting

One of the most important considerations in any cancer gene therapy strategy is the targeting of transgene expression to tumour cells. The ideal gene therapy vector can be administered systemically and will produce gene delivery to, and transgene expression within, a target population of cells, with minimal expression within normal, non-malignant cells. Current vectors are some distance from realising this goal, but a variety of techniques exist by which it may be achieved.

Direct injection

At the most crude level, it is possible to inject vectors directly into a single tumour nodule, thereby providing a level of tumour targeting. This method was widely employed in early clinical trials in, for example, malignant melanoma nodules and isolated metastases from distant primaries, as it maximises the delivery of vectors to one specific site. Although this technique was employed in one of the more successful phase I trials (Roth *et al.*, 1996), it is unlikely to be clinically useful since most cancers are widely metastatic and it is impractical directly to inject multiple tumour sites. Moreover, there is evidence that even careful intratumoral injection of virus can lead to some leaking into the systemic circulation (Toloza *et al.*, 1996).

Regional delivery

Some tumours remain localised within certain body cavities until very late in their natural history. Ovarian cancer, for example, usually remains within the peritoneal cavity, which would render it susceptible to the intraperitoneal delivery of both vectors and prodrugs if necessary.

Similarly, mesothelioma, an asbestos-induced primary malignancy of serosal surfaces, most often the pleura and peritoneum, almost invariably remains within that cavity for the duration of the disease and there is one published trial of local delivery of HSV *tk*/GCV in pleural mesothelioma (Sterman *et al.*, 1998). The theory of intraperitoneal chemotherapy is that high drug levels are achieved within the peritoneal cavity as well as adequate systemic levels, but there is evidence that the drug only penetrates a few cell layers (Markman, 1991) and viral penetration may be less. There is also evidence that chondroitin sulfate proteoglycans within malignant pleural effusions can inhibit retroviral gene transfer, although this inhibition may be avoided by pretreatment of the effusion with hyaluronidase (Batra *et al.*, 1997). It also appears that neutralising anti-adenovirus antibodies are present to high titre within the ascites of patients with ovarian cancer, which may also limit the usefulness of this mode of delivery *in vivo* (Stallwood *et al.*, 2000).

Another potentially exploitable feature of tumours is their macroscopic blood supply (rather than targeting neovasculature). Hepatic metastases of colorectal carcinoma reach the liver via the portal circulation, but, once established within the liver, derive their blood supply predominantly from the hepatic artery, such that it is possible to achieve an element of tumour-selective delivery by administering vectors and/or drugs via this artery (De Takats *et al.*, 1994). There are also reports that delivery of retroviral packaging cells to experimental colorectal carcinoma metastases within the liver can be achieved by injection of retroviral producer cells via the portal vein (Hurford *et al.*, 1995).

Tumour-specific vector binding

One of the keys to redirecting binding of any vector, viral or otherwise, is to identify specific cell surface molecules that are expressed exclusively or predominantly on one cell type and which are bound with high specificity and affinity by a known ligand (Russell, 1996). Currently, monoclonal antibodies are frequently employed to isolate such molecules and the overexpression of CA125 (MacDonald *et al.*, 1988) and folate-binding protein (Campbell *et al.*, 1991) in ovarian cancer has been identified in this way. However, the complexity of isolating and purifying monoclonal antibodies means that this technique is far from straightforward. Also, the fact that high-affinity binding does not always translate into efficient gene delivery means that there is currently no alternative to trial and error in the search for good potential targets. A different technique may be to employ peptide-displaying phages; this can be much more rapid than monoclonal antibody screening and can take place without any previous knowledge of cellular receptors (Russell, 1996). There have been reports of partially successful screening of peptide libraries to identify phages that have cell-specific binding characteristics (Barry *et al.*, 1996).

Retrovirus targeting

Retroviruses are frequently used for the gene delivery. The vast majority of retroviral vectors are based on the *Moloney murine leukemia virus* (MoMLV). The major determinant of the tropism of any retrovirus is the interaction of its envelope protein with specific cell-surface receptors and there are at least five classes of wild-type MoMLV envelope, the amphotropic, the ecotropic, the xenotropic, the dualtropic and the 10A1-MLV (Leverett *et al.*, 1998). By altering the envelope of a retrovirus, it may be possible to limit its binding to a specific cell population and hence target transgene delivery. The mechanisms that can be employed involve, for example, modifying preformed virions; it is possible to link biotinylated antibodies directed against the SU domain of the envelope and specific membrane markers via streptavidin. Alternatively, one can introduce small modifications into the retroviral envelopes, or indeed substitute the entire SU domain. Work in this latter area has revealed that some normal, wild-type envelope proteins must also be expressed for any normal envelope function to take place, which greatly complicates the targeting process. Finally, it is possible to add ligand-binding domains onto the envelope protein (Cosset and Russell, 1996).

It has been noticed in all attempts at re-directing retroviral tropism that, even if the virus–cell infection can be limited to a specific cell population, the efficiency with which fusion and entry occur is often greatly reduced (Schnierle and Groner, 1996). Nonetheless, there have been reports of successful incorporation of a ten-amino-acid collagen-binding domain into the MoMLV envelope protein which redirected virus binding to vascular lesions (Hall *et al.*, 1997) and the incorporation of the whole simian immunodeficiency virus (SIV) envelope into MoMLV-based vectors that only infect CD4+ human lymphocytes (Indraccolo *et al.*, 1998). One other technique that has been employed to alter the tropism of retroviruses is to co-incubate retroviruses with recombinant adenoviruses, which can result in infection of human cells by retroviruses expressing the ecotropic MoMLV envelope protein (Adams *et al.*, 1995).

Adenovirus targeting

As with retroviral vectors, the vast majority of adenoviral gene therapy vectors are derived from one virus strain, adenovirus type 5 (Ad 5). The normal mode of infection of target cells by Ad 5 is initiated by the binding of the high-affinity knob domain of the fibre protein to the recently identified coxsackie-adenovirus receptor (CAR) (Bergelson *et al.*, 1997), whilst internalisation requires interaction between an RGD amino acid motif on penton base proteins of the viral capsid and $\alpha_v\beta_3$ and $\alpha_v\beta_5$ integrins on the cell surface. The bound virus is then internalised via a clathrin-coated vesicle which becomes an endosome. The penton bases cause disruption of the endosome and the uncoated virus is released into the cytoplasm, where it migrates to the nuclear membrane, to which the viral core binds, releasing the DNA into the nucleus (Watkins *et al.*, 1997). The adenovirus receptor is expressed on a very wide range of cells, reflecting the relative ease with which adenoviruses can mediate gene transfer to many cell types. However, there is some evidence that CAR and α_V integrin expression, whilst necessary, is not absolutely sufficient for transgene expression after systemic delivery, implying that there may be other barriers to successful gene transfer with adenoviruses (Fechner *et al.*, 1999). One technique to limit adenovirus–cell interactions is to fuse a single-chain antifibre antibody (Ab) with a specific ligand, such as epidermal growth factor (EGF). The EGF receptor (EGFR) is overexpressed on a wide range of tumours cells and, following binding of the Ab-EGF fragment to recombinant Ad 5, virus infection is limited to EGFR-positive cells (Watkins *et al.*, 1997). A similar strategy has been employed to limit Ad 5 expression to Kaposi's sarcoma cells via the fibroblast growth factor receptor (Goldman *et al.*, 1997). Similarly, convalently linking biotin molecules to adenovirus molecules followed by biotinylated stem cell factor (the ligand for the c-kit receptor) permits dramatic increases in transgene expression in c-kit-positive haematopoietic cells (Smith *et al.*, 1999).

In order to avoid the structural complexity of these virus–ligand molecules, others have sought to integrate new motifs into the fibre protein itself. The simplest method is to include the RGD motif in the fibre knob region, which can increase the range of cell types that can be infected by adenoviruses (Reynolds *et al.*, 1999) and increase the level of transgene expression in cells that are otherwise resistant to adenoviral transfection (Staba *et al.*, 2000). Also, inclusion of the RGD motif in the hexon monomer protein can provide a pathway for infection that entirely bypasses the fibre knob protein (Vigne *et al.*, 1999). However, if cancer cell-specific motifs were introduced into the fibre region, it may prove difficult to propagate the adenovirus particles using traditional cell lines such as 293 or 911, if they lack the receptors for these novel motifs (Douglas *et al.*, 1999).

Tumour- or tissue-specific promoters

Many tumours are known to overexpress certain genes, and a representative list is presented in Table 5.2. If the expression of therapeutic genes can be linked to the transcriptional control regions of these genes, then expression of HSV *tk* or *E. coli* NTR, for example, can be limited to tumour cells, ensuring a degree of tumour selectivity. The promoter of the carcinoembryonic antigen (CEA) (Schrewe *et al.*, 1990) has been the focus of the greatest amount of research, most noticeably in the potential treatment of colorectal carcinoma (Huber *et al.*, 1993). It has been shown that colorectal xenografts expressing CEA-driven cytosine deaminase show partial, although not complete, regression upon treatment with 5-FC (Richards *et al.*, 1995). In a comparison of the CEA promoter and a constitutive cytomegalovirus (CMV) enhancer/chicken β actin promoter construct in adenoviruses in the treatment of human gastric cancer in nude mice, Lan and co-workers demonstrated tumour-specific *cd* expression both *in vitro* and *in vivo* with the CEA promoter, and markedly reduced hepatic toxicity with Ad CEA–*cd* compared with Ad CMV/β actin–*cd*. The Ad CMV/β actin–*cd* and Ad CEA–*cd* mice treated with 5-FC demonstrated similar increases in median survival compared with control mice. Interestingly, the mice that received Ad CMV/β actin–*cd* and placebo (PBS) had a modest increase in median survival compared with those that were treated with PBS alone without virus, implying that the virus alone mediated an antitumour effect (Lan *et al.*, 1997).

There are reports of the use of multiple alternative promoters to drive tumour- or tissue-specific expression, including tyrosinase in melanoma (Vile and Hart, 1993b), *MUC1* in breast and ovarian disease (Ring *et al.*, 1997) and c-*erb*B-2 in breast cancer (Pandha *et al.*, 1999). However, one of the intrinsic problems is that such promoters are less powerful than strong constitutive ones, such as the CMV immediate early, or the simian virus 40 large T-antigen promoters. In one study comparing CEA- and CMV-driven expression of NTR in the strongly CEA-positive pancreatic line SUIT2, 40 times as much CEA virus as CMV was required to achieve comparable degrees of cell sensitisation (S. Weedon, personal communication).

Table 5.2   Genes frequently overexpressed in specific tumours

Gene product	Tumour/tissue type
α-Fetoprotein	Hepatoma, teratoma
Carcinoembryonic antigen (CEA)	Colorectal, other gastrointestinal and lung carcinomas
c-*erb*B-2	Breast and gastrointestinal cancers
c-*erb*B-3	Breast cancer
c-*erb*B-4	Breast and gastric cancers
Tyrosinase, tyrosinase-related protein	Melanoma and melanocytes
Neuron-specific enolase	Small cell lung cancer
Prostate-specific antigen (PSA)	Prostate and prostate carcinoma
Folate-binding protein	Ovarian cancer
Polymorphic epithelial mucin (PEM)	Breast and ovarian cancers
Placental-like alkaline phosphatase (PLAP)	Ovarian and testicular cancers, seminoma
Calcitonin	Medullary carcinoma of thyroid
Thyroglobulin	Follicular thyroid cancer

One other potential problem with the use of tissue-specific promoters in adenoviral vectors lies in enhancer elements early in the E1
region, close to the packaging signal that cannot be excised from the
vector genome. These elements have been reported to override the tissue
specificity of the c-*erb*B-2 promoter in one first-generation adenoviral
vector. However, it is possible to restore tissue-specific expression of the
transgene by insulating the promoter–transgene cassette with sequences
that contain the stop signal from the bovine growth hormone gene
(Vassaux *et al.*, 1999).

Tumour-specific virus replication

The goal of a virus that replicates purely within tumours but not in surrounding non-tumour tissue is an appealing one, as it would allow the
local generation of vectors that could produce further gene transfer. This
could overcome many of the current problems of poor gene transfer *in
vivo*. If that virus were also able to lyse the tumour cells in which it was
replicating, it could be doubly effective. For this reason, investigation
has focused upon HSV and adenoviral vectors, which produce lytic
infection in the wild-type state.

Herpes simplex virus-based vectors

Vectors based on *Herpes simplex virus type 1* (HSV1) are attractive candidates for the transfection of intracranial disease given their natural tropism for neurological tissue. Their ability to travel in a retrograde direction suggests that it may be possible to deliver transgenes to the CNS from peripheral sites. A major disadvantage is that wild-type HSV1 produces rapidly fatal encephalitis. However, a series of mutant HSV-based vectors have been developed, most of which lack both copies of the gene for the neurovirulence factor ICP34.5. An ICP34.5-negative HSV mutant, 1716, was found to lyse F9 teratoma and actively cycling murine fibroblasts, but not contact inhibited fibroblasts (Brown *et al.*, 1994). Similarly, 1716 is capable of producing lytic infection in a variety of tumour cell lines (Kucharczuk *et al.*, 1997), but not normal tissue, nor the normal CNS tissue of the mouse (Randazzo *et al.*, 1995). Two early clinical trials using ICP34.5-negative HSV1 mutants in the treatment of recurrent glioblastoma multiforme have taken place, with minimal toxicity and some encouraging clinical results (Markert *et al.*, 2000; Rampling *et al.*, 2000).

Adenovirus-based vectors

Most conventional adenoviral vectors for gene therapy are deleted in the entire E1 region, such that they cannot replicate. The 55-kDa protein from the E1B region is thought to bind to and inactivate p53, thereby allowing virus replication. Thus, in normal cells, a virus which lacks this 55-kDa protein should not replicate, whilst in cells that lack functional p53 (e.g. tumour cells), the virus should be able to undergo replication and hence cause cell lysis. Since the original description of an E1B-deleted adenovirus, various groups have produced similar viruses. The most heavily marketed, called ONYX 015, has been tested both *in vitro* and *in vivo* in a variety of tumour models and has been shown to replicate lytically in p53-null and p53-mutant tumour cells, but not in normal, non-tumorous tissue (Heise *et al.*, 1997). However, there is also evidence that tumours with a normal *p53* gene are capable of sustaining lytic replication, implying that p53 status may not be the sole determinant of this effect of this virus (Goodrum and Ornelles, 1998; Turnell *et al.*, 1999). To corroborate this, other groups report that an Ad 5 deleted for both the 19-kDa and the 55-kDa E1B proteins is capable of lysing tumour cells with normal *p53* sequences and that this double negative virus induces greater lysis in *p53*-mutated or deleted tumour cells than wild-type Ad 5, again implying that the effect of this virus is determined by more than *p53* status (Duque *et al.*, 1998). Most recently, one poss-ible explanation for the replication of E1B 55 kDa-deleted adenoviruses in p53-positive tumour cells is the absence of p14/ARF. Tumour cells that are p14/ARF-negative have upregulated expression of MDM2, which in turn binds to and inhibits p53. The colorectal carcinoma cell line HCT116 is *p53*-positive, yet permits ONYX 015 replication. Following transfection of the p14/ARF gene, the ability of ONYX 015 to replicate within HCT116 cells is lost (McCormick, 2000).

Several clinical trials of ONYX 015 have been commenced. Initial results suggest that, whilst the injection of virus alone into p53-null head and neck tumours does not produce objective responses (Ganly *et al.*, 2000), the combination of virus and conventional chemotherapy can produce significant reduction in the volume of tumours that have failed to respond to conventional therapy (Khuri *et al.*, 2000).

Reovirus

The third virus that has potential for tumour-specific replication differs from either the herpes simplex or adenovirus vectors mentioned above, as it is the wild-type virus, rather than a deletion mutant, that is being utilised. Reoviruses are ubiquitous double-stranded RNA viruses that appear to produce no clinical symptoms in humans. However, in cells with an activated Ras pathway, either through direct mutations of Ras itself or through mutations of upstream activators of Ras, such as Her-2/c-*erb*B-2, infection with reovirus leads to a lytic cycle, producing death of the infected cell (Norman and Lee, 2000). Although Ras mutations themselves are found in only 30% of human tumours, mutations in Ras-activating elements can be found in up to 50% of other tumours (Norman and Lee, 2000). Reovirus infection of transformed murine fibroblasts and human glioblastoma cells at a multiplicity of infection of 10 infectious particles per cell can lead to cell death *in vitro* and regres-sion of established tumour nodules in murine models and this antitumour activity appears not to be affected by the presence of the anti-reovirus antibodies carried by up to 50% of adults (Coffey *et al.*, 1998).

Conclusions

One of the most persistent criticisms of gene therapy is that it has failed to live up to the not inconsiderable expectations made of it (Friedmann, 1989). This criticism has been heightened further by the death of a young patient in 1999 shortly after being injected with a recombinant adeno-viral vector (Editorial, 2000). However, in the defence of gene therapy for cancer, early clinical trials of any new treatment involve patients with recurrent and metastatic disease that is, by definition, refractory to current conventional therapy. Consequently, it is of little surprise that there have been few objective clinical responses in published trials. However, the degree of prior expectation has ensured that these results are heralded as a wholesale failure of gene therapy (Verma, 1994). There has also been more than a suggestion of *schadenfreude* in some quarters as poor results are announced. Gene therapy, especially as a treatment for malignant disease, is a technique in its infancy [an excuse that has been used for over a decade (Weatherall, 1988), but surely cannot be valid indefinitely] and it is very unlikely that any one gene therapy strategy will ever produce dramatic cures for all types of malignant disease. Much more likely, combined gene therapy strategies will be used in conjunction with existing modalities in the treatment of residual post-surgical disease. The introduction of vectors that can selectively replicate within tumour populations is a particularly exciting prospect, as it helps to overcome the main problem of all gene therapy studies, namely the very low rates of gene transfer *in vivo*.

The Varmus report in 1995 (reported in Wadman, 1995) was particularly damning about the poor design of clinical trials, which reduced the amount of useful information that was gleaned from any negative results. Therefore, future trials of gene therapy must be sophisticated in design with clear and distinct scientific endpoints if the potential of this exciting technology is to be realised.

References

Abdel-Wahab Z, Weltz C, Hester D, *et al.* (1997) A phase I trial of immunotherapy with interferon-gamma gene-modified autologous melanoma cells – monitoring the humoral immune response. *Cancer* 80: 401–412.

Adams R, Wang M, Steffen D, *et al.* (1995) Infection by retroviral vectors outside of their host range in the presence of replication-defective adenovirus. *J Virol* 69: 1887–1894.

Anlezark G, Melton R, Sherwood R, *et al.* (1992) The bioactivation of 5-(aziridin-1-yl)-2,4-dinitrobenzamide (CB 1954) – I: Purification and properties of a nitroreductase enzyme from *Escherichia coli* – a potential enzyme for antibody-directed enzyme prodrug therapy (ADEPT). *Biochem Pharmacol* 44: 2289–2295.

Arap W, Pasqualini R, Ruoslahti E (1998) Cancer treatment by targeted drug delivery to tumor vasculature. *Science* 279: 377–380.

Austin E, Huber B (1993) A first step in the development of gene therapy for colorectal carcinoma: cloning, sequencing and expression of *Escherichia coli* cytosine deaminase. *Mol Pharmacol* 43: 380–387.

Badie B, Goh C, Klaver J, *et al.* (1999) Combined radiation and p53 gene therapy of malignant glioma cells. *Cancer Gene Ther* 6: 155–162.

Bailey S, Hart I (1997) Nitroreductase activation of CB1954 – an alternative 'suicide' gene system (editorial). *Gene Ther* 4: 80–81.

Barry M, Dower W, Johnston S (1996) Toward cell-targeting gene therapy vectors: selection of cell binding peptides from random peptide presenting phage libraries. *Nat Med* 2: 299–305.

Baskar S, Ostrand-Rosenberg S, Nabavi N, *et al.* (1993) Constitutive expression of B7 restores immunogenicity of tumor cells expressing truncated major histocompatibility complex class II molecules. *Proc Natl Acad Sci USA* 90: 5687–5690.

Batra R, Olsen J, Hoganson D, *et al.* (1997) Retroviral gene transfer is inhibited by chondroitin sulfate proteoglycans/glycosaminoglycans in malignant pleural effusions. *J Biol Chem* 272: 11736–11743.

Beltinger C, Fulda S, Kammertoens T, *et al.* (1999) Herpes simplex virus thymidine kinase/ganciclovir-induced apoptosis involves ligand-independent death receptor aggregation and activation of caspases. *Proc Natl Acad Sci USA* 96: 8699–8704.

Benedetti S, Dimeco F, Pollo B, *et al.* (1997) Limited efficacy of the HSV-TK/GCV system for gene therapy of malignant gliomas and perspectives for the combined transduction of the interleukin-4 gene. *Hum Gene Ther* 8: 1345–1353.

Bergelson J, Cunningham J, Droguett G, *et al.* (1997) Isolation of a common receptor for coxsackie B and adenoviruses 2 and 5. *Science* 275: 1320–1323.

Blaese R, Culver K, Miller D, *et al.* (1995) T lymphocyte directed gene therapy for ADA⁻ SCID: initial results after 4 years. *Science* 270: 475–480.

Blau H, Khavari P (1997) Gene therapy: progress, problems, prospects. *Nat Med* 3: 612–613.

Bodmer W (1994) Cancer genetics. *Br Med Bull* 50: 517–526.

Boland M, Knox R, Roberts J (1991) The differences in kinetics of rat and human DT diaphorase result in a differential sensitivity of derived cell lines to CB1954 (5-(aziridin-1-yl)-2,4-dinitrobenzamide). *Biochem Pharmacol* 41: 867–875.

Brennand J, Konecki D, Caskey C (1983) Expression of human and chinese hamster hypoxanthine-guanine phosphoribosyl transferase cDNA recombinants in cultured Lesch-Nyhan and Chinese hamster fibroblasts. *J Biol Chem* 258: 9593–9596.

Bridgewater J, Springer C, Knox R, *et al.* (1995) Expression of the bacterial nitroreductase enzyme in mammalian cells renders them selectively sensitive to killing by the prodrug CB1954. *Eur J Cancer* 31A: 2362–2370.

Brown S, Harland J, MacLean A, *et al.* (1994) Cell type and cell state determine differential *in vitro* growth of non-neurovirulent ICP34.5 negative herpes simplex virus types 1 and 2. *J Gen Virol* 75: 2367–2377.

Browning M and Bodmer W (1992) MHC antigens and cancer: implications for T cell surveillance. *Curr Opin Immunol* 4: 613–618.

Brunda M, Luistro L, Warrier R, *et al.* (1993) Antitumour and antimetastatic activity of IL-12 against murine tumours. *J Exp Med* 178: 1223–1230.

Bui L, Butterfield L, Kim J, *et al.* (1997) *In vivo* therapy of hepatocellular carcinoma with a tumor-specific adenoviral vector expressing interleukin-2. *Hum Gene Ther* 8: 2173–2182.

Cai D, Mukhopadhyay T, Liu Y, *et al.* (1993) Stable expression of the wild type p53 gene in human lung cancer cells after retrovirus mediated gene transfer. *Hum Gene Ther* 4: 614–624.

Campbell I, Jones T, Foulkes W, *et al.* (1991) Folate binding protein is a marker for ovarian cancer. *Cancer Res* 51: 5329–5338.

Cannon J, Hamzeh F, Moore S, *et al.* (1999) Human herpesvirus 8-encoded thymidine kinase and phosphotransferase homologues confer sensitivity of ganciclovir. *J Virol* 73: 4786–4793.

Cao X, Ju D, Tao Q, *et al.* (1998) Adenovirus-mediated GM-CSF gene and cytosine deaminase gene transfer followed by 5-fluorocytosine administration elicit more potent antitumor response in tumor-bearing mice. *Gene Ther* 5: 1130–1136.

Cavallo F, Di Carlo E, Butera M, *et al.* (1999) Immune events associated with the cure of established tumors and spontaneous metastases by local and systemic interleukin 12. *Cancer Res* 59: 414–421.

Cella M, Sallusto F, Lanzavacchia A (1997) Origin, maturation and antigen presenting function of dendritic cells. *Curr Opin Immunol* 9: 10–16.

Chen S, Shine H, Goman J, *et al.* (1994) Gene therapy for brain tumors: regression of experimental gliomas by adenovirus-mediated gene transfer *in vivo*. *Proc Natl Acad Sci USA* 91: 3054–3057.

Chen S, Chen X, Wang Y, *et al.* (1995) Combination gene therapy for liver metastasis of colon carcinoma *in vivo*. *Proc Natl Acad Sci USA* 92: 2577–2581.

Chen S, Knox R, Wu K, *et al.* (1997) Molecular basis of the catalytic differences among DT-diaphorase of human, rat and mouse. *J Biol Chem* 272: 1437–1439.

Chong H, Todryk S, Hutchinson G, *et al.* (1998) Tumour cell expression of B7 co-stimulatory molecules and interleukin-12 or granulocyte-macrophage colony-stimulating factor induces a local antitumour response and may generate systemic protective immunity. *Gene Ther* 5: 223–232.

Clark A, Iwobi M, Cui W, *et al.* (1997) Selective cell ablation in transgenic mice expressing *E. coli* nitroreductase. *Gene Ther* 4: 101–110.

Cobb L, Connors T, Elson L, *et al.* (1969) 2,4-Dinitro-5-ethyleneiminobenzamide (CB1954): a potent and selective inhibitor of growth of the Walker carcinoma 256. *Biochem Pharmacol* 18: 1519–1527.

Coffey M, Strong J, Forsyth P, *et al.* (1998) Reovirus therapy of tumours with activated Ras pathways. *Science* 282: 1332–1334.

Cordier L, Duffour M-T, Sabourin J-C, *et al.* (1995) Complete recovery of mice from a pre-established tumor by direct intratumoral delivery of an adenovirus vector harboring the murine IL-2 gene. *Gene Ther* 2: 16–21.

Cortés M, de Felipe P, Martin V, *et al.* (1998) Successful use of a plant gene in the treatment of cancer in vivo. *Gene Ther* 5: 1499–1507.

Cosset F-L, Russell S (1996) Targeting retrovirus entry. *Gene Ther* 3: 946–956.

Culver K, Ram Z, Wallbridge S, *et al.* (1992) In vivo gene transfer with retroviral vector-producer cells for treatment of experimental brain tumours. *Science* 256: 1550–1552.

De Takats P, Kerr D, Poole C, *et al.* (1994) Hepatic artery chemotherapy for metastatic colorectal carcinoma. *Br J Cancer* 69: 372–378.

Dewey R, Morrissey G, Cowsill S, *et al.* (1999) Chronic brain inflammation and persistent herpes simplex virus thymidine kinase expression in survivors of syngeneic glioma treated by adenovirus-mediated gene therapy: implications for clinical trials. *Nat Med* 5: 1256–1263.

DiMaio J, Clary B, Via D, *et al.* (1994) Directed enzyme pro-drug gene therapy for pancreatic cancer. *Surgery* 116: 205–213.

Douglas J, Miller C, Kim M, *et al.* (1999) A system for the propagation of adenoviral vectors with genetically modified receptor specificities. *Nat Biotechnol* 17: 470–475.

Drabek D, Guy J, Craig R, *et al.* (1997) The expression of bacterial nitroreductase in transgenic mice results in specific cell killing by the prodrug CB1954. *Gene Ther* 4: 93–100.

Dranoff G, Jaffee E, Lazenby A, *et al.* (1993) Vaccination with irradiated tumor cells engineered to secrete murine granulocyte-colony stimulating factor stimulates potent and long lasting antitumor immunity. *Proc Natl Acad Sci USA* 90: 3539–3543.

Dranoff G, Soiffer R, Lynch T, *et al.* (1997) A phase I study of vaccination with autologous, irradiated melanoma cells engineered to secrete human granulocyte-macrophage colony stimulating factor. *Hum Gene Ther* 8: 111–123.

Du C, Fang M, Li Y, *et al.* (2000) Smac, a mitochondrial protein that promotes cytochrome c-dependent caspase activation by eliminating IAP inhibition. *Cell* 102: 33–42.

Duque P, Alonso C, Sanchez-Prieto R, *et al.* (1998) Antitumoral effect of E1B defective adenoviruses in human malignant cells. *Gene Ther* 5: 286–287.

Editorial (2000) Gene therapy – a loss of innocence. *Nat Med* 7: 1.

Ellem K, O'Rourke M, Johnson G, *et al.* (1997) A case report: immune responses and clinical course of the first human use of granulocyte/macrophage-colony-stimulating-factor-transduced autologous melanoma cells for immunotherapy. *Cancer Immunol Immunother* 44: 10–20.

Elshami A, Saavedra A, Zhang H, *et al.* (1996) Gap junctions play a role in the bystander effect of the herpes simplex virus thymidine kinase/ganciclovir system *in vitro*. *Gene Ther* 3: 85–92.

Evrard A, Cuq P, Ciccolini J, *et al.* (1999) Increased cytotoxicity and bystander effect of 5-fluorouracil and 5′-deoxyuridine-5-fluorouridine in human colorectal cancer cells transfected with thymidine phosphorylase. *Br J Cancer* 80: 1726–1733.

Favrot M, Coll J-L, Louis N, *et al.* (1998) Cell death and cancer: replacement of apoptotic genes and inactivation of death suppressor genes in therapy. *Gene Ther* 5: 728–739.

Fechner H, Haack A, Wang H, *et al.* (1999) Expression of coxsackie adenovirus receptor and alpha$_v$-integrin does not correlate with adenovector targeting in vivo indicating anatomical vector barriers. *Gene Ther* 6: 1520–1535.

Fife K, Bower M, Cooper R, *et al.* (1998) Endothelial cell transfection with cationic liposomes and herpes simplex thymidine kinase mediated killing. *Gene Ther* 5: 614–620.

Folkman J (1990) What is the evidence that tumors are angiogenesis dependent. *J Natl Cancer Inst* 82: 4–6.

Freeman S, Abboud C, Whartenby K, *et al.* (1993) The bystander effect: tumour regression when a fraction of the tumour mass is genetically modified. *Cancer Res* 53: 5274–5283.

Frei III E, Teicher B, Holden S, *et al.* (1988) Preclinical studies and clinical correlation of the effect of alkylating agents. *Cancer Res* 48: 6417–6423.

Friedlos F, Denny W, Palmer B, *et al.* (1997) Mustard prodrugs for activation by *Escherichia coli* nitroreductase in gene-directed enzyme prodrug therapy. *J Med Chem* 40: 1270–1275.

Friedlos F, Court S, Ford M, *et al.* (1998) Gene-directed enzyme prodrug therapy: quantitative bystander toxicity and DNA damage induced by CB1954 in cells expressing bacterial nitroreductase. *Gene Ther* 5: 105–112.

Friedmann T (1989) Progress towards human gene therapy. *Science* 244: 1275–1281.

Fueyo J, Gomez-Manzano C, Alemany R, *et al.* (2000) A mutant oncolytic adenovirus targeting the Rb pathway produces anti-glioma effect *in vivo*. *Oncogene* 19: 2–12.

Gagandeep S, Brew R, Green B, *et al.* (1996) Prodrug-mediated gene therapy: involvement of an immunological component in the bystander effect. *Cancer Gene Ther* 3: 83–88.

Ganly I, Kirn D, Eckhardt S, *et al.* (2000) A phase I study of Onyx-015, an E1B attenuated adenovirus, administered intratumorally to patients with recurrent head and neck cancer. *Clin Cancer Res* 6: 798–809.

Gilligan M, Knox P, Weedon S, *et al.* (1998) Adenoviral delivery of B7–1 (CD80) increases the immunogenicity of human ovarian and cervical carcinoma cells. *Gene Ther* 5: 965–974.

Gimmi C, Morrison B, Mainprice B, *et al.* (1996) Breast cancer associated antigen DF3/MUC1 induces apoptosis of activated human T cells. *Nat Med* 2: 1367–1370.

Goldman C, Rogers B, Douglas J, *et al.* (1997) Targeted gene delivery to Kaposi's sarcoma cells via the fibroblast growth factor receptor. *Cancer Res* 57: 1447–1451.

Goldman C, Kendall R, Cabrera G, *et al.* (1998) Paracrine expression of a native soluble vascular endothelial growth factor receptor inhibits tumor growth, metastasis and mortality rate. *Proc Natl Acad Sci USA* 95: 8795–8800.

Golumbek P, Hamzeh F, Jaffee E, *et al.* (1992) Herpes-simplex 1 virus thymidine kinase is unable to completely eliminate live, nonimmunogenic tumor cell vaccines. *J Immunother* 12: 224–230.

Goodrum F, Ornelles D (1998) p53 status does not determine outcome of E1B 55-kilodalton mutant adenovirus lytic infection. *J Virol* 72: 9479–9490.

Green N, Youngs D, Neoptolomos J, *et al.* (1997) Sensitization of colorectal and pancreatic cancer cell lines to the prodrug 5-(aziridin-1-yl)-2,4-dinitrobenzamide (CB1954) by retroviral transduction and expression of the *E. coli* nitroreductase gene. *Cancer Gene Ther* 4: 229–238.

Habib N (1997) Preliminary results of intratumoural plasmid p53 in patients with localised hepatocellular carcinoma. *Cancer Gene Ther* 4: 67.

Hall F, Gordon E, Wu L, *et al.* (1997) Targeting retroviral vectors to vascular lesions by genetic engineering of the MoMLV gp70 envelope protein. *Hum Gene Ther* 8: 2183–2192.

Heise C, Sampson-Johannes A, Williams A, *et al.* (1997) ONYX-015, an E1B gene attenuated adenovirus, causes tumor-specific cytolysis and antitumoral efficacy that can be augmented by standard chemotherapeutic agents. *Nat Med* 3: 639–644.

Herman J, Adler H, Aguilar-Cordova E, *et al.* (1999) *In situ* gene therapy for adenocarcinoma of the prostate: a phase I clinical trial. *Hum Gene Ther* 10: 1239–1249.

Hirama T, Koeffler H (1995) Role of cyclin-dependent kinase inhibitors in the development of cancer. *Blood* 86: 841–854.

Huang H, Yee J, Shew J, *et al.* (1988) Suppression of the neoplastic phenotype by replacement of the Rb gene in human cancer cells. *Science* 242: 1563–1566.

Huber B, Richards C, Krenitsky T (1991) Retroviral-mediated gene therapy for the treatment of hepatocellular carcinoma: an innovative approach for cancer therapy. *Proc Natl Acad Sci USA* 88: 8039–8043.

Huber B, Austin E, Good S, *et al.* (1993) *In vivo* antitumor activity of 5-fluorocytosine on human colorectal carcinoma cells genetically modified to express cytosine deaminase. *Cancer Res* 53: 4619–4626.

Huber B, Austin E, Richards C, *et al.* (1994) Metabolism of 5-fluorocytosine to 5-fluorouracil in human colorectal tumor-cells transduced with the cytosine deaminase gene – significant antitumor effects when only a small percentage of tumor-cells express cytosine deaminase. *Proc Natl Acad Sci USA* 91: 8302–8306.

Hughes B, Wells A, Bebok Z, *et al.* (1995) Bystander killing of melanoma cells using the human tyrosinase promoter to express the *Escherichia coli* purine nucleoside phosphorylase gene. *Cancer Res* 55: 3339–3345.

Hurford R, Dranoff G, Mulligan R, *et al.* (1995) Gene therapy of metastatic cancer by *in vivo* retroviral gene targeting. *Nat Genet* 10: 430–435.

Indraccolo S, Minuzzo S, Feroli F, *et al.* (1998) Pseudotyping of Moloney leukemia virus-based retroviral vectors with simian immunodeficiency virus envelope leads to targeted infection of human CD4+ lymphoid cells. *Gene Ther* 5: 209–217.

Izquierdo M, Martin V, de Felipe P, *et al.* (1996) Human malignant brain tumor response to herpes simplex thymidine kinase (HSVtk)/ganciclovir gene therapy. *Gene Ther* 3: 491–495.

Khuri F, Nemunatis J, Ganly I, *et al.* (2000) A controlled trial of intratumoral ONYX-015, a selectively-replicating adenovirus, in combination with cisplatin and 5-fluorouracil in patients with recurrent head and neck cancer. *Nat Med* 6: 879–885.

Kianmanesh A, Perrin H, Panis Y, *et al.* (1997) A distant bystander effect of suicide gene therapy: regression of nontransduced tumors together with a distant transduced tumor. *Hum Gene Ther* 8: 1807–1814.

Kikuchi T, Moore M, Crystal R (2000) Dendritic cells modified to express CD40 ligand elicit therapeutic immunity against pre-existing murine tumors. *Blood* 96: 91–99.

Kimura M, Tagawa M, Takenaga K, *et al.* (1997) Inability to induce the alteration of tumorigenicity and chemosensitivity of p53-null pancreatic carcinoma cell after transduction of wild-type p53 gene. *Anticancer Res* 17: 879–883.

Knowles M, Hohneker K, Zhou Z, *et al.* (1995) A controlled study of adenoviral vector mediated gene transfer in the nasal epithelium of patients with cystic fibrosis. *N Engl J Med* 333: 823–831.

Knox R, Boland M, Friedlos F, *et al.* (1988a) The nitroreductase enzyme in Walker cells that activates 5-(aziridin-1-yl)-2,4-dinitrobenzamide (CB 1954) to 5-(aziridin-1-yl)-4-hydroxylamino-2-nitrobenzamide is a form of NAD(P)H dehydrogenase (quinone) (EC 1.6.99.2). *Biochem Pharmacol* 37: 4671–4677.

Knox R, Friedlos F, Jarman M, *et al.* (1988b) A new cytotoxic, DNA interstrand crosslinking agent, 5-(aziridin-1-yl)-4-hydroxylamino-2-nitrobenzamide, is formed from 5-(aziridin-1-yl)-2,4-dinitrobenzamide (CB1954) by a nitroreductase enzyme in Walker carcinoma cells. *Biochem Pharmacol* 37: 4661–4669.

Knox R, Friedlos F, Sherwood R, *et al.* (1992) The bioactivation of 5-(aziridin-1-yl)-2,4-dinitrobenzamide (CB 1954) – II: a comparison of an *E. coli* nitroreductase and Walker DT diaphorase. *Biochem Pharmacol* 44: 2297–2301.

Kojima A, Hackett N, Ohwada A, *et al.* (1998) In vivo human carboxylesterase cDNA gene transfer to activate the prodrug CPT-11 for local treatment of solid tumors. *J Clin Invest* 101: 1789–1796.

Kokoris M, Sabo P, Adman E, *et al.* (1999) Enhancement of tumor ablation by a selected HSV-1 thymidine kinase mutant. *Gene Ther* 6: 1415–1426.

Kucharczuk J, Randazzo B, Chang M, *et al.* (1997) Use of a 'replication-restricted' herpes virus to treat experimental malignant mesothelioma. *Cancer Res* 57: 466–471.

Lan K, Kanai F, Shiratori Y, *et al.* (1997) *In vivo* selective gene expression and therapy mediated by adenoviral vectors for human carcino-embryonic antigen-producing gastric carcinoma. *Cancer Res* 57: 4729–4284.

Lane D (1995) p53 and human cancers. *Br Med Bull* 51: 31–44.

Lau K, Bicknell R (1999) Antiangiogenic gene therapy. *Gene Ther* 6: 1793–1795.

Leiden J (1995) Gene therapy – promises, pitfalls and prognosis. *N Engl J Med* 333: 871.

Leverett B, Farrell K, Eiden M, *et al.* (1998) Entry of the amphotropic murine leukaemia virus is influenced by residues in the putative second extracellular domain of its receptor, Pit2. *J Virol* 72: 4956–4961.

Lin P, Buxton J, Acheson A, *et al.* (1998) Antiangiogenic gene therapy targeting the endothelium-specific receptor tyrosine kinase Tie2. *Proc Natl Acad Sci USA* 95: 8829–8834.

Lodge P, Jones L, Bader R, *et al.* (2000) Dendritic cell-based immunotherapy of prostate cancer: immune monitoring of a phase II trial. *Cancer Res* 60: 829–833.

Loubiere L, Tiraby M, Cazaux C, *et al.* (1999) The equine herpes virus 4 thymidine kinase leads to a superior ganciclovir cell killing than the human herpes virus 1 thymidine kinase. *Gene Ther* 6: 1638–1642.

MacDonald F, Bird R, Stokes H, *et al.* (1988) Expression of CEA, CA125, CA19-9 and human milk fat globule membrane antigen in ovarian tumours. *J Clin Pathol* 41: 260–264.

Marais R, Spooner R, Light Y, *et al.* (1996) Gene-directed enzyme prodrug therapy with a mustard prodrug/carboxypeptidase G2 combination. *Cancer Res* 56: 4735–4742.

Markert J, Medlock M, Rabkin S, *et al.* (2000) Conditionally replicating herpes simplex virus mutant, G207, for the treatment of malignant glioma: results of a phase I trial. *Gene Ther* 7: 867–874.

Markman M (1991) Intraperitoneal chemotherapy. *Semin Oncol* 18: 248–254.

Matsuda K, Madoiwa S, Hasumi Y, *et al.* (2000) A novel strategy for tumor angiogenesis-targeted gene therapy: Generation of angiostatin from endogenous plasminogen by protease gene transfer. *Cancer Gene Ther* 7: 589–596.

McCormick F (2000) Design and development of oncolytic viruses. *41st Meeting American Association of Cancer Research, San Francisco.*

McNeish I, Green N, Gilligan M, *et al.* (1998) Virus directed enzyme prodrug therapy for ovarian and pancreatic cancer using retrovirally delivered *E. coli* nitroreductase and CB1954. *Gene Ther* 5: 1061–1069.

McNeish I, Tenev T, Bell S, *et al.* (2001) Herpes simplex virus thymidine kinase/ganciclovir-induced cell death is enhanced by co-expression of caspase-3 in human ovarian carcinoma cells. *Cancer Gene Ther* 8: 308–319.

Melcher A, Todryk S, Hardwick S, *et al.* (1998) Tumor immunogenicity is determined by the mechanism of cell death via induction of heat shock protein expression. *Nat Med* 4: 581–587.

Melton D, Konecki D, Brennand J, *et al.* (1984) Structure, expression and mutation of the hypoxanthine phosphoribosyl transferase gene. *Proc Natl Acad Sci USA* 81: 2147–2151.

Mesnil M, Piccoli C, Tiraby G, *et al.* (1996) Bystander killing of cancer cells by herpes simplex virus thymidine kinase gene is mediated by connexins. *Proc Natl Acad Sci USA* 93: 1831–1835.

Michael N, Brehm J, Anlezark G, *et al.* (1994) Physical characterisation of the *Escherichia coli* B gene encoding nitroreductase and its overexpression in *Escherichia coli* K12. *FEMS Microbiol Lett* 124: 195–202.

Mirjolet J-F, Barberi-Heyob M, Merlin J-L, *et al.* (1998) Thymidylate synthase expression and activity: relation to S-phase parameters and 5-fluorouracil sensitivity. *Br J Cancer* 78: 62–68.

Moolten F (1986) Tumor chemosensitivity conferred by inserted herpes thymidine kinase genes: paradigm for a prospective cancer control strategy. *Cancer Res* 46: 5276–5281.

Mullen C, Kilstrup M, Blaese R (1992) Transfer of the bacterial gene for cytosine deaminase to mammalian cells confers lethal sensitivity to 5-fluorocytosine: a negative selection system. *Proc Natl Acad Sci USA* 89: 33–37.

Mullen C, Coale M, Lowe R, *et al.* (1994) Tumors expressing the cytosine deaminase suicide gene can be eliminated in vivo with 5-fluorocytosine and induce protective immunity to wild-type tumor. *Cancer Res* 54: 1503–1506.

Mullen C, Petropoulos D, Lowe R (1996) Treatment of microscopic pulmonary metastases with recombinant autologous tumor vaccine expressing interleukin-6 and *Escherichia coli* cytosine deaminase suicide genes. *Cancer Res* 56: 1361–1366.

Nestle F, Alijagic S, Gilliet M, *et al.* (1998) Vaccination of melanoma patients with peptide- or tumor lysate-pulsed dendritic cells. *Nat Med* 4: 328–332.

Nicholson D (1999) Caspase structure, proteolytic substrates, and function during apoptotic cell death. *Cell Death Differ* 6: 1028–1042.

Niculescu-Duvaz I, Springer C (1997) Antibody-directed enzyme prodrug therapy (ADEPT): a review. *Adv Drug Del Rev* 26: 151–172.

Norman K, Lee P (2000) Reovirus as a novel oncolytic agent. *J Clin Invest* 105: 1035–1038.

O'Malley B, Chen S, Schwartz M, *et al.* (1995) Adenovirus-mediated gene therapy for head and neck squamous cell cancer in a nude mouse model. *Cancer Res* 55: 1080–1085.

Orkin S, Daddona P, Shewach D, *et al.* (1983) Molecular cloning of human adenosine deaminase gene sequences. *J Biol Chem* 258: 12753–12756.

Palmer K, Moore J, Everard M, *et al.* (1999) Gene therapy with autologous, interleukin 2-secreting tumor cells in patients with malignant melanoma. *Hum Gene Ther* 10: 1261–1268.

Pandha H, Martin L-A, Rigg A, *et al.* (1999) Genetic prodrug activation therapy for breast cancer: a phase I clinical trial of *erb*B-2-directed suicide gene expression. *J Clin Oncol* 17: 2180–2189.

Pardoll D (1998) Cancer vaccines. *Nat Med* 4: 525–531.

Peoples G, Goedegebuure P, Smith R, *et al.* (1995) Breast and ovarian cancer-specific cytotoxic T lymphocytes recognise the same HER2/neu-derived peptide. *Proc Natl Acad Sci USA* 92: 432–436.

Rainov N, Dobberstein K, Sena-Esteves M, *et al.* (1998) New prodrug activation gene therapy for cancer using cytochrome P450 4B1 and 2-aminoanthracene/4-ipomeanol. *Hum Gene Ther* 9: 1261–1273.

Ram Z, Culver K, Walbridge S, *et al.* (1993) *In situ* retroviral-mediated gene transfer for the treatment of brain tumors in rats. *Cancer Res* 53: 83–88.

Ram Z, Culver K, Oshiro E, *et al.* (1997) Therapy of malignant brain tumours by intratumoral implantation of retroviral vector-producer cells. *Nat Med* 4: 1354–1361.

Rampling R, Cruickshank G, Papanastassiou V, *et al.* (2000) Toxicity evaluation of replication-competent herpes simplex virus (ICP 34.5 null mutant 1716) in patients with recurrent malignant glioma. *Gene Ther* 7: 859–866.

Randazzo B, Kesari S, Gesser R, *et al.* (1995) Treatment of experimental intracranial murine melanoma with a neuroattenuated herpes simplex virus 1 mutant. *Virology* 211: 94–101.

Restifo N, Esquivel F, Asher A, *et al.* (1991) Defective presentation of endogenous antigens by a murine sarcoma – implications for the failure of an antitumor immune response. *J Immunol* 147: 1453–1459.

Reynolds P, Dmitriev I, Curiel D (1999) Insertion of an RGD motif into the HI loop of the adenovirus fiber protein alters the distribution of transgene expression of the systemically administered vector. *Gene Ther* 6: 1336–1339.

Ricciono T, Cirielli C, Wang X, *et al.* (1998) Adenovirus-mediated wild-type p53 overexpression inhibits endothelial cell differentiation *in vitro* and angiogenesis *in vivo*. *Gene Ther* 5: 747–754.

Richards C, Austin E, Huber B (1995) Transcriptional regulatory sequences of carcinoembryonic antigen: identification and use with cytosine deaminase for tumour-specific gene therapy. *Hum Gene Ther* 6: 881–893.

Ring C, Blouin P, Martin L-A, *et al.* (1997) Use of transcriptional regulatory elements of the *MUC1* and *ERBB2* genes to drive tumour-selective expression of a prodrug activating enzyme. *Gene Ther* 4: 1045–1052.

Riordan J, Rommens J, Kerem B, *et al.* (1989) Identification of the cystic fibrosis gene: cloning and characterization of the complementary DNA. *Science* 245: 1066–1073.

Roberts J, Friedlos F, Knox R (1986) CB1954 (2,4-dinitro-5-azirinyl benzamide) becomes a DNA interstrand crosslinking agent in Walker tumour cells. *Biochem Biophys Res Commun* 140: 1073–1078.

Rommens J, Iannuzzi M, Kerem B, *et al.* (1989) Identification of the cystic fibrosis gene – chromosome walking and jumping. *Science* 245: 1059–1065.

Rosenberg S, Packard B, Aebersold P, *et al.* (1988) Use of tumour infiltrating lymphocytes and interleukin-2 in the immunotherapy of patients with malignant melanoma. *N Engl J Med* 319: 1676–1680.

Rosenberg S, Yang J, Schwartzentruber D, *et al.* (1998) Immunologic and therapeutic evaluation of a synthetic peptide vaccine for the treatment of patients with metastatic melanoma. *Nat Med* 4: 321–327.

Roth J, Cristiano R (1997) Gene therapy for cancer: what have we done and where are we going? *J Natl Cancer Inst* 89: 21–39.

Roth J, Nguyen D, Lawrence D, *et al.* (1996) Retrovirus mediated wild type *p53* gene transfer to tumors of patients with lung cancer. *Nat Med* 2: 985–991.

Rubin J, Galanis E, Pitot H, *et al.* (1997) Phase I study of immunotherapy of hepatic metastases of colorectal carcinoma by direct gene transfer of an allogeneic histocompatibility antigen, HLA-B7. *Gene Ther* 4: 419–425.

Russell S (1996) Peptide-displaying phages for targeted gene delivery. *Nat Med* 2: 276–277.

Sacco M, Mangiarini L, Villa A, *et al.* (1995) Local regression of breast tumors following intramammary ganciclovir administration in double transgenic mice bearing *neu* oncogene and herpes simplex virus thymidine kinase. *Gene Ther* 2: 493–497.

Saleh M, Stacker S, Wilks A (1996) Inhibition of growth of C6 glioma cells *in vivo* by expression of antisense vascular endothelial growth factor sequence. *Cancer Res* 56: 393–401.

Salvadori S, Gansbascher B, Wenick I, *et al.* (1995) B7–1 amplifies the response to interleukin-2-secreting tumor vaccines *in vivo*, but fails to induce a response by naive cells *in vitro*. *Hum Gene Ther* 6: 1299–1306.

Samejima Y, Merulo D (1995) 'Bystander killing' induces apoptosis and is inhibited by forskolin. *Gene Ther* 2: 50–58.

Sauter B, Martinet O, Zhang W-J, *et al.* (2000) Adenovirus-mediated gene transfer of endostatin *in vivo* results in high level of transgene expression and inhibition of tumor growth and metastases. *Proc Natl Acad Sci USA* 97: 4802–4807.

Schmidt W, Schweighoffer T, Herbst E, *et al.* (1995) Cancer vaccines – the interleukin-2 dosage effect. *Proc Natl Acad Sci USA* 92: 4711–4714.

Schnierle B, Groner B (1996) Retroviral targeted delivery. *Gene Ther* 3: 1069–1073.

Schreiber M, Muller W, Singh G, *et al.* (1999) Comparison of the effectiveness of adenovirus vectors expressing cyclin kinase inhibitors p16^{INK4A}, p18^{INK4C}, p19^{INK4D}, p21$^{WAF1/CIP1}$ and p27^{KIP1} in inducing cell cycle arrest, apoptosis and inhibition of tumorigenicity. *Oncogene* 19: 1663–1676.

Schrewe H, Thompson J, Bona M, *et al.* (1990) Cloning of the complete gene for carcinoembryonic antigen: analysis of its promoter indicates a region conveying cell type-specific expression. *Mol Cell Biol* 10: 2738–2748.

Schuler G, Steinman R (1997) Dendritic cells as adjuvants for immune-mediated resistance to tumors. *J Exp Med* 8: 1183–1187.

Shand N, Weber F, Mariani L, *et al.* (1999) A phase 1–2 clinical trial of gene therapy for recurrent glioblastoma multiforme by tumor transduction with the herpes simplex thymidine kinase gene followed by ganciclovir. *Hum Gene Ther* 10: 2325–2335.

Sharma S, Wang J, Huang M, *et al.* (1996) Interleukin-7 gene transfer in non-small cell lung cancer decreases tumor proliferation, modifies cell surface molecule expression and enhances antitumor reactivity. *Cancer Gene Ther* 3: 302–313.

Sharma S, Miller P, Stolina M, *et al.* (1997) Multicomponent gene therapy vaccines for lung cancer: effective eradication of established murine tumors *in vivo* with interleukin-7/herpes simplex thymidine kinase-transduced autologous tumor and *ex vivo* activated dendritic cells. *Gene Ther* 4: 1361–1370.

Sheikh M, Rochefort H, Garcia M (1995) Overexpression of p21/waf1/cip1 induces growth arrest, giant cell formation and apoptosis in human breast carcinoma cell lines. *Oncogene* 11: 1899–1905.

Shinoura N, Murumatsa Y, Yoshida Y, *et al.* (2000) Adenovirus-mediated transfer of caspase-3 with Fas ligand induces drastic apoptosis in U-373MG glioma cells. *Exp Cell Res* 256: 423–433.

Shirakawa T, Gardner T, Kao C, *et al.* (1998) Ablative gene therapy treatment of human renal cell carcinoma: cytosine deaminase plus 5-fluorocytosine has superior bystander effect over thymidine kinase plus acyclovir. *J Urol* 159(5 SS): 558.

Simons J, Jaffee E, Weber C, *et al.* (1997) Bioactivity of autologous irradiated renal cell carcinoma vaccines generated by *ex vivo* granulocyte-macrophage colony-stimulating factor gene transfer. *Cancer Res* 57: 1537–1546.

Smith J, Keller J, Lohrey N, *et al.* (1999) Redirected infection of directly biotinylated recombinant adenovirus vectors through cell surface receptors and antigens. *Proc Natl Acad Sci USA* 96: 8855–8860.

Song W, Kong H, Carpenter H, *et al.* (1997) Dendritic cells genetically modified with an adenovirus vector encoding the cDNA for a model antigen induce protective and therapeutic antitumor immunity. *J Exp Med* 8: 1247–1256.

Sorscher E, Peng S, Bebok Z, *et al.* (1994) Tumor cell bystander killing in colonic carcinoma utilizing the *Escherichia coli* DeoD gene to generate toxic purines. *Gene Ther* 1: 233–238.

Specht J, Wang G, Do M, *et al.* (1997) Dendritic cells retrovirally transduced with a model antigen gene are therapeutically effective against established pulmonary metastases. *J Exp Med* 186: 1213–1221.

Srinivasula S, Ahmad M, MacFarlane M, *et al.* (1998) Generation of constitutively active recombinant caspases-3 and -6 by rearrangement of their subunits. *J Biol Chem* 273: 10107–10111.

Staba M-J, Wickham T, Kovesdi I, *et al.* (2000) Modifications of the fiber in adenovirus vectors increase tropism for malignant glioma models. *Cancer Gene Ther* 7: 13–19.

Stallwood Y, Fisher K, Gallimore P, *et al.* (2000) Neutralisation of adenovirus infectivity by ascitic fluid from ovarian cancer patients. *Gene Ther* 7: 637–643.

Sterman D, Treat J, Litsky L, *et al.* (1998) Adenovirus-mediated herpes simplex virus thymidine kinase/ganciclovir gene therapy in patients with localised malignancy: results of a phase I clinical trial in malignant mesothelioma. *Hum Gene Ther* 9: 1083–1092.

Sulitzeanu D (1993) Immunosuppressive factors in human cancers. *Adv Cancer Res* 60: 247–267.

Szary J, Missol E, Szala S (1997) Characteristics of cytosine deaminase-5-fluoro-cytosine system: enhancement of radiation cytotoxicity and bystander effect. *Cancer Gene Ther* 4: 307–308.

Tahara H, Lotze M (1995) Antitumor effects of interleukin-12 (IL-12): applications for the immunotherapy and gene therapy of cancer. *Gene Ther* 2: 96–106.

Tenev T, Marani M, McNeish I, *et al.* (2000) Caspase-3 overexpression sensitises ovarian cancer cells to proteasome inhibitors. *Cell Death Diff* 8: 256–264.

Thatcher N, Edwards R, Lemoine N, *et al.* (1999) The potential of acetaminophen as a prodrug in gene directed enzyme prodrug therapy. *Cancer Gene Ther* 7: 521–525.

Timmerman J, Levy R (1998) Melanoma vaccine: prim and proper presentation. *Nat Med* 4: 269–270.

Toloza E, Hunt K, Swisher S, *et al.* (1996) *In vivo* cancer gene therapy with a recombinant interleukin-2 adenovirus vector. *Cancer Gene Ther* 3: 11–17.

Topf N, Worgall S, Hackett N, *et al.* (1998) Regional 'pro-drug' gene therapy: intravenous administration of an adenoviral vector expressing the *E. coli* cytosine deaminase gene and systemic administration of 5-fluorocytosine suppresses growth of hepatic metastases of colon carcinoma. *Gene Ther* 5: 507–513.

Townsend S, Allison J (1993) Tumour rejection after direct co-stimulation of CD8+ T cells by B7 transfected melanoma cells. *Science* 259: 368–370.

Trinh Q, Austin E, Murray D, *et al.* (1995) Enzyme/prodrug gene therapy: comparison of cytosine deaminase/5-fluorocytosine *versus* thymidine kinase/ganciclovir enzyme prodrug systems in a human colorectal carcinoma line. *Cancer Res* 55: 4808–4812.

Tsao Y, Huang S, Chang J, *et al.* (1999) Adenovirus-mediated p21[WAF1/SDII/CIP1] gene transfer induces apoptosis of human cervical cancer cell lines. *J Virol* 73: 4983–4990.

Tubiana M, Malaise E (1976) Growth rate and cells kinetics in human tumours: some prognostic and therapeutic implications. In: Symington T, Carter R, eds. *Scientific Foundations of Oncology*. London: Heinemann, 126–136.

Turnell A, Grand R, Gallimore P (1999) The replicative capacities of large E1B-null group A and C adenoviruses are independent of the host cell p53 status. *J Virol* 73: 2074–2083.

Tuting T, Gambotto A, Baar J, *et al.* (1997) Interferon-alpha gene therapy for cancer: retroviral transduction of fibroblasts and particle-mediated transfection of tumor cells are both effective strategies for gene delivery in murine tumour cells. *Gene Ther* 4: 1053–1060.

Uckert W, Kammertons T, Haack K, *et al.* (1998) Double suicide gene (cytosine deaminase and herpes simplex virus thymidine kinase) but not single gene transfer allows reliable elimination of tumor cells *in vivo*. *Hum Gene Ther* 9: 855–865.

van der Eb M, Cramer S, Verouwe Y, *et al.* (1998) Severe hepatic dysfunction after adenovirus-mediated transfer of the herpes simplex virus thymidine kinase gene and ganciclovir administration. *Gene Ther* 5: 451–458.

Vassaux G, Hurst H, Lemoine N (1999) Insulation of a conditionally expressed transgene in an adenoviral vector. *Gene Ther* 6: 1192–1197.

Verhagen A, Ekert P, Pakusch M, *et al.* (2000) Identification of DIABLO, a mammalian protein that promotes apoptosis by binding to and antagonising IAP proteins. *Cell* 102: 43–53.

Verma I (1994) Gene therapy: hopes, hypes and hurdles. *Mol Med* 1: 3.

Vigne E, Mahfouz I, Dedieu J-F, *et al.* (1999) RGD inclusion in the hexon monomer provides adenovirus type 5-based vectors with a fiber knob-independent pathway for infection. *J Virol* 73: 5156–5161.

Vile R, Hart I (1993a) *In vitro* and *in vivo* targeting of gene expression of melanoma cell. *Cancer Res* 53: 962–967.

Vile R, Hart I (1993b) Use of tissue-specific expression of the herpes simplex virus thymidine kinase gene to inhibit growth of established murine melanomas following direct intratumoural injection of DNA. *Cancer Res* 53: 3860–3864.

Vile R, Nelson J, Castleden S, *et al.* (1994) Systemic gene therapy of murine melanoma using tissue specific expression of the *HSVtk* gene involves an immune component. *Cancer Res* 54: 6228–6234.

Vile R, Castleden S, Marshall J, *et al.* (1997) Generation of an anti-tumour immune response in a non-immunogenic tumour: HSVtk killing *in vivo* stimulates a mononuclear cell infiltrate and a Th1-like profile of intratumoural cytokine expression. *Int J Cancer* 71: 267–274.

Wadman M (1995) Hyping results 'could damage' gene therapy. *Nature* 378: 655.

Wagner R (1995) The state of antisense research. *Nat Med* 1: 1116–1118.

Wang Q, Stanley J, Kudoh S, *et al.* (1995) T cells infiltrating non-Hodgkin's B cell lymphomas show altered tyrosine phosphorylation pattern even though T cell receptor/CD3-associated kinases are present. *J Immunol* 155: 1382–1392.

Watkins S, Mesyanzhinov V, Lurochkina L, *et al.* (1997) The 'adenobody' approach to viral targeting; specific and enhanced adenoviral gene delivery. *Gene Ther* 4: 1004–1012.

Weatherall D (1988) The slow road to gene therapy. *Nature* 331: 13–15.

Weedon S, Green N, McNeish I, *et al.* (2000) Sensitisation of human carcinoma cells to the prodrug CB1954 by adenovirus vector-mediated expression of *E. coli* nitroreductase. *Int J Cancer* 86: 848–854.

Weinberg R (1995) The retinoblastoma protein and cell cycle control. *Cell* 81: 323–330.

Wortzel R, Philipps C, Schreiber H (1983) Multiple tumor-specific antigens expressed by a single tumor cell. *Nature* 304: 165–167.

Wygoda M, Wilson M, Davis M, *et al.* (1997) Protection of herpes simplex virus thymidine kinase transduced cells from ganciclovir mediated cytotoxicity by bystander cells: the 'Good Samaritan' effect. *Cancer Res* 57: 1699–1703.

Xu H-J, Zhou Y, Seigne J, *et al.* (1996) Enhanced tumor suppressor gene therapy via replication deficient adenovirus vectors expressing an N-terminal truncated retinoblastoma protein. *Cancer Res* 56: 2245–2249.

Yamabe K, Shimizu S, Ito T, *et al.* (1999) Cancer gene therapy using a pro-apoptotic gene, caspase-3. *Gene Ther* 6: 1952–1959.

Yang Z-Y, Perkins N, Ohno T, *et al.* (1995) The p21 cyclin-dependent kinase inhibitor suppresses tumorigenicity *in vivo*. *Nat Med* 1: 1052–1056.

Yin C, Knudson C, Korsmeyer S, *et al.* (1997) Bax suppresses tumorigenesis and stimulates apoptosis *in vivo*. *Nature* 385: 637–640.

6

Gene therapy for the treatment of cardiovascular diseases

Dharmesh J Vara, Mehregan Movassagh and Gavin Brooks

Cardiovascular diseases such as heart failure, angina, hypertension and coronary heart disease are responsible for 12 million deaths world-wide each year (American Heart Association, 2000). Indeed, over 50% of deaths in developed and developing countries result from cardiovascular disease, despite the fact that there has been a general decline in cardiovascular mortality due to improvements in the treatment of patients (American Heart Association, 2000).

One of the problems with cardiovascular diseases in general is that patients often remain asymptomatic in early disease and are unaware of the need to make changes to their lifestyles, such as to stop smoking, increase levels of exercise and eat a healthy diet, which could help to halt the progression of their disease. Unfortunately, it is only after the clinical manifestation of these diseases that treatment is initiated, by which time it has become established and invariably has caused a substantial degree of irreversible damage to the heart and the circulatory system. The majority of therapies currently available for the treatment of cardiovascular diseases do not cure the problem but merely treat the symptoms. Furthermore, many cardioactive drugs have serious side effects and have narrow therapeutic windows that can limit their usefulness in the clinic. Thus, the development of more selective and highly effective therapeutic strategies that would cure specific cardiovascular diseases would be of enormous benefit both to the patient and to those countries where healthcare systems are responsible for the care of an increasing number of patients.

In this chapter, we will overview specific diseases that affect the cardiovascular system and show how gene therapy has already had an impact on the treatment and prognosis of patients affected by such disorders.

Gene therapy for the failing heart

Heart failure

Heart failure is defined as the inability of the heart to maintain an adequate cardiac output to meet bodily requirements. It is a chronic and debilitating condition that often develops in those patients who have survived a significant heart attack. Approximately 0.4–2% of the populations of the United Kingdom, Scandinavia and the United States suffer from this condition (Dargie and McMurray, 1994). Data obtained from the Framingham Study has shown that congestive heart failure occurs in 1% of the population studied, aged between 50 and 59 years; a percentage that doubled with each subsequent decade (Nolan *et al.*, 1996). Recent annual mortality rates for severe heart failure have been estimated to be 30–40% (Lonn and McKelvie, 2000). In 1994, it was estimated that a staggering £360 million was to be spent by the National Health Service (NHS) in the UK each year in diagnosing and treating heart failure and that at least 5% of hospital admissions were for this condition (Dargie and McMurray, 1994). Heart failure itself is a collective term used to describe a number of different diseases as classified below.

Classification of heart failure

Heart failure can be classified in three ways:

1 *Acute versus chronic heart failure.* Acute heart failure is sudden in onset and is commonly caused by severe damage to the myocardium, e.g. following heart attack or cardiogenic shock. In contrast, chronic heart failure usually precipitates after years of continuous damage to the heart as a result of various diseases, e.g. coronary heart disease (Walker and Tan, 1997).
2 *Left- and right-sided heart failure.* Left-sided heart failure refers to symptoms that mainly show pulmonary congestion, whereas right-sided heart failure presents with congestion of blood in the systemic circulation (Walker and Tan, 1997).
3 *Systolic (forwards) versus diastolic (backwards) failure.* Systolic failure is characterised by a decrease in the contractility of the left ventricle that results in the inability of the heart to pump blood efficiently (Walker and Tan, 1997). Diastolic failure is characterised by an inability of the ventricle to relax when it is filling with blood; thus the left ventricle receives an inadequate volume of blood to supply the systemic circulation.

Causes of heart failure

There are numerous causes of heart failure known including:

- *Coronary heart disease (CHD)*. This remains the primary cause of heart failure (Lip *et al.*, 2000).
- *Hypertension*. Hypertension (defined as a systolic blood pressure (BP) of >160 mmHg and a diastolic BP of >90 mmHg) is a symptom of numerous chronic cardiovascular diseases leading to the formation of heart failure (Grundy *et al.*, 1998). Various studies have shown that heart failure is strongly correlated with hypertension. In the Framingham Heart Study, for example, 75% of the population of Framingham that had hypertension developed heart failure (Walker and Tan, 1997). Hypertension causes a pressure overload on the heart (usually the left ventricle), since the heart has to work harder to pump sufficient blood into the circulation. CHD and hypertension have been implicated in over 90% of cases of heart failure (Lip *et al.*, 2000).
- *Valve dysfunction*. Defective mitral and aortic valves cause a volume overload on the heart, causing blood to leak back into the left ventricle (Lin *et al.*, 1990; Grace *et al.*, 1993). This leads to a requirement for the heart to work harder to pump the necessary volume of blood around the body.
- *Myocardial infarction*. Heart function is seriously compromised following the death of myocardial tissue, e.g. as a result of myocardial infarction. Since mature cardiac myocytes are unable to divide, areas of necrotic and dead myocardial tissue are replaced by fibrous tissue that severely reduces the contractile function of the ventricle. This rapidly leads to a decrease in blood flowing to the systemic circulation.
- *Cardiomyopathy*. Myocardial function also can be compromised by a number of diseases that directly affect the contractility of the heart muscle. Such diseases are referred to as cardiomyopathies and are separated into three main categories (Grace *et al.*, 1993; Nolan *et al.*, 1996; Lip *et al.*, 2000): dilated cardiomyopathies, which are induced by certain chemicals (e.g. cobalt and drugs such as adriamycin); hypertrophic cardiomyopathies, which are induced by diseases such as hypertension and aortic valve disease; and restrictive cardiomyopathies, in which infiltration of the ventricular wall with substances such as amyloid and sarcoia cause the muscle to become rigid.

All of these conditions eventually lead to decreases in both systolic and diastolic functions of the heart. Ultimately, stroke volume (i.e. the volume of blood that the heart pumps per contraction) is reduced, leading to hypoperfusion of the bodily organs with blood. Arterial baroreceptors (pressure receptors) are able to detect such decreases in blood pressure to these organs and activate a number of compensatory mechanisms to restore normal organ blood perfusion, such as an increase in the force and rate of contraction and constriction of peripheral blood vessels (Nolan *et al.*, 1996). Two important compensatory mechanisms that aid organ perfusion and cardiac function following stress and heart failure are cardiac hypertrophy and the renin angiotensin system (RAS). These two mechanisms are described in detail below.

Cardiac hypertrophy

Development of the heart is markedly different to that of other organs within the body. Thus, whereas most cells of the body grow by classical cell division (hyperplasia), where one cell divides to form two identical daughter cells, this is not the case for mature mammalian cardiac myocytes that cannot divide but grow by the process of hypertrophy (an increase in cell size) (Li and Brooks, 1999). Although fetal and early neonatal mammalian cardiac myocytes can divide, a switch from hyperplastic growth to hypertrophic growth occurs shortly after birth (Brooks *et al.*, 1997). All subsequent growth of myocardial cells occurs by hypertrophy or cell enlargement. Although myocyte hypertrophy is a normal physiological response during development, it also occurs in response to stress or disease in the heart (e.g. hypertension and myocardial infarction). Such hypertrophic growth initially is beneficial for the patient and is commonly referred to as 'compensated hypertrophy'. However, growth is often uncontrolled because patients are unaware of their disease and, therefore, do not initiate therapy to control the condition at an early stage of disease progression. Thus, compensated hypertrophic growth can progress into 'decompensated hypertrophic' growth if the stress is prolonged or severe, where the resulting large size of the heart severely compromises cardiac function (Figure 6.1). In such cases, myocardial tissue cannot relax during diastole and this results in increased filling pressures. Consequently, stroke volume is severely reduced because ventricular space is taken up by growth of myocardial tissue in a concentric manner. Also, the lack of adequate myocardial perfusion to new areas of tissue leads to a less efficient working heart.

Decompensated hypertrophy remains a serious clinical problem in heart failure. Therapeutically, angiotensin-converting enzyme (ACE) inhibitors have been shown to halt, and even reverse, decompensated

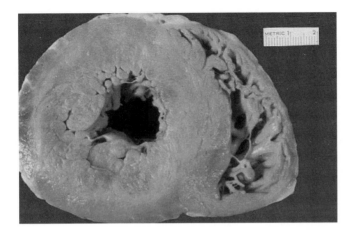

Figure 6.1   Cross-section through a hypertrophic human heart. Picture reproduced with the kind permission of Professor E C Klatt, Salt Lake City, USA.

hypertrophic growth, although no direct therapy currently exists that tackles this problem. However, recent research to investigate those mechanisms involved in hypertrophic growth are revealing specific molecules that could be targeted with gene therapy.

The renin-angiotensin system (RAS)

One of the major stimuli causing activation of the RAS system is a decrease in renal perfusion pressure. This causes renin to be released by the kidneys, which then converts angiotensinogen released by the liver to angiotensin I (AI) (Figure 6.2). AI is converted to angiotensin II (AII) by the action of ACE released from the lungs. ACE is responsible physiologically for causing cardiac hypertrophy, constriction of peripheral blood vessels and sodium and water retention, all of which increase tissue blood perfusion. Unfortunately, these responses also increase the workload on the failing heart and speed up failure of the myocardium. Numerous trials, such as the Study of Left Ventricular Dysfunction (SOLVD), Survival And Ventricular Enlargement (SAVE), Acute Infarction Ramipril Efficiency (AIRE) and Trandolapril Cardiac Evaluation (TRACE) trials, have shown that treatment with ACE inhibitors generally reduces the incidence of cardiac death and the need for hospitalisation of patients with heart failure (Pepine, 1997). In the SAVE trial, treatment with the ACE inhibitor captopril reduced mortality rates by 19%, cardiac death by 21%, development of severe heart failure by 37%

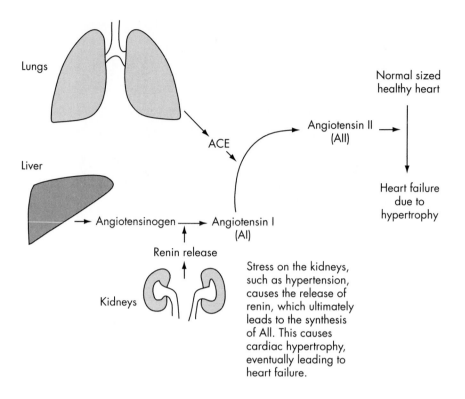

Figure 6.2 Diagram showing the cascade of physiological events leading to angiotensin II (AII) release and subsequent deleterious effects on the heart.

and hospitalisation by 22%. Clearly, the RAS system is an important target for the treatment of heart failure.

Current drug treatments for heart failure

The general aims for treating heart failure patients are to provide relief from symptoms, to reduce progression of the disease and to improve quality of life. A variety of pharmacological treatments are employed currently to achieve these goals.

Diuretics These compounds, which include bendrofluazide, frusemide and metolazone, act principally by promoting renal excretion of sodium and water, the consequence of which is a reduction in blood volume (Lonn and McKelvie, 2000). This in turn decreases the work performed by the heart as both pre-load and after-load are reduced (British National

Formulary, 2000). Diuretics are of particular value in treating patients with fluid retention, pulmonary congestion, raised jugular venous pressure, oedema and ascites. Unfortunately, they do cause a number of side effects including hypokalaemia, hypomagnesaemia and stimulation of the RAS due to naturesis, all of which can limit their use in therapy.

β-Blockers   A recent study, pooling results from three trials, showed that β-blocker therapy improves the New York Heart Association functional class of heart failure and also improves left ventricular ejection after three months of therapy. These agents (e.g. atenolol and carvedilol) act by blocking the β_1-adrenergic receptors on the heart, which causes a decrease in the rate and force of contraction of the myocardium. Trials such as the CIBIS-1 trial found that hospital admissions decreased by 34% in patients taking the drug bisoprolol (Lonn and McKelvie, 2000). Other trials have shown similar results for other β-blockers. As is the case with other pharmacological agents, β-blockers induce several side effects including hypotension, increased risk of heart failure and brady-arrythmias. However, these unwanted effects can be avoided by careful monitoring of patients (British National Formulary, 2000).

Cardiac glycosides   Digoxin is the most commonly used agent in this class of drugs. Its mode of action ultimately is to increase intracellular levels of calcium by blocking the Na^+K^+ ATPase pump in the heart, leading to a positive inotropic effect. Generally, digoxin is administered to patients with established atrial fibrillation. Studies have found no real beneficial effects on mortality rates of patients with heart failure, although hospital admission rates have been shown to decrease by 6% (Lonn and McKelvie, 2000). Despite this, digoxin does have a place in therapy for heart failure although it should be used with caution. Digoxin has a small therapeutic window and side effects such as cardiac arrythmias, anorexia, nausea and vomiting and neurological complaints can become problematic if patients are not carefully monitored (Nolan *et al.*, 1996).

ACE inhibitors   These drugs, which include captopril and enalapril, act on the RAS to prevent the conversion of angiotensin I (AI) to angiotensin II (AII). AII is known to be responsible for causing changes such as cardiac hypertrophy and vasoconstriction, all of which lead to heart failure. Numerous trials have proven the effectiveness of these compounds, for example the SOLVD trial showed that treatment with enalapril reduced total mortality rates by 35% (Lonn and McKelvie, 2000). Despite their usefulness, ACE inhibitors elicit a number of side effects including angio-oedema, cough, hyperkalaemia and syncope. This often limits their clinical use.

Although conventional treatments for heart failure are beneficial, they do not cure patients and most exhibit side effects that reduce their usefulness over the long term. Therefore, alternative strategies are required that would improve the prognosis of heart failure patients and might ultimately lead to a cure. Recently, gene therapy approaches have been investigated to try to improve the treatment of heart failure patients. The following sections provide an overview of the constructs and vectors that have been used for gene therapy in the heart and outline the clinical trials that have been initiated.

Vectors for myocardial gene therapy

Gene delivery to the myocardium can be achieved using a variety of vectors, including direct delivery of naked DNA by intracardiac injection, liposome complexes, and adenoviruses, adeno-associated viruses and lentiviruses. Despite the variety of vectors available, the choice of vector used to deliver genes to the myocardium requires careful consideration. To date, a number of effective methods have been employed for the delivery of therapeutic genes into the myocardium. Of these, the most direct method is the injection of naked DNA into the myocardium. Using this method, various groups have achieved effective gene transfer and stable transfection of the gene in myocardial cells. For example, Lin and co-workers (1990) injected plasmids encoding the β-galactosidase gene under the transcriptional control of the Rous sarcoma virus (RSV) promoter into adult myocytes present in the left ventricular wall (Lin *et al.*, 1990; Nabel, 1995). Expression of the β-galactosidase gene was observed up to four weeks post treatment. Buttrick *et al.* (1992) also achieved gene transfer of two different plasmids by direct intracardiac injection. The first of these plasmids encoded the chloramphenicol acetyltransferase reporter gene under the control of the RSV promoter and the second encoded the α-cardiac myosin heavy chain promoter fused to the firefly luciferase gene. Expression of both acetyltransferase and luciferase was localised to a 1–2 mm^2 region surrounding the injection site and was seen in 100% of rats from days 1 to 7 post injection. The expression of these molecules decreased with time such that expression was observed in only 60% of rat hearts from days 17 to 23 and in 30% from days 38 to 60 after injection. Interestingly, fusing both promoters into one plasmid with the luciferase reporter gene produced a construct that was expressed 20-fold more actively in the myocardium. von Harsdorf *et al.* (1993) showed a dose-dependent response for expression of chloramphenicol acetyltransferase that was under the transcriptional control of either β-myosin heavy chain or a promiscuous (mouse sarcoma virus) promoter (Nabel, 1995; von Harsdorf *et al.*, 1999). The concentration of plasmid DNA injected varied between 10 and 200 μg per injection site. In accordance with the results reported by Buttrick *et al.* (1992), chloramphenicol acetyltransferase activity was maximal at day 7, with subsequent decreases at days 14 and 21 post injection.

The most successful gene transfer approach for efficient delivery to myocardial cells is to use adenoviral vectors. The advantage of using adenovirus for gene delivery is that they can be produced in high titre, but more specifically, they can infect replicating and non-replicating cells (see Chapter 2) and, hence, can infect terminally differentiated cardiac myocytes (Yla-Herttuala and Martin, 2000). Unfortunately, adenoviruses do not integrate into the host genome and therefore transgene expression is usually transient. Also, these vectors induce strong immune responses that limit their effectiveness in clinical practice (Quinones *et al.*, 1996).

Molecular targets for myocardial gene therapy

Calcium metabolism

One strategy used to improve the contractility of the myocardium during heart failure has focused on modifying the handling of calcium during heart failure. Calcium influx through L-type calcium channels and its subsequent release from the sarcoplasmic reticulum (SR) is involved in the contraction of the heart. Therefore, levels of calcium in this organ need to be regulated tightly. During relaxation of the heart muscle, 75% of the intracellular calcium is re-accumulated in the SR by the action of the SR calcium ATPase (SERCA2a) pump, whereas the remaining 25% is excreted out of the cell by the sarcolemmal sodium/calcium exchanger. Phospholamban (PL) modulates the activity of the SERCA2a pump by inhibiting its function when in the unphosphorylated state. Once PL is phosphorylated, this inhibition is reversed. It is known that a decrease in the activity of the SERCA2a pump occurs concomitantly with an increase in PL expression in hypertrophied and failing hearts (Eizema *et al.*, 2000) and thus is believed to play a significant role in reducing myocardial contractility (Hajjar *et al.*, 2000). Eizema *et al.* (2000) showed that by using antisense gene therapy, they could reduce the expression of PL mRNA and protein and improve calcium handling in rat myocytes. In their experiments, the antisense strand of PL was cloned into an adenoviral vector prior to infection of myocytes. Endogenous PL mRNA was reduced to $30 \pm 7\%$ of baseline levels after 48 hours of infection. Similarly, expression of PL protein was reduced by $24 \pm 3\%$ 72 hours after infection. Electrophysiological studies revealed that there was an increased affinity of calcium for SERCA2a and, as a consequence, the time taken to recover 50% of the calcium current was reduced. This probably was due to a quick removal of intracellular calcium back to the SR store. Similar studies have been performed in human myocytes obtained from hearts in end-stage heart failure. These studies showed that infecting myocytes with the SERCA2a gene increased the expression of this pump in the SR and improved myocardial contractility. In addition, both contraction and relaxation velocity were restored to levels observed in non-failing hearts (Hajjar et al., 2000).

Work carried out by Schmidt et al. (2000) also targeted this pump in 26-month-old male Fisher rats. The SERCA2a gene was delivered globally to the myocardium of rats using an adenoviral vector and control animals received the reporter gene, β-galactosidase. Both systolic and diastolic function were measured to assess the success of treatment, and results showed that rate-dependent contractility and diastolic function in senescent hearts did improve with gene therapy.

Another method used to improve myocardial contractility is to modulate the activity of L-type calcium channels. Whereas L-type calcium channels are involved in maintaining normal contraction in healthy hearts, it has been proposed that such channels are defective in failing hearts, causing prolonged action potential duration and depressed contractility (Wei et al., 2000). Thus, Wei and co-workers (2000) used an adenoviral gene delivery system to express the β-subunit of the L-type channel in adult ventricular myocytes. A novel method was used to deliver the gene encoding the β-subunit; this consisted of a replication-deficient adenovirus with poly-L-lysine residues. This method was used in preference to normal adenoviral delivery since it takes less time than it would have taken to produce new recombinant particles, and also there is no limit on the size of genes that can be transfected. The method led to a 70% transfection efficiency of myocytes as determined from the expression of green fluorescent protein (GFP) that was encoded in the plasmid. Results from this study revealed that L-type calcium channel current density was enhanced by up to 3- to 4-fold in infected myocytes, even though only the β-subunit of the L-type channel was transfected and subsequently expressed.

Gene therapy for the RAS system

Untreated hypertension is a very important risk factor for the development of congestive heart failure and myocardial infarction. The RAS is thought to contribute to at least 10–30% of all cases of hypertension (Gelband *et al.*, 2000). Long-term detrimental effects such as cardiac hypertrophy are thought to result from the paracrine/autocrine secretion of AII from tissues such as the heart (Dostal and Baker, 1999). ACE inhibitors and the newer AII receptor antagonists have proved to be very successful at decreasing mortality rate in diseased patients, even though adverse side effects and problems such as a short duration of action limit their clinical use (Raizada *et al.*, 1999). Targeting various components of this system with a gene therapy approach has recently proved to be effective in treating hypertension and ultimately heart failure as will now be discussed.

Angiotensinogen (AGT) as a target   Tang *et al.* (1999) used an antisense gene therapy approach to control hypertension in rats. A 1.65-kb full-length rat AGT cDNA sequence was cloned into an adeno-associated virus vector (pTR-UF3) in the antisense orientation. A control plasmid also was generated where the cDNA was inserted in the sense direction. Each construct was placed under the transcriptional control of the CMV promoter and contained the GFP gene, which revealed a 50% transfection efficiency 48 hours post transfection in Reuber hepatoma cells. The antisense plasmid significantly reduced the amount of AGT secreted by 47.9% compared to the control. *In vivo* studies were then carried out in which adult spontaneously hypertensive rats (SHR) were injected with the antisense AGT plasmid at doses of 0.6 mg/kg, 1.5 mg/kg and 3 mg/kg. Systolic blood pressure was monitored for 9 days post injection and showed a dose-dependent fall by 12 ± 3 mmHg, 16.5 ± 2.2 mmHg and 22.5 ± 5.2 mmHg, respectively, compared with control.

ACE as a target   Inhibition of ACE activity would be another means by which the effects of the RAS system in disease could be ablated. Wang *et al.* (1999) generated retroviral vectors (LNSV) encoding the sense and antisense sequences of ACE. Initial *in vitro* experiments showed that infection of rat pulmonary artery endothelial cells (RPAECs) with the antisense vector caused a 75% decrease in ACE mRNA expression compared with those infected with the sense vector. Interestingly, the activity of the enzyme also decreased by 70% in cells infected with the antisense vector compared with controls. A study of AII receptors in RPAECs showed that these cells predominantly express the AT1 receptor subtype.

A Scatchard analysis of cells treated with the antisense vector showed an increase in receptor density. These receptors did not, however, show an increase in affinity for the ligands that bind them. *In vivo* experiments were carried out, in which 5-day-old WKY and SHR rats were injected with either the sense or antisense vectors. Blood pressure readings at 60 days of age were higher in SHR rats than in WKY rats. However, a decrease in blood pressure was seen in SHR rats treated with the antisense vector compared with rats treated with the sense vector whereas no such differences were seen in the WKY rats.

The importance of ACE in the development of cardiac hypertrophy was shown by Higaki and colleagues (2000). It had been documented previously that treatment with ACE inhibitors stops, and even regresses, cardiac hypertrophy; however, Higaki *et al.* (2000) showed that ACE plays a direct role in the development of hypertrophic growth. In a series of experiments, the human ACE gene within a liposomal vehicle was injected directly into the myocardium of male rats. Control animals were injected with the vehicle alone and another group of animals were injected with the ACE vector along with the ACE inhibitor perindopril. To measure the efficiency with which the transgene product had entered the myocardium, hearts were harvested 3 days after transfection and ACE activity measured. A 2-fold increase in ACE activity was observed in ACE-transfected cells compared with the control group. Furthermore, both the thickness and surface area of myocytes were significantly greater in the ACE-transfected group compared with the control group. Hypertrophy of myocytes was maintained for up to two weeks after transfection. The results of this study clearly show the importance of ACE in the pathogenesis of heart failure.

Targeting the cell cycle to inhibit decompensated cardiac hypertrophy

As stated above, cardiac hypertrophy is a common consequence of cardiovascular disease and, if left untreated, the uncontrolled growth of cardiac myocytes leads to a substantial decrease in myocardial function (decompensated hypertrophy). To date, conventional drug therapy has not targeted molecules specifically involved in the hypertrophic process: instead, therapy has been aimed at reducing the stimuli that cause hypertrophy. A more selective approach might be to target those molecules known to be involved in this growth process, such as mitogen-activating protein kinase (MAPK), calcineurin and cell cycle regulatory molecules, including the E2F transcription factors and cyclin-dependent kinases

(CDKs). Cardiac hypertrophy has been shown previously to involve a partial reactivation of the cell cycle machinery which allows myocytes to progress from the G_1 phase of the cell cycle through the S phase and arrest in G_2 (Li *et al.*, 1998; Li and Brooks, 1999; Figure 6.3). The E2F family of transcription factors are essential for cell cycle progression into the S phase of the cell cycle. Therefore, blocking the transcriptional activity of these factors might enable the extent of cardiac hypertrophy to be controlled such that hypertrophy is limited to compensated growth alone.

The importance of E2F transcription factors in the G_1 to S phase transition in cardiac muscle cells was investigated by Agah *et al.* (1997). These authors investigated the effects of adenoviral delivery of human E2F-1 in adult rat ventricular myocytes, both *in vitro* and *in vivo*. The results of this study showed that DNA synthesis was evoked in 19% of adult rat myocytes that were infected with E2F-1 compared with 0% of myocytes infected with a control virus. Importantly, there was no increase in cell number in the infected myocytes, which illustrates the fact E2F-1 promotes cell cycle progression past the S phase but is not able to push cells past to the M phase of the cell cycle.

von Harsdorf *et al.* (1999) also has showed that adenoviral delivery of E2F-1 into rat myocytes causes an increase of cells in the S phase from 1.2% to 23%. In accordance with the results of Agah *et al.* (1997), >90% of cells underwent apoptosis but this was rescued by co-expression of insulin-like growth factor 1 (IGF-1). It was postulated that IGF-1 led to the downregulation of p21 and p27 expression in these cells. This subsequently led to an increase in CDK 2, 4 and 6 activities, enabling cells to pass into the S phase.

Recent work from our laboratory has shown that specific E2F transcription factors are up-regulated during the development of hypertrophy in cultured 3-day old neonatal rat myocytes (unpublished). However, it still remains to be determined whether blocking the function of these transcription factors leads to an inhibition of hypertrophy.

Gene therapy for the vascular system

Whereas gene therapy for the treatment of myocardial disease currently is limited, greater success has been achieved in the vascular system. The following sections will address the major diseases of the vasculature and discuss recent gene transfer trials.

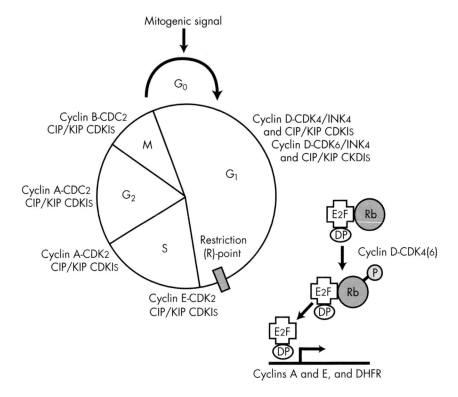

Figure 6.3 Diagram showing the mammalian cell cycle. The normal cell division cycle is subdivided into four distinct phases: two gap phases (G_1 and G_2) where RNA and protein synthesis occur, S phase (DNA synthesis) and M phase (mitosis, where the cell divides into two daughter cells). An additional gap phase, known as G_0, exists in some cell types that undergo a stage of quiescence where RNA and protein syntheses are minimal. Each phase of the cycle is under the control of specific positive [cyclin/cyclin-dependent kinase (CDK) complexes] and negative [inhibitor of CDK4 (INK) and/or CDK2 interacting protein (CIP) and CDK inhibitory protein (KIP) CDKIs] regulators that act in concert with each other to either promote or arrest cell cycle progression, depending on the relative levels of expression. Specific checkpoints are shown that act as surveillance systems to determine whether the cellular environment is favourable for continued progression through the cycle. The restriction point is a position of control that functions in late G_1. In order for a cell to pass the R point, cyclin D/CDK4(6) complexes need to be activated (e.g. following a mitogenic signal being received at the cell surface) to phosphorylate the retinoblastoma (Rb) protein that is normally found in a hypophosphorylated form bound to the transcription factor E2F. E2F itself comprises the subunits E2F and DP. Phosphorylation of Rb (shown as P) leads to its dissociation from E2F, the release of transcriptionally active E2F and the synthesis of genes necessary for S phase progression, e.g. cyclins A and E and dihydrofolate reductase (DHFR).

Coronary heart disease

In 1997, 953 110 Americans died from cardiovascular diseases (41.2% of all deaths) and coronary heart disease claimed the lives of 466 101 (48.9%) of these individuals. When compared with death from other causes, such as cancer, accidents and HIV (AIDS) in the same year, CHD stands out as the leading cause of death in America (American Heart Association, 2000). Indeed, data from the Framingham Study have revealed that one in two men and one in three women will develop CHD by the age of 40 years (Lloyd-Jones *et al.*, 1999). Clearly, early diagnosis and effective treatment of this condition is of paramount importance if we are to save lives and lessen the burden of healthcare costs. Conventional drug therapy for the treatment of CHD only provides relief from symptoms, but does not provide a cure. Atherosclerosis is the primary cause of CHD leading to heart attack, stroke and peripheral vascular disease and it has been estimated to cause 40–50% of deaths in America, Western Europe and Japan (Ross, 1993). Atherosclerosis is the term used to describe the development of an atheromatous lesion on the luminal surface of a blood vessel which leads to its narrowing. Clinical manifestation of this disease often presents as ischaemic heart disease and peripheral vascular disease, where narrowing occurs to such an extent that blood flow to the myocardium and muscles in the extremities is severely compromised. Modern pharmaceutical therapies are aimed at increasing blood flow to ischaemic areas to control symptoms of these diseases. Unfortunately, disease progression in a large number of patients occurs to such an extent that surgical intervention including bypass surgery, angioplasty and stenting often is required. These procedures initially provide great relief for patients but, unfortunately, are limited in their efficacy by natural body mechanisms that cause re-closure of the treated vessels (called restenosis), and ultimately failure of treatment.

Future therapies need to focus on obtaining a cure for these conditions, for instance, by targeting the molecules involved in disease development. Gene therapy offers some hope for the treatment of certain diseases of the vascular system, some of which will be discussed in the following sections.

Atherosclerosis

Atherosclerosis is a progressive disease that starts early in life. Indeed, when autopsied, the coronary vessels of young children start to show the deposition of fat along the walls of blood vessels from the age of 10 years onwards. The consequences of this fat deposition are only seen in mid-to-late life, and usually manifest themselves as coronary artery disease resulting from a reduced blood supply and ischaemia. Peripheral vascular disease, myocardial infarction and stroke are other consequences of atherosclerosis.

A number of risk factors have been identified for the development of atherosclerosis and CHD:

- *Dietary fat* intake is believed to be an important factor in the development of CHD. Thus, low levels of high-density lipoprotein (HDL) co-existing with high triglyceride and total cholesterol levels have been associated with an increased risk of coronary events (Jousilahti *et al.*, 1999; Ascherio *et al.*, 1996; Jeppesen *et al.*, 1997).
- *Body mass index (BMI)* has a positive association with CHD. Findings from a study by Jousilahti et al (1996) showed that an increase in body weight of 1 kg increased the risk of CHD mortality by 1–1.5%.
- *Gender* plays a role in the incidence of CHD. Men develop CHD earlier than women, and generally have a higher incidence of disease (Jousilahti *et al.*, 1999; Kiechl and Willeit, 1999; Lloyd-Jones *et al.*, 1999). It is believed that this difference is due to hormonal differences between males and females. Thus, oestrogen, the predominant hormone in females, is believed to have important cardio-protective properties, possibly as a result of its effect on glucose metabolism (Kiechl and Willeit, 1999).
- *Physical inactivity* has been shown to increase the incidence of CHD, especially in middle-aged and older men (Wannamethee *et al.*, 2000).
- *Ageing* increases the absolute risk of CHD in both sexes, with most new-onset CHD cases presenting after the age of 65 years (Grundy *et al.*, 1998; Kiechl and Willeit, 1999).
- *Smoking* has been recognised as a powerful risk factor for both CHD and myocardial infarction (Jousilahti *et al.*, 1999). In 1990, a staggering 180 000 deaths in the United States from CHD were related to smoking (Cooper *et al.*, 2000). Autopsy studies have shown that smoking accelerates plaque development, and hence increases the incidence of coronary events (Grundy *et al.*, 1998).
- *Diabetes mellitus* is believed to increase the risk of developing CHD (Grundy *et al.*, 1998). Patients with diabetes mellitus often have associated risk factors such as hypertension, low HDL levels and high triglyceride levels (Cooper *et al.*, 2000). Recent evidence suggests that

lowering all such risk factors is extremely important in treating CHD in diabetic patients (Cooper *et al.*, 2000).

Development of atherosclerotic plaques

The precise mechanism(s) for atheroma development is not yet fully understood; however, several theories have been proposed. The 'response to injury' hypothesis is one such proposal, originally put forward by Ross and Glomset (1976) and later consolidated by Ross (1993). This theory states that damage to the endothelium leads to endothelial dysfunction. Damage can occur from a number of sources such as toxins, mechanical stress or virus particles. Once the endothelium is damaged, LDL–cholesterol can enter the blood vessel wall, where it deposits in the intima and becomes oxidised by a process that is not clearly understood. Concomitant with this oxidation, the expression of adhesion molecules such as vascular cell adhesion molecule 1 (VCAM-1) and intracellular adhesion molecule 1 (ICAM-1) on the damaged endothelial surface allow circulating monocytes and lymphocytes to dock and then enter the vessel wall. Once inside, the monocytes gorge themselves on the oxidised LDL–cholesterol and form bodies called foam cells. Foam cells then release various cytokines that promote proliferation of vascular smooth muscle and connective tissue, which leads to the formation of an advanced atheroma.

Symptoms very rarely occur early in plaque formation, but over a period of years the size of the plaque increases. In fact symptoms only are seen when approximately 75–80% of the lumen is occluded (Figure 6.4) when anginal pains would occur during exercise.

Vascular diseases associated with defects in lipid metabolism

As stated above, the incidence of CHD increases dramatically with increased plasma LDL–cholesterol levels. Indeed, a variety of conditions exist where lipid metabolism is defective and this often leads to abnormal plasma lipid levels. Examples of such disorders include:

- *Familial hypercholesterolaemia.* This disorder has an incidence of 1 per 500 and is an autosomal dominant condition, where there is a mutation in the LDL receptor that prevents it from taking up and utilising plasma LDL and cholesterol. Patients usually have serum LDL and cholesterol levels that are 4- to 7-fold higher than the normal range.

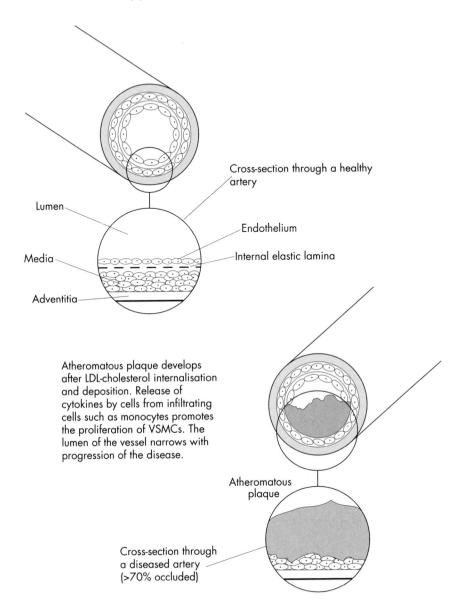

Cross-section through a healthy artery

Lumen

Endothelium

Media

Internal elastic lamina

Adventitia

Atheromatous plaque develops after LDL-cholesterol internalisation and deposition. Release of cytokines by cells from infiltrating cells such as monocytes promotes the proliferation of VSMCs. The lumen of the vessel narrows with progression of the disease.

Atheromatous plaque

Cross-section through a diseased artery (>70% occluded)

Figure 6.4 Cross-section through a healthy and a diseased artery.

- *Familial defective apoB-100.* This also has an incidence of 1 per 500. It is an autosomal dominant condition where the apoB-100 is defective due to a mutation that prevents the LDL receptor binding efficiently to LDL. Hypercholesterolaemia results, with an increase in the incidence of cardiovascular disease.

- *Familial-combined hyperlipidaemia.* This has an incidence as high as 3–5 per 1000. Numerous lipids are elevated in this disease, including very-low-density lipoprotein (VLDL), LDL or both. Diagnosis can be made because patients usually have an abnormal cholesterol-to-apoB ratio of greater than 1.3. Also, diagnosis can be confirmed when LDL–apoB levels are greater than 130 mg/dl of plasma. Some patients have normal LDL–cholesterol levels but elevated levels of LDL–apoB (>130 mg/dl). This gives the appearance of no real lipid metabolism dysfunction; however, there is an increase in the rate of VLDL–apoB synthesis, which can lead to premature heart disease.

- *Familial dysbetalipoproteinaemia.* This has an incidence of 1 per 5000 and is characterised by the presence of defective apoE on circulating lipids. Patients usually have elevated cholesterol and triglyceride (ratio of 1 : 1) and an elevated plasma–triglyceride ratio of >0.3 (normal ratio would be <0.3). Patients develop hyperlipidaemia and have an increased risk of premature CHD and peripheral vascular disease.

Current drug therapies for treating disorders of lipid metabolism

Currently, a number of therapeutic agents are used to regulate lipid levels in patients with hyperlipidaemia. One such group is the anion-exchange resins (e.g. cholestyramine), which act by binding to bile acids and preventing their reabsorption (British National Formulary, 2000). This then causes the liver to convert more cholesterol to bile, thereby increasing cholesterol metabolism. Another group of drugs is the clofibrate group, which decrease serum triglycerides. The statins also are used to reduce cholesterol synthesis in the liver, by blocking the cholesterol-synthesising activity of 3-hydroxy-3-methylglutaryl coenzyme A (HMG CoA) reductase enzyme. Indeed, studies such as the West of Scotland Coronary Prevention Study (WOSCOPS) (Shepherd *et al.*, 1995), the Helsinki Heart Study (Frick *et al.*, 1987) and the Cholesterol And Recurrent Event (CARE) study (Sacks *et al.*, 1996) have shown that these compounds reduce LDL–cholesterol, raise HDL–cholesterol and reduce coronary events in patients. Unfortunately, agents such as the statins and clofibrate group have dangerous side effects, including rhabdomyolysis, whilst the anion-exchange resins interfere with the absorption of fat-soluble vitamins and have numerous gastrointestinal side effects. Whilst they provide some benefit to patients, the underlying condition still remains. One way to improve treatment is to target those molecules that are defective in the lipid metabolic pathway in order to cure various lipid disorders. Over the past few decades, genetic manipulation of these molecules has provided some hope of more effective treatments, which will now be discussed.

Gene therapy for atherosclerosis

Apolipoprotein E (apoE)

A number of targets in the lipid metabolism pathway have been identified and are the subject of current research. For example, apolipoprotein E (apoE) is very important for the clearance of plasma lipoproteins. Genetic disorders where this protein is defective, such as familial dysbetalipoproteinaemia (see above), increase the incidence of CHD and peripheral vascular disease. ApoE is expressed in a number of tissues and various cell types such as tissue macrophages, but the majority of apoE is synthesised in the liver. It has been proposed that secretion of apoE from the arterial wall might protect against the formation of atherosclerosis. The mechanism by which this protective effect is exerted is not really known; however, a number of possibilities have been proposed including:

1 the promotion of cholesterol efflux from cholesterol-loaded macrophages in the arterial wall;
2 the facilitation of reverse cholesterol transport from the arterial wall;
3 the induction of remnant uptake through ApoE dependent pathways; and
4 local effects on inflammation, platelet aggregation, and leukocyte activation or growth factor sequestration.

To test this protective mechanism, Hasty *et al.* (1999) used an apoE-expressing retrovirus and infected apoE-deficient bone marrow which was then transplanted into apoE–/– recipient mice. Three weeks after transplantation, apoE was found to be expressed and was detected in plasma associated with lipoproteins at 0.5% to 1% of normal levels. Cholesterol levels were not affected. Two age groups of mice were used in this study to determine the stage of lesion formation at which apoE was important. The younger group of mice had early forming lesions, which were at the foam cell stage, whereas the older set of mice had more advanced lesions. The main conclusion from this study was that arterial macrophage secretion of apoE can delay lesion formation, but only at the early stages of lesion formation (i.e. at the foam cell stage). Measuring the aortic lesion areas in the different groups of mice demonstrated this clearly, since mice expressing either human or murine apoE had lesions that were 2- to 7-fold smaller than controls. For the older group of mice the experimental group had a lesion area of 186 282 ± 97 333 μm^2 versus 183 168 ± 88 771 μm^2 for the control group, showing no statistical difference. However, the younger group of experimental mice given murine or human apoE compared with their controls showed a significant decrease in lesion area (4847 ± 2410, 5294 ± 2868 and 12 837 ± 7166 μm^2, respectively).

In another study by Desurmont *et al.* (2000), apoE-deficient nude mice were infected with an adenovirus encoding human apoE cDNA. Using this approach, human apoE was detected in serum 4 days after injection and levels peaked at day 21. Expression of ApoE was maintained for at least four months after infection. When the lipoprotein metabolism profiles were studied, cholesterol levels dramatically decreased from 591 ± 85 mg/dl at day 0 to 97 ± 7 mg/dl at day 21 (in mice given 10^9 pfu). These levels were maintained for five months, with a slow rise in levels after six months. Mice given smaller doses of the adenovirus encoding the human apoE (5×10^8 pfu) also showed a significant decrease in cholesterol levels (513 ± 40 mg/dl at day 0 to 84 ± 6 mg/dl at day 21) but hypercholesterolaemia reappeared earlier. Triglyceride levels also decreased in mice injected with 10^9 pfu of the apoE adenovirus from 222 ± 45 mg/dl at day 0 to 93 ± 11 mg/dl at day 21. Again these levels were maintained for five months with an increase in levels in the sixth month. In mice that received a smaller dose of apoE virus (5×10^8 pfu), a decrease in triglyceride levels was observed from 145 ± 15 mg/dl at day 0 to 110 ± 12 mg/dl at day 21, but hypertriglyceridaemia reappeared between three and four months after injection

When the distribution of cholesterol in lipoproteins was investigated in these mice, elution profiles showed that cholesterol was primarily transported on VLDL–LDL lipoproteins in untreated animals. However, 21 days following apoE delivery, cholesterol content in the VLDL–LDL fractions decreased, with a concomitant increase in HDL–cholesterol levels.

Histological analyses of the atherosclerotic lesions showed that at 17 weeks of age (when mice received the virus), lesions were at the fatty streak stage. Macrophage foam cells were present underneath the endothelial layers and lesions had a mean size of 220 ± 37 mm^2. During the experimental period a 6-fold increase in lesion size was seen in the control group (1172 ± 255 mm²). However, a dose-dependent decrease in lesion size was seen in the treatment groups with lesion sizes of 147 ± 76 and 28 ± 6 mm² in mice treated with 5×10^8 and 10^9 pfu of virus, respectively. In fact the lesion sizes in mice treated with 10^9 pfu of virus represented only 13% of the size of the lesion that was present at the beginning of the experiment and only 2.2% of lesion size in normal control mice of the same age, 28 weeks after injection (Desurmont *et al.*, 2000).

LCAT – a target for gene therapy

Patients with familial hypercholesterolaemia usually have LDL–cholesterol levels that are elevated 2- to 6-fold above those found in healthy individuals. These patients also have an accompanying decrease in HDL levels. To reverse this phenotype, an enzyme called lecithin:cholesterol acyltransferase (LCAT) can be targeted (Brousseau *et al.*, 2000). LCAT is a glycoprotein that plays an important role in the transport of cholesterol from peripheral tissues to the liver for catabolism, a process called reverse cholesterol transport. It has been shown that overexpression of human LCAT (hLCAT) in New Zealand white rabbits reduces LDL–cholesterol levels whilst at the same time increasing HDL levels.

Apolipoprotein A-1 regulates the activation of LCAT. Once activated, LCAT catalyses the esterification of free cholesterol, which then appears on HDL molecules. The cholesterol esters and triglycerides are then transferred to acceptor lipoproteins, such as VLDL, LDL, chylomicrons and remnants of chylomicrons, VLDL and LDL. These acceptor lipoproteins are then endocytosed in the liver via the LDL receptor, and the cholesterol subsequently catabolised.

The effects of LCAT overexpression on diet-induced atherosclerosis were investigated by Hoeg *et al.* (1996). In studies carried out by this group, transgenic rabbits overexpressing the human LCAT enzyme were fed either a 0.3% cholesterol-rich diet or normal chow diet. Initial results from the study showed that transgenic animals have significantly higher LCAT activity than control (1593 ± 101 nmol/ml/h compared with 101 ± 11 nmol/ml/h, respectively). Cholesterol profiles later revealed that total cholesterol and non-HDL–cholesterol rose by 19-fold and 127-fold, respectively, in control animals fed on the cholesterol diet in comparison with transgenic animals that only observed increases of 2-fold and 11-fold, respectively. HDL–cholesterol levels were maintained 5-fold higher in transgenic animals for the duration of the experiment compared with controls. A sensitive indicator of clinically detectable atherosclerosis in humans is the total cholesterol-to-HDL–cholesterol ratio, which increased by more than 12-fold in control animals fed on the cholesterol diet. In comparison, transgenic rabbits showed less than a 2-fold increase in this ratio, which subsequently remained below 5, a ratio that provides an average risk of atherosclerosis in humans. The potential protective role of LCAT over-expression was assessed 17 weeks after the start of the experiment when animals were harvested and lesion size and intima/media (I/M) ratios were determined. Sudan IV lipid droplet staining of lesions in the aortas of control animals revealed a $35 \pm 7\%$ covering by atherosclerotic plaque, in comparison with transgenic animals that only had a $5 \pm 1\%$ covering. Also, foam cell formation, cellular proliferation and an increase in I/M of 0.4 ± 0.1 were seen in control animals. No significant cellular proliferation or foam cell formation was seen in transgenic rabbits, although an increase in I/M ratio was observed (0.03 ± 0.01), which was significantly lower than that for control animals. Overexpressing LCAT led to an 85–90% reduction in diet-induced atherosclerosis in these animals.

The role of apolipoprotein A-I in atherosclerosis formation was studied by Plump *et al.* (1994), who generated transgenic mice deficient in apoE and overexpressing human apoA-I (hapoA-I). Animal populations were divided into three groups based on their plasma hapoA-I levels: (1) apoE–/–, (2) apoE–/–, low expressing (low) hapoA-I (<200 mg/dl), and (3) apoE–/–, high expressing (high) hapoA-I (>200 mg/dl). Human apoA-I levels were 153 ± 26 mg/dl in the low expressing group, whereas in the high expressing group levels were determined to be 275 ± 50 mg/dl. HDL–cholesterol levels were also significantly elevated in animals highly expressing hapoA-I compared with control and low expressing hapoA-I animals. No significant differences were seen in total cholesterol and non-HDL–cholesterol in either groups.

At four months of age, animals were analysed for proximal aortic atherosclerosis, a time point in development where extensive fatty streak development is known to occur for apoE-deficient mice fed on a chow diet. Those animals highly expressing the hapoA-I protein had a mean lesion area of 470 ± 825 μm^2, which were significantly smaller than control animals (apoE–/–) with lesion areas of $22\ 964 \pm 23\ 030$ μm^2. At eight months, a similar trend was still seen in lesion size for the animals.

Ischaemic heart disease and angina

The myocardium receives its blood supply from two major vessels, the left and right coronary arteries which arise from the aorta at the sinuses of Valsalva (Bern and Levy, 1993). The left coronary artery then divides into the left anterior descending artery which supplies the majority of the left ventricle and septum with blood, and the left circumflex artery. As described above, atherosclerosis leads to the narrowing of blood vessels by the formation of an atheromatous plaque. In 1997, it was estimated that ischaemic heart disease would cost the National Health Service (NHS) of the UK £1.4 billion in healthcare and would kill over 150 000 people the following year (Crossman, 1997). The majority of patients first experience symptoms of disease when more than 70% of the lumen becomes occluded, at which point the oxygen and nutrient demands of the myocardium far outweigh their supply, usually during periods of exertion (e.g. exercise). Unfortunately, sudden cardiac death is the first sign of disease for many patients (Walker and Tan, 1997); however, most patients with established disease experience anginal pain as the principal symptom.

Classification of angina

Angina pectoris can be divided into three distinct clinical syndromes: chronic stable angina, unstable angina and variant angina pectoris.

Chronic stable angina

This is the most common form of angina. Pain often is precipitated by physical exertion, usually lasts for a few minutes and subsides upon rest. The duration and frequency of pain felt by patients has allowed further classification of chronic stable angina as shown in Table 6.1 (Nolan et al., 1996).

Table 6.1 Canadian Cardiovascular Society classification of angina

Class	Canadian Cardiovascular Society Classification
I	Angina occurs with strenuous physical activity
II	Symptoms occur with activity
III	Symptoms occur with ordinary activity
IV	Symptoms inhibit ordinary activity

Modified from Nolan et al. (1996).

Unstable angina

Various different types of syndrome can be classed under this description, including new onset angina, pre-infarction angina, crescendo angina, coronary insufficiency and impending myocardial infarction (Nolan *et al.*, 1996). Unstable angina presents in one of three ways: (1) as prolonged pain (>20 minutes) at rest; (2) as recent onset of angina (in the previous 1–2 months), where pain is felt following minimal exertion; or (3) as chronic stable angina, which seems to be occurring more frequently and persists for a longer duration of time than a normal episode of established stable angina. Pain usually is provoked by less exertion than in other forms of angina.

Variant angina pectoris (Prinzmetal's angina)

In this condition, coronary artery spasm critically restricts blood flow to the myocardium, causing ischaemia in the affected areas and hence pain. Atherosclerosis may or may not be a component of this condition. Typically, pain usually follows a circadian rhythm, being worst at midnight and at around 8 a.m. (Nolan *et al.*, 1996).

Current medical treatment for angina

Once the type of angina has been diagnosed, the correct treatment has to be initiated to control the condition. The general aims of drug therapy for all types of angina are to decrease the workload on the heart, increase coronary perfusion and increase cardiac reserve. Various groups of drugs are employed for these tasks, all of which act by different mechanisms.

Nitrates

The primary action of these compounds is to increase coronary blood flow by dilating the coronary vasculature. They also act on the venous system and this, in turn, reduces pre-load, thereby decreasing the work demand of the heart. At high doses they also reduce after-load by causing arterial dilatation. Unfortunately, these compounds cause many side effects due to their powerful vasodilatory properties, such as headaches, dizziness (due to hypotension), facial flushing and reflex tachycardia (British National Formulary, 2000).

Beta-blockers

These compounds act by decreasing the rate and force of contraction of the heart, which in turn reduces myocardial workload. Coronary perfusion also is improved as the heart spends longer in diastole. Beta-blockers have many dangerous side effects such as bradycardia, sinus arrest, atrioventricular node block, decreased left ventricular function, bronchoconstriction, fatigue, depression, nightmares, sexual dysfunction and intensification of diabetes mellitus (British National Formulary, 2000).

Calcium entry blockers (CEBs)

CEBs prevent the entry of calcium into vascular smooth muscle cells, which reduces the excitation–contraction coupling of these cells. The consequence of this is a decrease in coronary and peripheral vascular resistance, with a subsequent increase in coronary blood flow. Myocardial contraction is decreased, as is heart rate, leading to a decrease in workload by the myocardium. Flushing, headache, dizziness, peripheral oedema and depression of myocardial contractility are the main side effects of these compounds (British National Formulary, 2000).

Nicorandil

This compound is a powerful vasodilator of the arterial and venous systems. It is used for the treatment of angina when other treatments cannot be used (British National Formulary, 2000).

Angiogenesis

Even though drug therapy plays a critical role in controlling the symptoms of patients with angina, it does not provide a cure. A more powerful approach to treating ischaemic heart disease would be to generate new blood vessels in hypoxic areas of the myocardium. In fact, hypoxia is a natural stimulus for angiogenesis; however, this endogenous response is not sufficient to restore blood flow to the levels necessary for normal myocardial function following an infarct or ischaemic heart tissue. Extensive research in this field has armed us with significant knowledge about the molecules involved in this process. Fibroblast growth factor (FGF) and vascular endothelial growth factor (VEGF) are angiogenic factors that have shown some benefit in clinical practice (Bauters, 1997; Carmeliet, 2000; Leiden, 2000). Acidic-FGF (aFGF), also known as FGF-1, and basic-FGF (bFGF) are important angiogenic factors that are known to stimulate vessel formation. Of the four different isoforms of the VEGF family that have been isolated ($VEGF_{121}$, $VEGF_{165}$, $VEGF_{189}$ and $VEGF_{206}$), $VEGF_{165}$ and $VEGF_{121}$ have been used in clinical trials to induce angiogenesis in humans. The following section summarises some of these trials.

Acidic-fibroblast growth factor (FGF-1)

In a recent study by Fernandez *et al.* (2000), mice overexpressing FGF-1 were generated to determine the role of this molecule in the developing coronary system. To generate these transgenic mice, a 2.2-kb fragment of DNA containing the 3' untranslated sequence of human FGF-1 was ligated between the SV40 large intron and the 2.2-kb mouse myosin light chain 2v (MLC2v) promoter (L7). Another construct also was created where the cytomegalovirus (CMV) enhancer was added upstream from the MLC2v promoter (L1). These constructs were then injected into the male pronucleus of murine CD2F1 zygotes and transferred into pseudopregnant females. Western blot analysis revealed a 1.8-fold increase in protein expression in the transgenic mice compared with wild-type animals. Immunoconfocal microscopy studies showed that FGF-1 was in the extracellular matrix in both the wild-type (WT) and transgenic (TR) mice, but there was a marked increase in the amount of protein detected in the TR versus WT mice. Anatomical and histomorphological studies showed no major differences between the WT and TR mice; even the density of coronary capillaries did not differ statistically. Interestingly, increases in the number of arterial branches were seen in both TR groups of mice (T1 = 1.5-fold and T7 = 1.4-fold) compared with WT animals.

Importantly, *ex vivo* haemodynamic studies showed that coronary blood flow was significantly higher in the L1 TR group compared with WT mice. This trend was observed at each of four different blood pressures tested, with a 1.25-fold increase in blood flow compared with controls at the highest pressure of 142 mmHg. In order to ensure that the vasoactivity of the vessels was not responsible for the differences in blood flow, dissected hearts were perfused with 0.01% adenosine which caused maximal dilation of the vessels. Previously, it had been shown that animals such as the rat have a predetermined growth potential of their vessels: after the development of a defined number of branches, arterial growth stops. In contrast, this study has shown that, at least in mice, overexpression of FGF-1 can change the growth pattern of arterial branches, and might, therefore, provide a good approach for inducing angiogenesis by gene therapy.

Often, patients with severe CHD and normal left ventricular function have normal baseline blood flow. Usually angiogenesis is aimed at promoting vessel growth in areas of myocardial ischaemia in these patients. Safi *et al.* (1999) determined whether angiogenesis also could be induced in non-ischaemic areas of the myocardium. To accomplish this, a replicating deficient adenovirus encoding secreted acidic-FGF_{1-154} (AdCMV.sp + $aFGF_{1-154}$) was injected into the marginal branch of the left circumflex coronary artery of male New Zealand white rabbits, each receiving 1×10^9 pfu. Other rabbits were injected with either a control vector containing the *E. coli lacZ* gene (AdCMV.NLS β-gal), which codes for β-galactosidase (each receiving 1×10^9 pfu), or normal saline.

Animals were then sacrificed at days 1, 5, 12 or 15 after injection and tissue collected for analysis. Northern blot analyses showed that aFGF mRNA was overexpressed up to 12 days post injection in those rabbits that received the FGF expressing vector. Expression did, however, fall to baseline levels at day 15. Importantly, aFGF was not expressed at the mRNA level in either control group.

Once transgene expression had been established, protective effects in regions of myocardium prone to myocardial infarction needed to be determined. To induce such conditions, the left circumflex marginal artery was occluded with a surgical suture for 20 minutes. Interestingly, a 50% reduction in the risk region of the left ventricle from infarction was observed in aFGF-treated vessels compared with hearts from control animals, which was attributed to the growth of resistance coronary vessels and capillaries.

The important issue of uncontrolled systemic effects of the adenovirus also was addressed in this experiment. Arteriole length density was evaluated in apical and basal regions of the left ventricle in rabbits receiving the aFGF-expressing vector. No difference was found in these regions when compared with the control rabbits, which confirms that the vector had a very localised effect.

Vascular endothelial growth factor (VEGF)

A report published by Rosengart *et al.* (1999) summarised the results of a phase I clinical trial that used an adenovirus gene transfer vector expressing the $VEGF_{121}$ cDNA to induce therapeutic angiogenesis in the myocardium of patients with significant coronary artery disease (Simons *et al.*, 2000). In this study, the extent of CHD in 21 men and women aged between 18 and 85 years was assessed according to a number of clinical parameters. Fifteen people were assigned to receive the $VEGF_{121}$-expressing vector as an adjunct to coronary artery bypass grafting (CABG) (group A), whilst six people received sole $VEGF_{121}$ therapy (group B). Each individual from both treatment groups received ten injections of the $VEGF_{121}$-expressing vector (100 μl per injection) at, and around, sites of ischaemia (determined by ^{99m}Tc sestamibi perfusion scans with or without adenosine). A total of five different doses of vector were given to patients in group A, ranging from 4×10^8 to 4×10^{10} pfu, with three patients being assigned to each dose. Each patient in group B received a total dose of 4×10^9 pfu. Unfortunately, two patients in group A died perioperatively and two patients died postoperatively (receiving $4 \times 10^{8.5}$ and 4×10^{10} pfu). Neither of the postoperative deaths were deemed to have occurred as a consequence of the therapy. A further sudden death occurred in a patient receiving a vector dose of 4×10^{10} pfu, the cause of which was not known. Various safety parameters were monitored in each patient to detect any adverse effects of treatment, of which there were none.

Results from the above trial revealed that all individuals in group A showed improvements in the class of angina they had. However, as the $VEGF_{121}$ therapy was given as an adjunct to CABG, improvements cannot definitively be attributed to the $VEGF_{121}$ therapy. More importantly, all six members of group B showed a decrease in angina classification 30 days post injection compared with their status before therapy initiation. Angiograms of patient hearts were reviewed by three independent cardiologists, who evaluated the area of myocardium that was injected with the vector. Rentrope scores were given to the hearts and the majority of patients in group A showed improvements in filling of epicardial vessels.

In a separate phase I clinical trial, $VEGF_{165}$ was delivered to the myocardium of patients suffering from severe myocardial ischaemia (Losordo *et al.*, 1998; Simons *et al.*, 2000). $VEGF_{165}$ gene transfer was performed in five patients, all of whom had functional class 3 or 4 exertional angina, were refractory to maximum medical therapy, and had areas of visible underperfused myocardium and multivessel occlusive coronary artery disease. All five patients were injected with 125 μg of a eukaryotic expression vector encoding the human $VEGF_{165}$ isoform under the control of a CMV promoter ($phVEGF_{165}$), directly into the myocardium. After treatment, all five patients experienced a decrease in anginal severity and frequency. This improvement in condition began to take effect between 10 and 30 days after gene transfer. Surprisingly, angina was completely abolished in two patients. General improvements in conditions meant that glyceryl nitrate use for the whole group decreased from 7.7 ± 1.4 to 1.4 ± 1 tablet per day, 60 days post gene transfer. SPECT-sestamibi imaging of the myocardium also showed that the mean number of normally perfused segments per patient increased from 6.0 ± 1.1 before gene transfer to 8.0 ± 0.7, again 60 days post therapy, and coronary angiography studies also showed evidence for improved collateral flow into ischaemic areas of the myocardium in all five patients. Thus, VEGF gene therapy holds promise for the future treatment of ischaemic heart disease.

Surgical treatments for angina

When medical intervention has had no impact on the treatment of angina, surgical intervention often is the next method used to treat this condition. The following is a list of the procedures used to achieve revascularisation of the myocardium:

- coronary artery bypass grafting (CABG)
- percutaneous transluminal coronary angioplasty (PTCA)
- atherectomy
- intracoronary stent placement with PTCA.

Figure 6.5 shows how PTCA works and the potential for using double balloon catheters to deliver therapeutic agents to the site of damage. Unfortunately, the success rates of these procedures are always limited by the restenosis that for some procedures such as PTCA are known in up to 40% of cases.

Restenosis

Both PTCA, first carried out in 1978 by Gruentzig, and aortacoronary saphenous vein graft implantation, first carried out in a human by Garret and colleagues in 1967, have proved to be very effective in revascularising the ischaemic heart. Unfortunately, a staggering 40% of patients can develop restenosis within one year of the procedure (Ferns and Avades, 2000). In comparison, 15% of patients who have aortocoronary saphenous vein grafts develop occlusions in their grafts one year post surgery

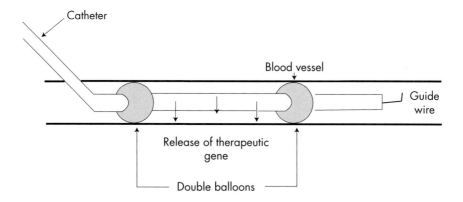

Figure 6.5   Use of a double-balloon catheter to deliver a therapeutic gene to a specific region of the blood vessel wall.

(Motwani and Topol, 1998). Only 60% of grafts remain patent 10 years after surgery, and of these, only 50% do not develop significant stenoses. Clearly, the problem of restenosis greatly limits the effectiveness of both procedures. The mechanism of restenosis is not well understood; however, current research into this phenomenon is arming us with information that has begun to be utilised in the development of more effective therapies.

Pathogenesis of restenosis

Restenosis can be precipitated by a number of events. The following is a general step-by-step description of what is believed to occur following PTCA leading to restenosis:

1 Recoil of the vessel wall might occur following PTCA leading to closure of the vessel.
2 An insult to an area of vessel, e.g. by PTCA, leads to disruption of the endothelium. Platelet adhesion and activation occurs, which permits thrombus formation. Accumulation of other cells, such as neutrophils, monocytes, lymphocytes, tissue macrophages and residual endothelial cells, occurs at this site. A host of mediators, such as platelet factor 4, platelet-derived growth factor (PDGF), interleukin 1, acidic and basic fibroblast growth factors, 5-HT, thrombin, thrombospondin, angiotensin II and transforming growth factor β (TGFβ), are released by these cells.
3 Once released, these mediators act as powerful chemoattractants that promote the migration of vascular smooth muscle cells (VSMCs) into

the intimal layer. VSMC proliferation occurs, leading to intimal thickening and a subsequent decrease in lumen diameter.
4 Further narrowing of the vessel occurs by on-going atherosclerosis of the vessel.

Current medical treatments for restenosis

As stated above, up to 40% of patients undergoing PTCA develop restenosis within 12 months of intervention, and current treatments for restenosis have limited success and include PTCA, CABG and atherectomy. Other potential treatments have been investigated, including targeting the thrombus that forms following PTCA.

Trials such as the EMPAR study (Cairns et al., 1996), the FACT study (Lablanche et al., 1997) and the ERA trial (Faxon et al., 1994) have used various anticoagulants post surgery to inhibit thrombus formation; however, this approach does not appear to protect patients against the development of restenosis. Inhibition of the intimal hyperplasia of VSMCs is another approach that has been identified. Low-dose radiation administered to the site of PTCA has been shown significantly to inhibit intimal thickening in a dose-dependent manner (Waksman et al., 1995). Trials such as the PREVENT (Proliferation Reduction with Vascular Energy Trial) have shown that low-dose radiation therapy might play an important role in combination with other therapies in successfully treating restenosis (Raizner et al., 2000).

In-stent stenosis

The use of stents (expandable mesh-like scaffolds) as a method to hold a balloon-dilated vessel lumen open following PTCA has increased substantially in recent years. Indeed, it was estimated that approximately one million stents were to be used in PTCA procedures in 1999 in the UK (Sigwart, 1999). Approximately 50–90% of PTCA procedures are followed by intracoronary stenting, depending on the clinical centre, and in 1996, of the 20 500 PTCA procedures carried out in the UK, half were followed by stenting (Gandhi and Dawkins, 1999). A number of major clinical benefits are gained from coronary stenting following PTCA, such as an increased luminal diameter, limited vascular recoil, reduced vascular remodelling and a smoother coronary lumen than angioplasty alone (Gandhi and Dawkins, 1999). Stents are usually metallic in composition, and form a mesh-like network that maintains a constant outward pressure on the wall of the lumen (Kraiss and Clowes, 1997). Despite benefiting the clinical outcome of PTCA procedures (restenosis rates are reduced to 15–25% of interventions when a stent is used), the effectiveness of stents is greatly reduced by the formation of in-stent stenosis, especially when multiple stents are used (Kraiss and Clowes, 1997). Indeed, the number of patients presenting with in-stent stenosis is increasing such that more than 20% of patients who receive a stent are likely to be affected within 3–6 months of treatment. One of the major mechanisms responsible for in-stent stenosis is hyperproliferation of VSMCs that probably accounts for more than 99% of cases.

Current medical treatments for in-stent stenosis

In-stent stenosis is notoriously difficult to treat. The aim of current therapies has been to prevent the uncontrolled proliferation of VSMCs in the intimal layer. A number of approaches have been taken such as the use of radioactive stents that reduce the ability of cells to divide. Trials such as the BETA WRIST (Washington Radiation for In-Stent restenosis Trial) (Waksman *et al.*, 2000) have shown that beta radiation slows down the rate of clinical in-stent stenosis. Antiproliferative agents such as angiopeptin also have been shown to reduce in-stent stenosis significantly by inhibiting neointimal hyperplasia.

Other approaches have looked at coating stents with non-thrombogenic materials, such as phosphorylcholine, resulting in a decline of in-stent stenosis rates by 20% (Sigwart, 1999).

Gene therapy for restenosis and in-stent stenosis

Undoubtedly, more research is needed before an effective therapy can be found to treat restenosis and in-stent stenosis. The following section will overview a variety of molecules that have been targeted by gene therapy to control this phenomenon.

Targeting the cell cycle machinery

The expressions and activities of specific cell cycle regulatory molecules recently have been targeted in VSMCs in an attempt to control restenosis. One of the first molecules to be targeted in this way was the retinoblastoma (Rb) protein (see Figure 6.3). In an experiment carried out by Chang *et al.* (1995), cDNA encoding a mutant form of the Rb protein was transferred into damaged rodent and porcine arteries *in vivo*. This mutant form of the protein could not be inhibited by phosphorylation and so constantly maintained an inhibitory activity on cellular growth. Expression of this mutant Rb protein led to a decrease in the intima-to-media (I/M) ratio by 42% and 47% in rat and porcine arteries, respectively.

In another experiment, Chang *et al.* (1995) infected injured rat carotid arteries with an adenoviral vector encoding the cyclin dependent kinase inhibitor (CDKI) gene, *p21*. When overexpressed *in vivo*, *p21* reduced the I/M ratio by 46% at 20 days post injury compared with control values. Furthermore, VSMCs were arrested in the G_0/G_1 phase of the cell cycle in *p21*-treated vessels.

Luo *et al.* (1999) performed a similar experiment to that described above but used lower titres of adenoviral *p21*. They observed reduced intimal thickening by 58% in a rat model of balloon injury compared with control animals.

Overexpression of the CDK inhibitory protein in balloon-injured rat carotid arteries also reduced the I/M ratio by 49% (Chen *et al.*, 1997).

All of these studies demonstrate that restenosis is slowed down significantly by overexpressing negative regulators of the cell cycle and they highlight the potential importance of targeting cell cycle molecules for the treatment of restenosis.

Morishita *et al.* (1995) showed that E2F transcription factors play a role in the development of certain cardiovascular diseases and that benefits could be gained by inhibiting their action. In this study, the activity of E2F in VSMCs was blocked using a double-stranded 14-mer oligonucleotide that had E2F-binding sites. Quiescent VSMCs were stimulated with serum, and gel shift analyses performed to show an increase in E2F–DNA binding activity. Following transfection of the cells with E2F decoy, this binding was abolished and led to a decrease in proliferation of the cells, as well as a decrease in the expression of E2F-dependent genes, namely c-*myc*, *cdc2* and *PCNA*, as determined by RT-PCR. These results were in contrast to those obtained with a missense decoy oligonucleotide that did not have sequences that would allow E2F to bind, which showed no reduction in growth or in the induction of these genes. Further experiments looked at the effects of the E2F decoy in balloon-injured rat carotid arteries. In accordance with the *in vitro* studies, there was a marked decrease in c-*myc*, *cdc2* and *PCNA* mRNA expressions.

Interestingly, the inhibitory effects of the E2F decoy on neo-intimal growth were maintained for up to eight weeks following transfection and the effect was shown to be dose-dependent.

Recently, Mann *et al.* (1999) reported the encouraging results of a phase I clinical trial (PREVENT) using an E2F decoy oligonucleotide in patients who had undergone bypass surgery. Autologous vein grafts are prone to neo-intimal hyperplasia due to changes in systemic blood pressures at their new site and this commonly leads to rejection of the vein within 12 months of grafting. Mann *et al.* (1999) investigated the effects of blocking the activity of the transcription factor E2F-1 with a 14-mer E2F decoy oligodeoxynucleotide. A total of 41 patients were recruited into this trial, 16 of whom were not given any gene therapy, 17 patients received the E2F decoy nucleotide and 17 received a scrambled oligonucleotide sequence.

The surgical procedure involved harvesting viable veins from the patients in order to replace damaged infra-inguinal atherosclerosed veins. Prior to these veins being transferred into the patient, they were transfected with the oligonucleotide sequences under 300 mmHg pressure. Control veins were handled similarly without oligonucleotide transfection. This method led to a transfection efficiency of 89% and the inhibition of the expression of E2F-regulated growth genes in grafted veins that received the E2F decoy compared with those transfected with the scrambled nucleotide sequence. Importantly, VSMC growth in the E2F decoy-transfected veins was reduced significantly compared with control and scrambled oligonucleotide-transfected veins. One month following treatment, 12 patients in the control group were found to have high-grade stenotic lesions whereas in the E2F decoy group, 3 out of 15 patients underwent revision and none had a critical stenosis at 12 months.

Promoting cell death

It has been well documented that DNA and general cellular damage can induce *p53*-mediated apoptosis or cell death. Yonemitsu *et al.* (1998) showed that by delivering *p53* to areas of balloon-injured carotid arteries in rabbits, intimal thickness could be decreased significantly. Cell proliferation and differentiation also were shown to be impaired.

Scheinman *et al.* (1999) also showed that neo-intimal thickening could be reduced in a dose-dependent manner by delivering wild-type *p53* via an adenoviral vector. Intimal thickness was reduced by 47%, 51% and 96% with increasing doses of the adenoviral-delivered vector $(8 \times 10^9, 1.6 \times 10^{10}$ and 8×10^{10} pfu/ml, respectively) thereby demonstrating that the promotion of apoptosis in VSMCs by gene therapy can limit the formation of restenosis.

Inhibition of intracellular signal transducers

Ras and Raf are serine/threonine kinases that are activated following mitogenic stimulation by growth factors, e.g. platelet-derived growth factor (PDGF). They promote the release of transcription factors in the nucleus through a cascade of interactions with other molecules. Cioffi *et al.* (1997) constructed antisense oligonucleotides to A-Ras and C-Raf and inhibited the proliferation of VSMCs *in vitro*.

A dominant-negative construct of H-ras was created by Ueno *et al.* (1997). Hyperplasia of the intimal layer was reduced by 81% after delivery of this construct to balloon-injured rat carotid arteries.

Nitric oxide

Nitric oxide (NO) has important functions in the vascular system since it prevents the adhesion of platelets to the vessel wall and to other cell types as well as inhibiting VSMC proliferation. NO is normally produced by endothelial cells, but following balloon injury the endothelial layer is often damaged, resulting in loss of NO production. This can be overcome by delivering endothelial nitric oxide synthase (eNOS) gene to the damaged vessels, allowing NO to be synthesised again and the protective effect returned. This approach was described by von der Layen *et al.* (1995), who used hemagglutinating virus of Japan (HVJ) liposomes to deliver eNOS to balloon-injured rat carotid arteries. A 70% reduction in I/M ratio was observed using this approach.

Another enzyme that can produce NO is iNOS (inducible nitric oxide synthase). The advantages of using iNOS for producing NO are that it is not dependent on calcium and that levels are sustained. Studies have been carried out in which iNOS has been introduced at sites of injury and shown to inhibit intimal hyperplasia. Shears *et al.* (1998) infected rat carotid arteries with iNOS using an adenovirus, leading to a 97% reduction in intimal hyperplasia.

Stroke: prevalence and mortality

As stated above, cardiovascular disease is the leading cause of death in the UK, accounting for well over 250 000 or 40% of all deaths in 1998 (Petersen *et al.*, 2000). After CHD, stroke is the most prominent cause of death, leading, in 1998, to more than 65 000 (about a quarter) of all deaths reported in the UK (Petersen *et al.*, 2000). In the United States, about 600 000 people suffer from stroke annually (or one person every 53 seconds!) of whom approximately one quarter die as a direct result (Cromie, 2000; American Stroke Association, 2000). Overall, stroke is the third leading cause of death in industrialised countries and is the major cause of long-term disability (American Stroke Association, 2000).

Types of stroke

The World Health Organization has defined stroke as 'an acute neurological dysfunction of vascular origin with sudden (within seconds) or at least rapid (within hours) occurrence of symptoms and signs corresponding to the involvement of a focal region of the brain' (World Health Organization, 1989). If the symptoms of stroke disappear within 24 hours, the stroke is termed a transient ischaemic attack (TIA); however, if the signs and symptoms persist for longer, the event is termed a 'complete stroke' (Reynolds, 1996). Stroke is broadly categorised into two groups: ischaemic and haemorrhagic stroke.

Ischaemic stroke

More than 80% of all strokes are due to ischaemic stroke (Rosamond *et al.*, 1999) which occurs as a consequence of blockage of a major artery supplying the brain (Figure 6.6). This usually is initiated by either a thrombus (a stationary clot formed in a blood vessel) or, more commonly, when an embolus (a clot that is formed elsewhere but travels through the bloodstream) becomes lodged in a cerebral artery that already has been narrowed substantially due to atherosclerosis. Commonly, the blockage results in a TIA, that is a period of inadequate blood perfusion to the appropriate region of the brain, resulting in an acute episode of focal neurological deficits. This can lead to periods of dizziness, double vision, inability to speak or a sudden physical weakness, but usually lasts less than 24 hours and more commonly for only a few minutes. Patients suffering from a TIA are at a higher risk of suffering a complete stroke. Complete stroke occurs when there is a period of inadequate cerebral perfusion, depriving the brain of glucose and oxygen and leading to the death of brain cells. This can result in permanent neurological damage.

Haemorrhagic stroke (cerebral haemorrhage)

The reported incidence of this type of stroke is far lower than that for ischaemic stroke (less than 1 in 5 strokes have been reported to be haemorrhagic); however, it is fatal in about 38% of cases (compared with only 8% in ischaemic stroke) (Rosamond *et al.*, 1999). Correct diagnosis is vital since the underlying cause and treatment of cerebral haemorrhage is markedly different to that required for treatment of ischaemic stroke. Cerebral haemorrhagic stroke occurs as a result of bleeding in the brain and is secondary to subarachnoid haemorrhage (SAH) or to intracerebral haemorrhage. SAH usually occurs as a result of rupture of an aneurysm leading to bleeding into the fluid-filled subarachnoid space between the brain and the skull. Intracerebral haemorrhage is bleeding into the parenchyma of the brain and often occurs as a result of rupture of arteries due to chronic hypertension. This type of haemorrhage leads to production of a focal haematoma, leading to an increase in local pressure. This may cause further local bleeding and an increase in the haematoma size, resulting in local ischaemia.

Bleeding in the brain can either directly lead to death of adjacent brain cells, due to build-up of pressure in the area, or indirectly cause death as a result of the diminishing blood supply that hinders normal circulation to the affected region.

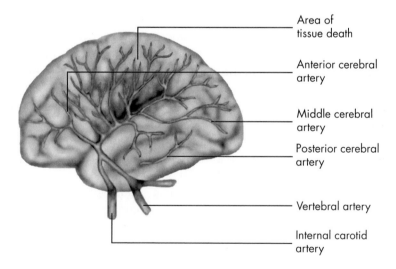

Figure 6.6 Diagram showing the major arteries supplying the brain. Blockage of these arteries can cause stroke (from Anon, 2000).

Diagnosis and current treatments for stroke

Diagnosis

As mentioned earlier, the correct diagnosis of the type of stroke is very important since the treatment for one form is quite different to treatment of the other. For instance, in haemorrhagic stroke the aim is to minimise further haemorrhage, which can be achieved by promoting clotting of blood; however, this treatment could be detrimental, and even fatal, if the stroke is ischaemic in nature, since further clotting would contribute to the progression of ischaemia (Reynolds, 1996).

The clinical manifestation and symptoms of stroke are wide ranging and dependent on the site of haemorrhage or infarction and the part of the brain affected. Neurological symptoms include impairment of speech, balance, vision, movement and touch sensation. Haemorrhagic stroke usually occurs suddenly and the subsequent increase in the intracranial pressure leads to typical symptoms, including severe headache, vomiting and rapid loss of consciousness. However, it is far more difficult to distinguish between mild to moderate haemorrhagic stroke and ischaemic stroke purely based on clinical symptoms. Use of a computerised tomography (CT) scan greatly assists in correct diagnosis and enables the two major types of stroke to be distinguished (Reynolds, 1996).

Current treatments

Antiplatelet agents, such as aspirin (which also inhibits thromboxane A_2), and intravenous administration of the anticoagulant heparin have been widely prescribed to treat the after-effects of ischaemic stroke, to prevent thrombus formation and hence decrease the size of the infarct. Although the therapeutic benefits of these agents have not yet been fully evaluated, results from two large independent clinical trials have played a major role in defining current treatments administered to patients who have suffered this type of stroke (International Stroke Trial Collaborative Group, 1997; CAS Trial Collaborative Group, 1997). These trials demonstrate that the use of aspirin in early ischaemic stroke produces a small, but real, reduction of nine deaths or recurrent strokes per 1000 patients treated for the first few weeks (CAS Trial Collaborative Group, 1997). However, results from these trials did not provide conclusive evidence that heparin administration produces any net long-term clinical benefit when used early in acute stroke (Sandercock and Counsell, 1997).

Other current treatments include use of thrombolytics, such as streptokinase, to dissolve existing thrombi. However, results from three separate clinical trials using this drug were disappointing and the investigations had to be terminated early due to intracranial bleeding and increased mortality in the treatment group (Reynolds, 1996). Calcium channel blockers, such as nimodipine, have been shown to be effective in increasing cerebral blood flow (American Nimodipine Study Group, 1992).

Some therapeutic benefit might be provided by reducing the influx of calcium into neurons and hence the subsequent damage by administration of N-methyl-D-aspartate (NMDA) receptor antagonists such as ketamine. Other treatments currently under investigation are use of oxpentifylline, a drug that decreases the viscosity of blood; the prostaglandin epoprostenol, thought to inhibit a specific stage in the ischaemic cascade; and monosialogangliosides, such as GM-1 ganglioside, that are believed to reduce neurotoxicity due to excitatory amino acids. In addition, opioid antagonists such as naloxone have been used, as it has been argued that the release of endorphin neurotransmitters during acute ischaemic stroke contributes to membrane damage (Reynolds, 1996).

Other novel drugs, yet to be approved by the FDA, might offer additional therapeutic benefits. In a clinical trial named PROACT II, recombinant prourokinase (a clot-dissolver), proved effective for patients suffering from severe stroke as a result of blockage of the middle cerebral artery, even when administered 6 hours post onset of symptoms (3 hours being the golden therapeutic window) (Furlan et al., 1999). In yet another clinical trial (Sherman et al., 2000) involving 500 patients, there was a 24% improvement in recovery from stroke in patients administered a clot-dissolving drug called ancrod, derived from the venom of the pit viper, compared with patients given an inactive substance (Furlan et al., 1999). Current treatment for haemorrhagic stroke is dependent upon whether the damage is in the subarachnoid or intracerebral region (Figure 6.6). Thus, for SAH, it is important to maintain the plasma volume to prevent cerebral ischaemia by increasing the fluid intake to around 3 l/day (Reynolds, 1996). Calcium channel blockers, such as nimodipine, also are commonly administered. Other treatments that have proved beneficial include administration of a lipid peroxidation inhibitor, trilazad (Reynolds, 1996). The use of antifibrinolytic drug therapy, such as tranexamic acid, has been shown to reduce the risk of re-bleeding, although the overall outcome was not much improved (van Gijn and Rinkel, 2001).

In the case of intracerebral haemorrhage, it is vital to reduce systolic blood pressure to below 170 mmHg, by using drugs such as β-receptor blockers, e.g. labetalol. Surgical drainage of the haematoma also is carried out to minimise intracranial pressure (Reynolds, 1996).

Gene therapy for stroke

Gene therapy offers the possibility of introducing genes, and therefore restoring function, into host cells where there is a mutation in that particular gene (see Chapter 1). However, one must bear in mind that stroke and other cardiovascular diseases are not single gene disorders. If this were the case, as in cystic fibrosis, the introduction of the mutated/ defective gene would provide a good chance for recovery from the disease. However, by identifying the genes that are associated with an increased risk of stroke, gene therapy could potentially improve prognosis for patients by decreasing the severity of symptoms and could even prevent the occurrence of stroke.

The adult brain is a fully differentiated organ and it generally is accepted that, except in specific regions, it lacks the regenerative capacity of some other organs of the body, such as the liver or skin. Neurogenesis in the brain has been reported only to occur in the subventricular zone (SVZ), in the wall of the lateral ventricle where new interneurons are generated for the olfactory bulb, and also in the subgranular zone of the dentate gyrus, giving rise to granule neurons (Bjorklund and Lindvall, 2000). This apparent lack of neurogenesis in other regions of the brain, such as the neurocortex, is pernicious, since necrosis of neurons in this region occurs as a result of stroke or inadequate blood supply to the cerebrum, leading to permanent damage. This lack of neurogenesis is most likely due to an arrest in the cell cycle of these cells. Hence, it might be possible to re-initiate the proliferative capacity of these neurons by modulating the expression of specific genes that regulate the cell cycle machinery in such cells. Interestingly, Magavi and collaborators recently reported that, in the neurocortex of the adult mouse, there is a continuous formation of new non-neuronal cells (Magavi *et al.*, 2000). When these investigators destroyed a subset of pyramidal neurons, they observed that 1–2% of new cells in the damaged neurocortex were neurons. These results raise the exciting possibility that the brain has the latent capacity for self-repair; however, the limited neurogenic response and the lack of evidence for functional recovery requires further investigation (Magavi *et al.*, 2000).

Gene transfer into the brain

Cerebral vasospasm, which occurs following haemorrhagic stroke, contributes immensely to the morbidity and mortality of patients. Delivery of genes that could aid vasodilatory function to the cerebral blood vessels, could prove useful in the treatment, or even prevention, of cerebral vasospasm. Muhonen *et al.* (1997) showed that delivery of a recombinant adenovirus via intracisternal injection was a possible route of gene delivery into the brain and demonstrated that the subarachnoid blood did not prevent transgene expression. These investigators used a double-haemorrhage intracranial-injection model to induce vasospasm in mongrel dogs. Their findings showed that intracisternal injection of a recombinant adenovirus expressing the β-galactosidase reporter gene resulted in expression of β-galactosidase in the cerebral blood vessels, cortex and the overlying meninges, even in the presence of cisternal blood (Muhonen *et al.*, 1997). This suggests that gene therapy in the brain may be a viable approach for the treatment of neurological disorders such as stroke.

Genes involved in stroke

Table 6.2 summarises some of the genes proposed to be involved in stroke.

Cyclin-dependent kinases (CDKs) as therapeutic targets for stroke

Cell cycle progression is controlled in a careful and orderly manner by a series of cell cycle-dependent molecules in both a positive and negative manner (see Figure 6.3) (Brooks and La Thangue, 1999). The positive regulators of the cell cycle are composed of complexes formed between a regulatory subunit, named a cyclin, and its respective CDK, and they promote progression of the cell cycle and proliferation. Distinct CDKs regulate the progression of different phases of the cell cycle (see Figure 6.3). The negative regulators exert their effect by binding specifically to various cyclin–CDK complexes. The cyclin–CDK heterodimers in the G_0/G_1 phase of the cell cycle, specifically CDK4/6–cyclin D1, exert their function through the phosphorylation of various members of the pocket protein family, such as pRb and p107. Following hyperphosphorylation of pRb/p107 by these CDKs, their repression of a family of transcription factors called E2F is abrogated. The release of 'free E2F' leads to the transcription of genes that are necessary for progression of the cell cycle.

Table 6.2 Genes implicated as potential therapeutic targets in stroke and their likely mode of action

Defective/ targeted gene	Possible mechanism	Animal model/ studied species	References
G$_1$/S phase cell cycle molecules	Inhibit cell cycle progression	Rats Mice	Osuga et al., 2000 Macmanus et al., 1999
ANP	Lowers blood pressure	Rats Human	Rubattu et al., 1999a Rubattu et al., 1999b; Lin et al., 1999
eNOS	Relaxation of cerebral arteries	Dogs	Reynolds, 1996
IL-1ra	Inhibits IL-1 receptor	Rat Mice	Betz et al. 1995; Relton and Rothwell, 1992 Yang et al., 1997
NAIP	Protects against neuronal apoptosis	Rat	Xu et al., 1997
hFIX	Regulates blood coagulation capacity	Human	Kurachi et al. 1999; Kurachi and Kurachi, 2000

Interestingly, it has been reported that CDKs might have functions beyond regulating the progression of the cell cycle, and there is evidence suggesting that a signalling pathway involving CDKs could play a role in the death of neurons evoked by ischaemia (Osuga et al., 2000). Thus, Osuga et al. (2000) induced focal cerebral ischaemia in rats by occluding the middle cerebral artery, followed by an immediate occlusion of both common carotid arteries for 30 minutes, prior to reperfusion. These authors also examined the effect of flavopiridol, a CDK inhibitor, by administering the drug to a subset of rats, 24 hours prior to focal cerebral ischaemia. The results showed that activation of the CDK4/6–pRb pathway occurred in dying neurons adjacent to the focal ischaemia and that intracerebroventricular administration of flavopiridol dramatically decreased both the infarction volume and the number of dead cells as indicated by a positive TUNEL (Terminal deoxynucleotidyl transferase biotin-dUTP Nick End Labeling) test. It was concluded that activation of CDKs, especially CDK4/6, is required for the death of adult neurons in this *in vivo* model of ischaemia-induced stroke. Additional evidence confirms the role of this pathway in neuronal death. Earlier reports by the same group demonstrated that dominant negative DP-1, the hetero-dimeric partner of E2Fs, protects against neuronal death (Osuga *et al.*, 2000). It also has been reported that the average infarct volume in E2F–/– homozygous mice was on average 24% less than that in E2F+/– heterozygous mice that received the same ischaemic insult (Macmanus *et al.*, 1999). Additionally, cultured neurons of E2F-1-deficient mice have been reported to be resistant to death by β-amyloid and to ischaemic damage (Osuga *et al.*, 2000).

Altogether, these results indicate that a CDK-mediated pathway might play a significant role in neuronal death caused by ischaemic stroke, and further research might offer potential therapeutic targets for the treatment of stroke-induced neuronal injury. Gene therapy could offer a novel therapeutic approach, if the specific genes that play a crucial role in stroke are identified. In such cases, either dominant negative constructs, decoy oligonucleotides or even deleted mutants of a particular gene (e.g. CDK4/6, E2F, DP or pRb) could be targeted to neurons to offer protection against the deleterious effects of stroke.

Atrial natriuretic peptide (ANP)

ANP is a hormone that lowers blood pressure by relaxing blood vessels and increasing excretion of sodium ions. Rubattu and colleagues (1999a,b) identified two point mutations in the regulatory and coding regions of this gene in stroke-prone, spontaneously hypertensive rats (SPSHR) compared with stroke-resistant, spontaneously hypertensive rats (SHR). Additionally, a lower brain ANP expression was reported in the SPSHRs compared with the SHRs in the absence of any differences in blood pressure (Rubattu *et al.*, 1999a).

In a separate study, the same group took advantage of the Physicians Health Study (1989), which has been ongoing since 1982, and selected 696 participants, 348 of whom had suffered from strokes. They identified a molecular variant of the ANP gene which was responsible for a valine to methionine substitution in the pro-ANP peptide. This mutation was strongly associated with the occurrence of stroke. Together with the results obtained from the animal model study of stroke-prone rats (Rubattu *et al.*, 1999a), these authors suggested that molecular variants of ANP might represent an independent risk factor for cerebrovascular accidents in humans (Rubattu *et al.*, 1999b).

Lin and colleagues (1999) investigated delivery of the ANP gene via the adenovirus route into salt-sensitive rats and reported that three weeks after delivery of this gene, only 17% of rats died of stroke compared with 54% of control animals. Although this 69% reduction in stroke deaths seems encouraging, it was not a long-term effect since the transformed viruses were ejected from the body (Lin *et al.*, 1999).

eNOS

The relaxation mediated by nitric oxide synthase in cerebral arteries has been shown to be impaired as a result of SAH (Faraci and Brian, 1994). Onoue *et al.* (1998) investigated the effects of delivering the recombinant endothelial nitric oxide synthase (eNOS) gene, using adenovirus-mediated gene transfer, into canine basilar artery following experimental SAH (Onoue *et al.*, 1998). These investigators obtained rings of basilar arteries from control dogs and dogs exposed to SAH and incubated them with replication-deficient adenovirus vectors encoding both bovine eNOS and *E. coli* β-galactosidase. Twenty-four hours later, the expression and function of the recombinant gene was examined using immuno-histochemical staining and β-galactosidase protein measurements. eNOS function was determined by measuring isometric tension in the isolated rings. The results of this study suggested that the expression of the recombinant proteins was increased in cerebral arteries, affected by SAH and that local production of nitric oxide led to at least a partial restoration of the NO-dependent relaxation (Onoue *et al.*, 1998). Although these results appear encouraging, further research is required to determine whether delivery of the recombinant eNOS gene can enhance NOS relaxation in cerebral arteries in an *in vivo* model and, if so, whether it can decrease the detrimental effects of haemorrhagic stroke.

Interleukin 1 receptor antagonist protein (IL-1ra)

It has been reported that the occlusion of the middle cerebral artery in rats leads to overexpression of interleukin 1 (IL-1) (Touzani *et al.*, 1999) and direct injection of interleukin 1 receptor antagonist protein (IL-1ra) into the cerebral ventricles has been shown to attenuate ischaemic injury in the brain (Relton and Rothwell, 1992). Betz *et al.* (1995) investigated the effects of adenovirus-mediated overexpression of IL-1ra on the extent of ischaemic brain injury in a rat model of stroke (Betz *et al.*, 1995). They used a replication-deficient recombinant adenovirus vector carrying the human cDNA for IL-1ra to examine whether brain injury could be attenuated in rats that had undergone permanent focal ischaemia. Although the route of administration of vector was via intraventricular injection, these authors achieved an effective concentration of IL-1ra in brain and cerebrospinal fluid. The cerebral infarct volume of a group of six rats that had undergone 24 hours of permanent middle cerebral artery occlusion was reduced by 64% in animals that had received recombinant adenovirus carrying the IL-1ra compared with other groups that received either a saline injection or a recombinant adenovirus carrying the β-galactosidase gene (Betz *et al.*, 1995).

In a separate study, this same group used a recombinant adenovirus vector to deliver the cDNA encoding human IL-1ra to the brains of control mice and mice suffering from brain oedema formation and infarction after permanent focal ischaemia (Yang *et al.*, 1997). Using an immunoassay procedure, these authors confirmed successful over-expression of IL-1ra protein in the brains of mice 5 days after injection with IL-1ra recombinant adenovirus compared with control mice that were injected with saline alone (the expression of IL-1ra protein was sustained in the experimental group up to 13 days post injection – the last time point of the experiment). On the fifth day following injection, the middle cerebral artery was occluded for 24 hours and the occurrence of oedema was confirmed by determining the brain:water content and histology to obtain a quantitative value for infarct size. The results indicated a significant decrease in brain oedema and also cerebral infarct volume in mice injected 5 days earlier with recombinant vector carrying the IL-1ra cDNA compared with vector carrying just a β-galactosidase gene or injected with saline alone. They concluded that adenoviral vectors are effective vectors for gene therapy for stroke and, importantly, provided further evidence for the role played by IL-1 in cerebral ischaemia (Yang *et al.*, 1997).

Neuronal apoptosis inhibitory protein (NAIP)

Xu and his collaborators (1997) examined the role of the protein neuronal apoptosis inhibitory protein (NAIP) in protecting against ischaemic brain damage (Xu *et al.*, 1997). NAIP inhibits apoptosis in a number of cell lines and its overexpression has been shown to protect against apoptotic death induced by a variety of triggers (Liston *et al.*, 1996). Xu *et al.* (1997) demonstrated that in a rat model of induced transient forebrain ischaemia, the levels of this protein were elevated 'selectively' in the neurons of rats that were particularly resistant to the injurious effects of this treatment. To examine whether the elevated levels of NAIP may provide some protection against ischaemic brain damage, the endogenous levels of neuronal NAIP were increased using two different methods and the level of ischaemic brain damage examined in such animals compared with animals with endogenous levels of NAIP. Both methods of induction of NAIP protein, via either intracerebral injection of an adenovirus vector carrying the NAIP gene or administration of the bacterial alkaloid K252a, resulted in a significant reduction in observed ischaemic damage in the rat hippocampus (Xu et al., 1997). The results of this study suggest that delivery of the NAIP gene might prove a useful approach for treatment of, or protection from, ischaemic brain damage.

Other potential candidate genes involved in stroke

Recently, other novel genes have been identified that might play a role in the susceptibility or occurrence of stroke. One group of such candidate genes are genetic elements involved in the regulation of the human blood coagulation factor IX (hFIX) gene. The clotting ability in humans increases rapidly soon after birth and continues during development. Coagulation capacity of the newborn is only 40–45% that of a young adult and it continues to increase during adulthood, until by old age it is almost twice as high as that in a young adult (Sweeney and Hoernig, 1993). Kurachi and his collaborators (1999) have studied the genetic mechanism of age-regulation of hFIX. They identified two critical age-regulated genetic elements, AE5' and AE3', near to, and within, the gene for hFIX. These two elements function together to produce the steady increase in the capacity of blood to coagulate and help to explain the molecular mechanism involved in this process (Kurachi and Kurachi, 2000).

Further studies are required to determine whether a mutation in these genetic elements leads to an increased susceptibility to stroke and also whether it would be feasible to modulate the age-related clotting ability in humans, by manipulation of these genetic elements, to attenuate the risk of stroke in susceptible populations.

Summary and conclusions

In summary, research into the use of gene therapy for the treatment of cardiovascular diseases is ever growing. In this chapter we have highlighted some exciting advances that have been made in this field that in some instances have already provided great benefits for patients' health where conventional therapy had not been successful. It is clear that there has been more success in treating diseases of the vascular system than for myocardial disease. For example, treatment of ischaemic heart disease with FGF and VEGF has already proved to be very beneficial for human volunteers when conventional therapy has not worked. Due to the growth characteristics of myocytes, treatment of myocardial diseases with a gene therapy approach poses more of a challenge to researchers. However, advances in gene delivery technology will ultimately allow us to deploy effective therapies to their site of action in the myocardium and enable us overcome this obstacle. The future use of gene therapy in the cardiovascular system seems evermore feasible with an enormous potential for treating and, more importantly, curing conditions that will affect the majority of humans.

References

Agah R, Kirshenbaum L A, Abdellatif M, *et al.* (1997) Adenoviral delivery of E2F-1 directs cell cycle reentry and p53-independent apoptosis in postmitotic adult myocardium *in vivo. J Clin Invest* 100: 2722–2728.

American Heart Association (2000) International cardiovascular disease statistics. http://www.americanheart.org/statistics/cvd.html (accessed May 2000).

American Nimodipine Study Group (1992) Clinical trial of nimodipine in acute ischaemic stroke. *Stroke* 23(1): 3–8.

American Stroke Association (2000) American Stroke Association home page. http://www.strokeassociation.org/ (accessed May 2000).

Anon (2000) Stroke. http://onhealth.com/conditions/resource/conditions/item,47570.asp (accessed on 30th June 2000).

Ascherio A, Rimm E B, Giovannucci E L, *et al.* (1996) Dietary fat and risk of coronary heart disease in men: cohort follow up study in the United States. *BMJ* 313: 84–90.

Bauters C (1997) Growth factors as a potential new treatment for ischemic heart disease. *Clin Cardiol* 20 (Suppl. 2): II-52–57.

Bern R M, Levy M N (1993) *The Cardiovascular System.* St Louis: Mosby.

Betz, A L, Yang G Y, Davidson B L (1995) Attenuation of stroke size in rats using an adenoviral vector to induce overexpression of interleukin-1 receptor antagonist in brain. *J Cereb Blood Flow Metab* 15: 547–551.

Bjorklund A, Lindvall O (2000) Self-repair in the brain. *Nature* 405: 892–895.

British National Formulary (2000) *British National Formulary.* London: British Medical Association, Royal Pharmaceutical Society of Great Britain.

Brooks G, La Thangue N B (1999) The cell cycle and drug discovery: the promise and the hope. *Drug Discov Today* 4: 455–464.

Brooks G, Poolman R A, McGill C J, Li J M (1997) Expression and activities of cyclins and cyclin-dependent kinases in developing rat ventricular myocytes. *J Mol Cell Cardiol* 29: 2261–2271.

Brousseau M E, Kauffman R D, Herderick E E, *et al.* (2000) LCAT modulates atherogenic plasma lipoproteins and the extent of atherosclerosis only in the presence of normal LDL receptors in transgenic rabbits. *Arterioscler Thromb Vasc Biol* 20: 450–458.

Buttrick P M, Kass A, Kitsis R N, *et al.* (1992) Behavior of genes directly injected into the rat heart *in vivo*. *Circ Res* 70: 193–198.

Cairns J A, Gill J, Morton B, *et al.* (1996) Fish oils and low-molecular-weight heparin for the reduction of restenosis after percutaneous transluminal coronary angioplasty. The EMPAR Study. *Circulation* 94: 1553–1560.

Carmeliet P (2000) Fibroblast growth factor-1 stimulates branching and survival of myocardial arteries: a goal for therapeutic angiogenesis? *Circ Res* 87: 176–178.

CAS Trial Collaborative Group (1997) CAST: randomised placebo-controlled trial of early aspirin use in 20 000 patients with acute ischaemic. *Lancet* 349(9066): 1641–1649.

Chang M W, Barr E, Seltzer J, *et al.* (1995) Cytostatic gene therapy for vascular proliferative disorders with a constitutively active form of the retinoblastoma gene product. *Science* 267: 518–522.

Chen D, Krasinski K, Sylvester A, *et al.* (1997) Downregulation of cyclin-dependent kinase 2 activity and cyclin A promoter activity in vascular smooth muscle cells by p27(KIP1), an inhibitor of neointima formation in the rat carotid artery. *J Clin Invest* 99: 2334–2341.

Cioffi C L, Garay M, Johnston J F, *et al.* (1997) Selective inhibition of A-Raf and C-Raf mRNA expression by antisense oligodeoxynucleotides in rat vascular smooth muscle cells: role of A-Raf and C-Raf in serum-induced proliferation. *Mol Pharmacol* 51: 383–389.

Cooper R, Cutler J, Desvigne-Nickens P (2000) Trends and disparities in coronary heart disease, stroke, and other cardiovascular diseases in the United States: findings of the national conference on cardiovascular disease prevention. *Circulation (Online)* 102: 3137–3147.

Cromie W J (2000) Gene linked to stroke is found. *The Harvard University Gazette*.

Crossman D (1997) The future of the management of ischaemic heart disease. *BMJ* 314: 356–359.

Dargie H J, McMurray J J (1994) Diagnosis and management of heart failure. *BMJ* 308: 321–328.

Desurmont C., Caillaud J M, Emmanuel F, *et al.* (2000) Complete atherosclerosis regression after human ApoE gene transfer in ApoE-deficient/nude mice. *Arterioscler Thromb Vasc Biol* 20: 435–442.

Dostal D E, Baker K M (1999). The cardiac renin-angiotensin system: conceptual, or a regulator of cardiac function? *Circ Res* 85: 643–650.

Eizema K, Fechner H, Bezstarosti K, *et al.* (2000) Adenovirus-based phospholamban antisense expression as a novel approach to improve cardiac contractile dysfunction: comparison of a constitutive viral versus an endothelin-1-responsive cardiac promoter. *Circulation* 101: 2193–2199.

Faraci F M, Brian J E (1994) Nitric oxide and the cerebral circulation. *Stroke* 25: 692–703.

Faxon D P, Spiro T E, Minor S, *et al.* (1994) Low molecular weight heparin in prevention of restenosis after angioplasty. Results of Enoxaparin Restenosis (ERA) Trial. *Circulation* 90: 908–914.

Fernandez B, Buehler A, Wolfram S, *et al.* (2000) Transgenic myocardial overexpression of fibroblast growth factor-1 increases coronary artery density and branching. *Circ Res* 87: 207–213.

Ferns G A, Avades T Y (2000) The mechanisms of coronary restenosis: insights from experimental models. *Int J Exp Pathol* 81: 63–88.

Frick M H, Elo O, Haapa K, Heinonen O P, *et al.* (1987) Helsinki Heart Study: primary-prevention trial with gemfibrozil in middle-aged men with dyslipidemia. Safety of treatment, changes in risk factors, and incidence of coronary heart disease. *N Engl J Med* 317: 1237–1245.

Furlan A, Higashida R, Wechsler L, *et al.* (1999) Intra-arterial prourokinase for acute ischemic stroke. The PROACT II study: a randomized controlled trial. Prolyse in Acute Cerebral Thromboembolism. *JAMA* 282: 2003–2011.

Gandhi M M, Dawkins K D (1999) Fortnightly review: intracoronary stents. *BMJ* 318: 650–653.

Gelband C H, Katovich M J, Raizada M K (2000) Current perspectives on the use of gene therapy for hypertension. *Circ Res* 87: 1118–1122.

Grace A A, Hall J A, Schofield P M (1993) *Cardiology*. Edinburgh: Churchill Livingstone.

Grundy S M, Balady J G, Criqui M H, *et al.* (1998) Primary prevention of coronary heart disease: guidance from Framingham: a statement for healthcare professionals from the AHA Task Force on Risk Reduction. American Heart Association. *Circulation* 97: 1876–1887.

Hajjar R J, del Monte F, Matsui T, Rosenzweig A (2000) Prospects for gene therapy for heart failure. *Circ Res* 86: 616–621.

Hasty A H, Linton M F, Brandt S J, *et al.* (1999) Retroviral gene therapy in ApoE-deficient mice: ApoE expression in the artery wall reduces early foam cell lesion formation. *Circulation* 99: 2571–2576.

Higaki J, Aoki M, Morishita R, *et al.* (2000) *In vivo* evidence of the importance of cardiac angiotensin-converting enzyme in the pathogenesis of cardiac hypertrophy. *Arterioscler Thromb Vasc Biol* 20: 428–434.

Hoeg J M, Santamarina-Fojo S, Berard A M, *et al.* (1996) Overexpression of lecithin: cholesterol acyltransferase in transgenic rabbits prevents diet-induced atherosclerosis. *Proc Natl Acad Sci USA* 93: 11448–11453.

International Stroke Trial Collaborative Group (1997) The International Stroke Trial (IST): a randomised trial of aspirin, subcutaneous heparin, both, or neither among 19 435 patients with acute ischaemic stroke. *Lancet* 349: 1569–1581.

Jeppesen J, Hein H O, Suadicani P, Gyntelberg F (1997) Relation of high TG-low HDL cholesterol and LDL cholesterol to the incidence of ischemic heart disease. An 8-year follow-up in the Copenhagen Male Study. *Arterioscler Thromb Vasc Biol* 17: 1114–1120.

Jousilahti P, Tuomilehto J, Vartiainen E, *et al.* (1996) Body weight, cardiovascular risk factors, and coronary mortality. 15-year follow-up of middle-aged men and women in eastern Finland. *Circulation* 93: 1372–1379.

Jousilahti P, Vartiainen E, Tuomilehto J, Puska P (1999) Sex, age, cardiovascular risk factors, and coronary heart disease: a prospective follow-up study of 14 786 middle-aged men and women in Finland. *Circulation* 99: 1165–1172.

Kiechl S, Willeit J (1999) The natural course of atherosclerosis. Part II: vascular remodeling. Bruneck Study Group. *Arterioscler Thromb Vasc Biol* 19: 1491–1498.

Kraiss L W, Clowes A W (1997) Response of the arterial wall to injury and intimal hyperplasia. In: Sidawy A N, Sumpio B E, DePalma R G, eds. *The Basic Science of Vascular Disease*. Armonk, New York: Futura Publishing Company Inc.

Kurachi K, Kurachi S (2000) Genetic mechanisms of age regulation of blood coagulation: factor IX model. *Arterioscler Thromb Vasc Biol* 20: 902–906.

Kurachi S, Deyashiki Y, Takeshita J, Kurachi K (1999) Genetic mechanisms of age regulation of human blood coagulation factor IX. *Science* 285: 739–743.

Lablanche J M, McFadden E P, Meneveau N, *et al.* (1997) Effect of nadroparin, a low-molecular-weight heparin, on clinical and angiographic restenosis after coronary balloon angioplasty: the FACT study. Fraxiparine Angioplastie Coronaire Transluminale. *Circulation* 96: 3396–3402.

Leiden J M (2000) Human gene therapy: the good, the bad, and the ugly. *Circ Res* 86: 923–925.

Li J M, Brooks G (1999) Cell cycle regulatory molecules (cyclins, cyclin-dependent kinases and cyclin-dependent kinase inhibitors) and the cardiovascular system; potential targets for therapy? *Eur Heart J* 20: 406–420.

Li J M, Poolman R A, Brooks G (1998) Role of G1 phase cyclins and cyclin-dependent kinases during cardiomyocyte hypertrophic growth in rats. *Am J Physiol* 275(3 Part 2): H814–822.

Lin H, Parmacek M S, Morle G, *et al.* (1990) Expression of recombinant genes in myocardium *in vivo* after direct injection of DNA. *Circulation* 82: 2217–2221.

Lin K F, Chao J, Chao L (1999) Atrial Natriuretic Peptide gene delivery reduces stroke-induced mortality rate in Dahl salt-sensitive rats. *Hypertension* 33(1 Part 2): 219–224.

Lip G Y, Gibbs C R, Beevers D G (2000) ABC of heart failure: aetiology. *BMJ* 320: 104–107.

Liston P, Roy N, Tamai K, *et al.* (1996) Suppression of apoptosis in mammalian cells by NAIP and a related family of IAP genes. *Nature* 379: 349–353.

Lloyd-Jones D M, Larson M G, Beiser A, Levy D (1999) Lifetime risk of developing coronary heart disease. *Lancet* 353: 89–92.

Lonn E, McKelvie R (2000) Drug treatment in heart failure. *BMJ* 320: 1188–1192.

Losordo D W, Vale P R, Symes J F (1998) Gene therapy for myocardial angiogenesis: initial clinical results with direct myocardial injection of phVEGF165 as sole therapy for myocardial ischemia. *Circulation* 98: 2800–2804.

Luo Z, Sata M, Nguyen T, *et al.* (1999) Adenovirus-mediated delivery of fas ligand inhibits intimal hyperplasia after balloon injury in immunologically primed animals. *Circulation* 99(14): 1776–1779.

Macmanus J P, Koch C J, Walker J M, Zurakowski B (1999) Decreased brain infarct following focal ischemia in mice lacking the transcription factor E2F1. *Neuroreport* 10: 2711–2714.

Magavi S S, Leavitt B R, Macklis J D (2000) Induction of neurogenesis in the neurocortex of adult mice. *Nature* 405: 951–955.

Mann M J, Whittemore A D, Donaldson M C, *et al.* (1999) *Ex-vivo* gene therapy of human vascular bypass grafts with E2F decoy: the PREVENT single-centre, randomised, controlled trial. *Lancet* 354: 1493–1498.

Morishita R, Gibbons G H, Horiuchi M, *et al.* (1995) A gene therapy strategy using a transcription factor decoy of the E2F binding site inhibits smooth muscle proliferation *in vivo*. *Proc Natl Acad Sci USA* 92: 5855–5859.

Motwani J G, Topol E J (1998) Aortocoronary saphenous vein graft disease: pathogenesis, predisposition, and prevention. *Circulation* 97: 916–931.

Muhonen M G, Ooboshi H, Welsh M J, *et al.* (1997) Gene transfer to cerebral blood vessels after subarachnoid hemorrhage. *Stroke* 28: 822–829.

Nabel E G (1995) Gene therapy for cardiovascular disease. *Circulation* 91: 541–548.

Nolan P E, Raehl J C L, Zarembski D G (1996) Congestive heart failure. In: Herfindal E T, Gourley D R, eds. *Textbook of Therapeutics: Drugs and Disease Management*. Philadelphia: Williams and Wilkins, 729–763.

Onoue H, Tsutsui M, Smith L, *et al.* (1998) Expression and function of recombinant endothelial nitric oxide synthase gene in canine basilar artery after experimental subarachnoid hemorrhage. *Stroke* 29: 1959–1966.

Osuga H, Osuga S, Wang F, *et al.* (2000) Cyclin-dependent kinases as a therapeutic target of stroke. *Proc Natl Acad Sci USA* 97: 10254–10259.

Pepine C J (1997) Potential role of angiotensin-converting enzyme inhibition in myocardial ischemia and current clinical trials. *Clin Cardiol* 20 (11 Suppl. 2): II-58–64.

Petersen S, Rayner M, Press V (2000) Coronary heart disease statistics, British Heart Foundation promotion research group. http: //www.dphpc.ox.ac.uk/bhfhprg/stats/2000/index.html (accessed May 2000).

Physicians' Health Study (1989) Final report on the aspirin component of the ongoing Physicians' Health Study. Steering Committee of the Physicians' Health Study Research Group. *N Engl J Med* 321: 129–135.

Plump A S, Scott C J, Breslow J L (1994) Human apolipoprotein A-I gene expression increases high density lipoprotein and suppresses atherosclerosis in the apolipoprotein E-deficient mouse. *Proc Natl Acad Sci USA* 91: 9607–9611.

Quinones M J, Leor J, Kloner R A, *et al.* (1996) Avoidance of immune response prolongs expression of genes delivered to the adult rat myocardium by replication-defective adenovirus. *Circulation* 94: 1394–1401.

Raizada M K, Katovich M J, Wang H, *et al.* (1999) Is antisense gene therapy a step in the right direction in the control of hypertension? *Am J Physiol* 277(2 Part 2): H423–432.

Raizner A E, Oesterle S N, Waksman R, *et al.* (2000) Inhibition of restenosis with beta-emitting radiotherapy: Report of the Proliferation Reduction with Vascular Energy Trial (PREVENT). *Circulation* 102: 951–958.

Relton J K, Rothwell N J (1992) Interleukin-1 receptor antagonist inhibits ischaemic and excitotoxic neuronal damage in the rat. *Brain Res Bull* 29: 243–246.

Reynolds J E F (1996) *Martindale: The Extra Pharmacopoeia*. London: Royal Pharmaceutical Society.

Rosamond W D, Folsom A R, Chambless L E, *et al.* (1999) Stroke incidence and survival among middle-aged adults: 9-year follow-up of the Atherosclerosis Risk in Communities (ARIC) cohort. *Stroke* 30: 736–743.

Rosengart T K, Lee L Y, Patel S R, *et al.* (1999) Angiogenesis gene therapy: phase I assessment of direct intramyocardial administration of an adenovirus vector expressing VEGF121 cDNA to individuals with clinically significant severe coronary artery disease. *Circulation* 100: 468–474

Ross R, Glomset J A (1976) The pathogenesis of atherosclerosis (first of two parts). *N Engl J Med* 295: 369–377.

Ross R (1993) The pathogenesis of atherosclerosis: a perspective for the 1990s. *Nature* 362: 801–809.

Rubattu S, Lee-Kirsch M A, DePaolis P, *et al.* (1999a) Altered structure, regulation and function of the gene encoding the Atrial Natriuretic Peptide in the stroke-prone spontaneously hypertensive rat. *Circ Res* 85: 900–905.

Rubattu S, Ridker P, Stampfer M J, *et al.* (1999b) The gene encoding Atrial Natriuretic Peptide and the risk of human stroke. *Circulation* 100: 1722–1726.

Sacks F M, Pfeffer M A, Moye L A, *et al.* (1996) The effect of pravastatin on coronary events after myocardial infarction in patients with average cholesterol levels. Cholesterol and Recurrent Events Trial investigators. *N Engl J Med* 14: 335: 1001–1009.

Safi J, DiPaula A F, Riccioni T, *et al.* (1999) Adenovirus-mediated acidic fibroblast growth factor gene transfer induces angiogenesis in the nonischemic rabbit heart. *Microvasc Res* 58: 238–249.

Sandercock P, Counsell C (1997) Interpretation of IST and CAST stroke trials. *Lancet* 350: 440–443.

Scheinman M, Ascher E, Levi G S, *et al.* (1999) p53 gene transfer to the injured rat carotid artery decreases neointimal formation. *J Vasc Surg* 29(2): 360–369.

Schmidt U, del Monte F, Miyamoto M I, *et al.* (2000) Restoration of diastolic function in senescent rat hearts through adenoviral gene transfer of sarcoplasmic reticulum Ca(2+)-ATPase. *Circulation* 101: 790–796.

Shears L L, Kibbe M R, Murdock A D, *et al.* (1998) Efficient inhibition of intimal hyperplasia by adenovirus-mediated inducible nitric oxide synthase gene transfer to rats and pigs in vivo. *J Am Coll Surg* 187(3): 295–306.

Shepherd J, Cobbe S M, Ford I, *et al.* (1995) Prevention of coronary heart disease with pravastatin in men with hypercholesterolemia. West of Scotland Coronary Prevention Study Group. *N Engl J Med* 333: 1301–1307.

Sherman D G, Atkinson R P, Chippendale T, *et al.* (2000) Intravenous ancrod for treatment of acute ischemic stroke: the STAT study: a randomized controlled trial. Stroke Treatment with Ancrod Trial. *JAMA* 283: 2395–2405.

Sigwart U (1999) Prevention of restenosis after stenting. *Lancet* 354: 269–270.

Simons M, Bonow R O, Chronos N A, *et al.* (2000) Clinical trials in coronary angiogenesis: issues, problems, consensus: an expert panel summary. *Circulation* 102: E73–86.

Sweeney J D, Hoernig LA (1993) Age-dependent effect on the level of factor IX. *Am J Clin Pathol* 99: 687–688.

Tang X, Mohuczy D, Zhang Y C, *et al.* (1999) Intravenous angiotensinogen antisense in AAV-based vector decreases hypertension. *Am J Physiol* 277 (6 Part 2): H2392–2399.

Touzani O, Boutin H, Chuquet J, Rothwell N (1999) Potential mechanisms of interleukin-1 involvement in cerebral ischaemia. *J Neuroimmunol* 100(1–2): 203–215.

Ueno H, Yamamoto H, Ito S, *et al.* (1997) Adenovirus-mediated transfer of a dominant-negative H-ras suppresses neointimal formation in balloon-injured arteries *in vivo. Arterioscler Thromb Vasc Biol* 17: 898–904.

van Gijn J J, Rinkel J G (2001) Subarachnoid haemorrhage: diagnosis, causes and management. *Brain* 124 (Part 2): 249–278.

von der Leyen H E, Gibbons G H, Morishita R *et al.* (1995) Gene therapy inhibiting neointimal vascular lesion: *in vivo* transfer of endothelial cell nitric oxide synthase gene. *Proc Natl Acad Sci USA* 92: 1137–1141.

von Harsdorf R., Li P F, Dietz R (1999) Signaling pathways in reactive oxygen species-induced cardiomyocyte apoptosis. *Circulation* 99: 2934–2941.

Waksman R, Robinson K A, Crocker I R, *et al.* (1995) Intracoronary low-dose beta-irradiation inhibits neointima formation after coronary artery balloon injury in the swine restenosis model. *Circulation* 92: 3025–3031.

Waksman R, Bhargava B, White L, *et al.* (2000) Intracoronary beta-radiation therapy inhibits recurrence of in-stent restenosis. *Circulation* 101: 1895–1898.

Walker J M, Tan L B (1997) Cardiovascular disease. In: Souhami R L, Moxham J, eds. *Textbook of Medicine*, 3rd edn. Edinburgh: Churchill Livingstone, 381–506.

Wang H, Katovich M J, Gelband C H, *et al.* (1999) Sustained inhibition of angiotensin I-converting enzyme (ACE) expression and long-term antihypertensive action by virally mediated delivery of ACE antisense cDNA. *Circ Res* 85: 614–622.

Wannamethee S G, Shaper A G, Walker M (2000) Physical activity and mortality in older men with diagnosed coronary heart disease. *Circulation* 102: 1358–1363.

Wei S K, Colecraft H M, DeMaria C D, *et al.* (2000) Ca^{2+} channel modulation by recombinant auxiliary beta subunits expressed in young adult heart cells. *Circ Res* 86: 175–184.

World Health Organization (1989) Stroke-1989, recommendations on stroke prevention, diagnosis, and therapy: report of the WHO task force on stroke and other cerebovascular disorders. *Stroke* 20: 1407–1431.

Xu D G, Crocker S J, Doucet J P, *et al.* (1997) Elevation of neuronal expression of NAIP reduces ischemic damage in the rat hippocampus. *Nat Med* 3: 997–1004.

Yang G Y, Zhao Y J, Davidson B L, Betz A L (1997) Overexpression of interleukin-1 receptor antagonist in the mouse brain reduces ischemic brain injury. *Brain Res* 751: 181–188.

Yla-Herttuala S, Martin J F (2000) Cardiovascular gene therapy. *Lancet* 355: 213–222.

Yonemitsu Y, Kaneda Y, Tanaka S, *et al.* (1998) Transfer of wild-type p53 gene effectively inhibits vascular smooth muscle cell proliferation *in vitro* and *in vivo*. *Circ Res* 82: 147–156.

7

Gene therapy for AIDS and other infectious diseases

A John Frater, Sarah J Fidler and Myra O McClure

By the end of the twentieth century over 34.3 million people were esti-mated to be living with HIV-1 infection (Pisani *et al.*, 2000). The epi-demic has stimulated one of the most intensive research efforts in history and has revolutionised our understanding of retroviral pathogenesis and treatment. An understanding of the viral replication cycle in patients, and the enzymes necessary for particle regeneration [reverse transcrip-tase (RT), protease and integrase] led to the emergence of designer drugs to inhibit these enzymes and viral replication. By late 1995 protease inhibitors (PIs) were available in the clinic, and the combination of these drugs with the reverse transcriptase inhibitors (RTIs) led to the era of 'Highly Active AntiRetroviral Therapy' (HAART). Current UK guide-lines suggest that three drugs should be taken simultaneously: two nucleoside reverse transcriptase inhibitors (e.g. zidovudine, stavudine, didanosine or lamivudine) and either a non-nucleoside reverse tran-scriptase inhibitor (e.g. nevirapine or efavirenz) or a protease inhibitor (e.g. saquinavir, ritonavir, indinavir or nelfinavir) (BHIVA Writing Com-mittee, 2000). Virological and immunological success on HAART trans-lates into clinical benefit. The number of opportunistic infections (apart from non-Hodgkin's lymphoma) (Ledergerber *et al.*, 1999) and the number of AIDS-related deaths in industrialised countries have fallen since the introduction of this therapy (Palella *et al.*, 1998). HAART is expensive, however, and the continents that have the greatest need for it, such as Africa and Asia, where the majority of infections occur, have no access to therapy.

The nucleoside reverse transcriptase (RT) inhibitors (NRTI) were the first class of drugs to be used to inhibit the HIV-1 RT enzyme. They act as analogues to natural host deoxynucleoside triphosphates (dNTPs) which, when incorporated by viral RT cause chain termin-ation. The non-nucleoside RT inhibitors (NNRTI) (e.g. nevirapine, delavirdine and efavirenz) act as non-competitive inhibitors of RT and, although potent, induce early resistance. These drugs bind to a specific binding site associated with codons 100–108 and 181–190 of HIV-1 *RT* which are, correspondingly, the sites for the major resistance mutations. HIV-1 aspartyl protease is a homodimeric, 99-amino-acid peptide that acts in the late stages of the viral life cycle to produce post-translational cleavage of the large Gag-Pol polyprotein. If this enzyme is inhibited, only non-infectious particles can be released from an infected cell. The protease inhibitors (PI) were heralded as a major breakthrough in HIV-1 therapy and, in combination with RT inhibitors, are able to reduce replication of HIV-1 in plasma to levels undetectable by current techniques.

Monotherapy and dual therapy with RT inhibitors were associated with rapid failure and the resurgence of viral replication, as demonstrated in the Concorde (Concorde Coordinating Committee, 1994) and Delta (Delta Coordinating Committee, 1999) clinical trials, respectively. Although the most common HAART regime constitutes two nucleoside reverse transcriptase inhibitors (NRTIs) to be given in conjunction with a PI or NNRTI, there is growing evidence that two NRTIs could be combined with a third NRTI, such as abacavir (Hervey and Perry, 2000). Licensed therapies and those still in research stages are listed in Table 7.1.

Despite HAART, some patients infected with HIV-1 'fail' therapy (Hirsh *et al.*, 1998). Failure, in this context, is defined as an inability to achieve undetectable levels of viral RNA in plasma on therapy, or a rebound in plasma viraemia after undetectable levels have been achieved. 'Undetectability' is defined as a 'viral load' (VL) of less than 50 viral RNA copies per ml of plasma, which is the threshold limit of detection of the Chiron 3.0 bDNA assay (Emeryville, USA). One major reason for continued viral replication in the presence of drug is the development of resistant strains (Condra *et al.*, 1996).

HIV-1 can produce mutations, which are advantageous to the virus and that result from the infidelity of the reverse transcriptase (RT) enzyme and the lack of $3'-5'$ exonuclease activity, a proofreading function common in mammalian polymerase enzymes which repairs incorrectly synthesised DNA. Among retroviruses, the HIV-1 RT has one of the highest known mutation rates. *In vitro* studies on purified HIV-1 RT have estimated the error rate to be one nucleoside base in every 3.4×10^5 (Roberts *et al.*, 1988, 1989; Mansky and Temin, 1995). When this mutation rate is combined with a replication rate of 10 billion new virions each day (Ho *et al.*, 1995), it can be calculated that every possible single point mutation is created each day in one infected person.

Table 7.1 Drugs designed to inhibit HIV-1

Site of action	Drug class	Drug
Reverse transcriptase	Nucleoside analogues	Zidovudine (AZT/ZDV) Didanosine (ddI) Zalcitabine (ddC) Stavudine (D4T) Lamivudine (3TC) Abacavir (ABC) DAPD/DXG[a] FTC[a]
	Nucleotide analogues	Tenofovir (bis POC-PMPA)[a]
	Non-nucleoside analogues	Nevirapine (NEV) Delavirdine (DLV) Efavirenz (EFV) F-ddA[a] MKC-442[a] Capravarine (AG-1549)[a] DPC 961,[a] DPC963[a]
Protease	Protease inhibitors	Saquinavir (Hard and Soft Gel) (SQV) Ritonavir (RTN) Nelfinavir (NEL) Indinavir (IND) Amprenavir Tipranavir[a] ABT-378/r[a] BMS-232,632[a] DMP450[a] DPC681/684[a]
gp41	Fusion inhibitor	T-20[a] T-1249[a]
CXCR-4/CCR5	Entry inhibitors	

The table indicates those drugs that comprise the majority of HAART regimes, currently prescribed.
[a]Drugs still in research stages, under trial or not fully licensed at time of writing. These are either under laboratory investigation or are available through clinical trials or 'expanded access' programmes regulated by pharmacists.

Resistance is not the only reason for the failure of anti-retroviral therapies. Other explanations include difficulty with adherence to complex drug regimes, intra- and extracellular pharmacological factors and interactions with other medications. For these reasons alternative means of viral inhibition need to be explored. Gene therapy offers a number of potentially valuable strategies. In addition, HAART can never eradicate HIV-1 from the body. Although HAART can reduce the VL to undetectable levels [originally leading to the belief that viral replication was completely inhibited and that HIV-1 infection could be cured with 3 years of therapy (Ho, 1997)], it is now appreciated that despite undetectable virus in the plasma, replication is occurring in other body sanctuaries such as the lymph nodes (Finzi *et al.*, 1997; Wong *et al.*, 1997; Hoetelmans, 1998). In addition, replication-competent proviral DNA is detectable, even when RNA was not (Chun *et al.*, 1997). These findings reversed the premature optimism concerning a cure for AIDS, and perspectives changed to those of managing a life-long chronic condition.

In order to appreciate the failure of HAART to eradicate HIV-1, and why alternative approaches are required to do so, we need to consider the HIV-1 life cycle (Figure 7.1). The HIV-1 particle attaches to its target cell via the viral gp120/gp41 envelope complex and the cellular CD4 receptor together with a second co-receptor (CCR5 or CXCR4). The internalised virion releases its two copies of genomic RNA, which are reverse transcribed to DNA by the viral RT. This DNA is incorporated at random into the host chromosome by the viral integrase. Establishing integration is the cornerstone of chronic HIV-1 infection. The infected cell may now rest inactively, or may be immediately triggered into the production of new virions. In the latter case, viral DNA is transcribed by the cellular machinery either into full-length RNA which is assembled into new virions, or into spliced RNA which is transcribed into viral proteins for enzymatic and regulatory function. Virions are assembled in the cell cytoplasm, and bud through the plasma membrane to initiate a new cycle of replication. This life cycle offers a number of sites for possible intervention with gene therapy.

HIV-1 is a complex retrovirus, the genome of which includes six accessory genes, as well as the standard retroviral *gag*, *pol* and *env* structural genes. The genomic structure of HIV-1 is described in Figure 7.2. As discussed later in the chapter, these genes provide targets for a number of genetic approaches designed to inhibit replication, in particular the transcription-activating *tat* and RNA transport/splicing regulating *rev* genes.

This chapter will be divided into three sections. First, different gene therapy approaches will be explained. HIV-1 has been the prototype organism for gene therapy directed against infectious disease and, therefore, the second section will be devoted to some of the approaches used specifically to target HIV-1 infection. Finally, in the third section, attempts at applying gene therapy to other infectious conditions will be explored.

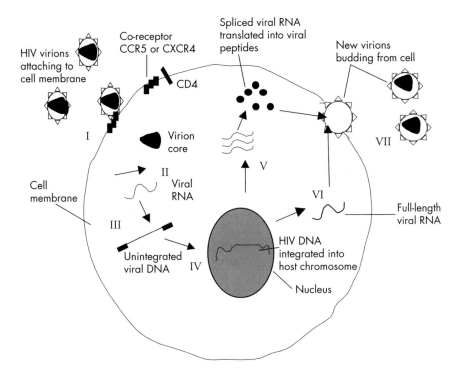

Figure 7.1   HIV life cycle. The infecting HIV virion binds to the cell membrane (I), releasing viral RNA into the cell cytoplasm (II). The RNA is reverse transcribed (III) to DNA which enters, and becomes integrated, into the cell nucleus (IV). The viral genome then either (V) is transcribed and translated into viral peptides, or (VI) is transcribed into a full-length single-stranded RNA copy. New virions are then formed as viral peptides and nucleic acid reassemble at the cell membrane, prior to budding and the formation of new infectious particles (VII).

Gene therapy techniques

It is over 10 years since Rosenberg *et al.* (1990) first transferred a gene into human lymphocytes using a viral vector (*Moloney murine leukemia virus*), as a means of treating melanoma. Early excitement has been tempered by the length of time it has taken for gene therapy to evolve from the laboratory into the clinic. Although there are still no licensed therapies for any disease, by the end of 1999 there were 238 ongoing gene therapy clinical trials in the United States. Of these, only 21 were devoted to HIV-1 infection, the majority being in the field of oncology (Morgan and Blaese, 1999).

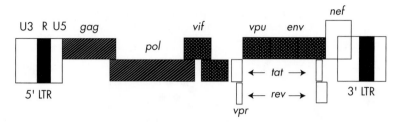

Gene	Function
gag	Encodes for nucleocapsid core proteins
pol	Encodes for reverse transcriptase, integrase, protease and RNase
vif	Promotes viral infectivity
vpr	Nuclear targeting
vpu	Required for virion budding
env	Encodes for the surface-coat proteins
tat	Amplifies viral gene expression
rev	Regulates structural gene expression
nef	Enhances viral infectivity

Figure 7.2   HIV-1 genomic structure. The 5′ and 3′ long terminal repeat (LTR) sequences contain binding sites for host transcription factors. The function of the three structural (*gag, pol* and *env*) and six accessory genes are summarised.

Control of infectious diseases by gene therapy can be approached in one of two ways: either by directing therapy against the infecting organism or by stimulating the host immune response. These will be dealt with separately.

Gene therapy directed against the infecting organism

Antisense oligonucleotides

Negative-stranded oligonucleotides can be used to bind, by standard Watson–Crick base pairing, to target genes (usually RNA). Both RNA and DNA (Stein and Cheng, 1993) have been used as antisense constructs, although the former have proved more successful (Bordier *et al.*, 1992; Morvan *et al.*, 1993). The antisense RNA–target RNA duplex is inactivated either through enzymatic digestion or by physical interference with target transcription or translation sites. Antisense RNA can be administered directly to the patient (although the backbone needs to be stabilised to prevent digestion), or alternatively, intracellular expression can be achieved using methods such as retroviral vectors (Gervaix *et al.*, 1997; Mautino and Morgan, 2000). A stoichiometric disadvantage of antisense RNA is the high expression required to successfully bind to all target RNA. A major advantage is the lack of immunogenicity of antisense constructs, such that the oligonucleotides and the cells producing them will not be destroyed by the host immune response. As we shall see later, this is a major problem with peptide-based gene therapy.

Ribozymes

Antisense RNA alone is often not potent enough to produce complete inhibition *in vivo* (Smythe and Symonds, 1995). An enzymatic moiety can be included in the antisense oligonucleotide, which will cleave the target RNA once the RNA–RNA duplex has formed (Christoffsen, 1997; Persidis, 1997). These enzymatic RNA strands are called 'ribozymes' and are divided broadly into the 'hammerhead' and 'hairpin' types (Sun *et al.*, 1997). The former have a unique secondary structure located centrally, which cleaves RNA strands at G-U-X (where X represents A, C or U), although other nucleotides may replace the G. Hairpin ribozymes have a different secondary structure which cleaves at C-U-G (Perriman *et al.*, 1992; Lian *et al.*, 1999).

Ribozymes have a number of advantages over antisense oligonucleotides (Sarver *et al.*, 1990). They have a much greater specificity for binding as a result of their enzymatic function, they are effective at lower concentrations as they remain functional post cleavage and can be used again on subsequent targets. Moreover, they are generally short oligonucleotides, facilitating the inclusion of many copies within one vector. As with antisense, they are not immunogenic, but they are at risk from RNase degradation.

RNA decoys

RNA decoys are positive-stranded sense oligonucleotides which mimic essential regulatory sequences (Graham and Maio, 1990; Sullender *et al.*, 1990, 1991; Lee *et al.*, 1992; Lisziewicz *et al.*, 1993). They bind to specific *trans*-activating proteins and, thereby, prevent binding of these proteins to their natural RNA targets. As a result RNA decoys can be used to prevent RNA transcription. As with the other nucleotide-based approaches, immunogenicity is not a problem, but there is the stoichiometric problem of providing enough decoy RNA for complete inhibition. In addition, decoy RNA does not remove or inactivate the target gene and may, therefore, be ineffective in the long term. Specificity may also present a problem, resulting in side effects from binding to cellular regulatory peptides.

Dominant-negative mutants: trans-dominant proteins

Viral structural and regulatory proteins are targets for inhibition by therapeutic peptides which are active *in trans* (Pearson *et al.*, 1990; Bevec *et al.*, 1992; Hope *et al.*, 1992; Liu *et al.*, 1994). Work originally performed on *Herpes simplex virus* (HSV) (Friedman *et al.*, 1988) and *Cytomegalovirus* (CMV) (Baltimore, 1988) demonstrated that modification of viral proteins into inactive mutant forms can inhibit replication either by direct competition for substrates or co-factors, or by binding with the viral peptide to form inactive complexes (Herskowitz, 1987).

A disadvantage of *trans*-dominant peptides, as with all protein-based gene therapy, is that immune responses may be induced in the host that target and destroy the proteins and the vector-expressing cell. In addition, there is a stoichiometric disadvantage based on the fact that the therapy is acting post integration and, therefore, with less than 100% efficacy; viral DNA will persist, permitting ongoing replication.

Intrabodies and protein sequestration

Efforts to utilise neutralising antibodies to inhibit HIV-1 cell entry are limited by the heterogeneity of the *env* gene, resulting in a lack of cross-reactivity between isolates. A more effective technique is the use of antibodies to cause protein sequestration (Chen *et al.*, 1994; Mhashilkar *et al.*, 1995, 1997; Levin *et al.*, 1997; Rondon *et al.*, 1997; Marasco *et al.*, 1999). Retention signals have been identified which trap the synthesised peptide permanently within the endoplasmic reticulum (ER) of the host cell, thereby preventing its use in viral replication. Intracellular antibodies can be manipulated to act in the same way as retention signals. Single-chain antibodies (intrabodies) are developed by cloning the light and heavy chain genes from a hybridoma that produces an antibody to the peptide of interest (Marasco *et al.*, 1999). When these genes are expressed within an infected cell they produce a single-chain antibody consisting of a heavy-chain region to target the intrabody to the ER and a heavy-light chain variable region, which is peptide-specific. As the intrabody cannot be secreted from the cell due to its attachment to the ER, the target peptide will also be trapped and will, therefore, be unavailable to perform its viral function (Marasco *et al.*, 1999).

Suicide genes

As an alternative to targeting the infectious organism, 'suicide genes' are designed to produce the death of the infected cell (Mullen, 1994). Some methods utilise genes to express lethal peptides activated by a viral promoter region. Examples include the use of the diphtheria toxin A-chain (Harrison *et al.*, 1992), the HSV thymidine kinase gene (Oldfield *et al.*, 1993) and the cytosine deaminase gene (Huber *et al.*, 1993). The diphtheria toxin gene kills infected cells directly, while the latter two activate and increase the effectiveness of cytotoxic agents. Although they have the potential to inhibit viral replication, suicide genes are also potentially harmful to the host in inducing the death of functionally important cells.

Gene therapy designed to manipulate the immune response

Background

The immune response to an infection can be manipulated either to stimulate a memory response to a pathogen prior to anticipated infection (prophylactic vaccination), or to enhance the failing response to a concurrent infection (therapeutic vaccination). An understanding of the mechanism of action of an immune response is necessary in order to appreciate the role of gene therapy interventions.

An effective immune response can differentiate 'self' from 'non-self', and uses a number of effector systems to destroy and remove 'non-self' (i.e. pathogens) from the body. In order to produce an immune response, foreign peptides are recognised as such by means of the major histocompatibility complex (MHC). Foreign antigen is processed intracellularly into 9–20mer peptide fragments (epitopes), which bind specifically to the MHC and are presented to immune effector cells. If the peptide is presented in conjunction with an MHC class I molecule a cytotoxic T lymphocyte (CTL) immune response is triggered, whereas if an MHC class II molecule is used the CD4 'helper' T-cell pathway is triggered. Generally, peptides that are synthesised endogenously are expressed via MHC class I, and those that are derived from the cytoplasm or extracellular space are presented via class II. A key to successful therapeutic immunotherapy is to ensure that vaccine peptides generate identical epitopes to those seen in natural infection.

Modern vaccination technology now encompasses genetic techniques. Historically, the first vaccines, such as Jenner's cowpox vaccine, enhanced the protective immune response by utilising cross-recognition of key immunogenic antigens expressed in a harmless infectious agent, thereby initiating immunological memory. The next stage was to alter virulent organisms to render them non-pathogenic, whilst retaining their immunogenic properties. Pathogens could be inactivated by heat or by chemical processes ('fixed inactivated') or remain alive, but weakened (live attenuated). The classic examples of these are the Salk and Sabin polio vaccines, respectively. The former are safe to use but lose immunogenicity in their preparation, whereas the latter stimulate a greater immune response, but carry the risk of reversion to a pathogenic strain.

Genetic manipulation of pathogens has permitted the production of recombinant viral proteins for use in vaccines (such as the hepatitis B surface antigen vaccine) which produce a strong immune response without the risks associated with live organisms. Disadvantages of these vaccines are that large-scale peptide production is problematic and there is a small risk of a mutant pathogen being refractory to the induced immune response.

The use of directly synthesised peptides for vaccination has been limited by the inability to replicate epitopes presented during infection. For example, the protein vaccines aimed against the HIV-1 envelope protein resulted in neutralising antibodies, CTL activity and CD4 activity *in vitro*, but have failed to protect animal models infected with field isolates.

Vaccines employing gene-based therapy

Transfer of plasmid-based DNA into cells allows *de novo* intracellular synthesis of immunogenic viral peptides, and this should more accurately mimic natural infection. This technique was first demonstrated when intramuscular injection of saline containing DNA plasmid into mice produced persistent expression, albeit at low levels, of a marker gene (Wolff *et al.*, 1990). The method was expanded using DNA encoding the influenza A nucleoprotein; injection into mice produced a specific CTL response and protected the animals from subsequent injections with lethal doses of influenza A (Ulmer *et al.*, 1993). These 'naked DNA' vaccines appear to overcome the strain-specific limitations of the earlier peptide-based vaccines. Intramuscular injection of DNA vaccines has since been used in murine and other animal models to produce both humoral and cell-mediated responses to parasitic, viral and bacterial pathogens. More recently, there has been success with prevention of clinical AIDS in rhesus monkeys by cytokine-augmented DNA vaccination (Barouch *et al.*, 2000).

DNA vaccination, therefore, has a number of advantages, including the expression of the antigen in its natural state, the ease of production of DNA compared with peptide and the advantage of administering the vaccine into cells that do not constitute the final target. Previous concerns over the low levels of gene expression have been countered with data showing that, in fact, low expression levels may induce stronger Th1-type immune responses, which are associated with viral clearance.

Therapeutic gene-based immunotherapy

In a healthy individual the immune response to infection is usually optimal, with little room for enhancement. As a result therapeutic immunotherapy has received little attention. However, there are certain conditions, such as rabies and hepatitis B, in which post-exposure vaccination has proved effective. Infection with HIV-1 is an example of a condition where the immune system is not functioning maximally, and therefore has been considered for therapeutic vaccination. The adoptive transfer of genetically altered autologous effector CTLs has been viewed as the most promising approach, particularly as the therapy should theoretically work in the immunocompromised (Riddell and Greenberg, 1995).

The technique was first described with the transfer of CMV-specific CTL clones into mice (Baenziger *et al.*, 1986). CTLs were harvested, and then infected and expanded *in vitro* before being re-introduced into the original mouse. The result was protection against CMV challenge, even in the presence of CMV pneumonia. When the same experiment was performed in humans, persistent enhancement of a CMV-specific immune response was demonstrated, but without evidence of improved clinical outcome (Greenberg *et al.*, 1991; Riddell *et al.*, 1991).

Gene therapy for HIV-1 infection

All currently available drugs for the treatment of HIV-1 infection inhibit either the RT or protease enzymes critical for viral replication. Although these drugs have increased life expectancy and reduced morbidity, ongoing viral replication can be demonstrated in patients with unde-tectable levels of plasma viraemia (Wong *et al.*, 1997). The nature of the HIV-1 life cycle, including integration into the host genome, means that no current interventions can eradicate HIV-1 infection. HIV-1 has there-fore been targeted as a key area for gene therapy research, and is the classic example of anti-infectious gene therapy (Bunnell and Morgan, 1998). This section will explore some of the ways gene therapy has been used to inhibit HIV-1 replication, looking at antiviral and immuno-modulatory strategies.

Antiviral gene therapy directed against HIV-1

Antisense RNA

Antisense RNA constructs have been used both pre and post integration to inhibit virion integration and production, respectively. Initial approaches targeted the HIV-1-specific long terminal repeat (LTR) to inhibit viral production (Vickers *et al.*, 1991). The TAR-directed anti-sense molecules inhibited *trans*-activation in a sequence-dependent fashion in a cell culture model, inhibiting HIV-1 replication in both acute and chronically infected viral assays. Constructs directed against *tat*, *rev*, *vpu* and *gag* have had limited success (Stein and Cheng, 1993). Particu-lar genomic areas of increased activity include a 1-kb fragment in *gag* and a 562-bp fragment in *tat-rev* (Rittner and Sczakiel, 1991).

The inhibitory effect of antisense molecules may be overcome by increasing the viral 'multiplicity of infection' (MOI), highlighting one of the essential stoichiometric disadvantages of antisense therapy, whereby large numbers of RNA construct need to be expressed for long periods in order to inhibit replication successfully. One solution to this problem is to include a viral promoter region to increase intracellular RNA levels, and this technique has been successful at inhibiting the 'transactivation response' gene of HIV-1 (Sullenger *et al.*, 1990, 1991).

Ribozymes

As described above, the effect of antisense RNA is enhanced by the hybridisation of enzymatic ribozyme molecules. Ribozymes have been effective at reducing the protein expression of the HIV-1 *gag*, *rev*, *tat*, *vif* and *integrase* genes (Sarver *et al.*, 1990; Heidenreich and Eckstein, 1992; Rossi *et al.*, 1992; Sun *et al.*, 1994; Tabler *et al.*, 1994; Kuwabara *et al.*, 1996). The first use of 'hammerhead' ribozymes showed decreased p24 production, following introduction into culture of a hammerhead ribozyme directed against the *gag* gene (Sarver *et al.*, 1990). 'Hairpin ribozymes' have been used to inhibit the 5′ leader sequences of HIV-1 and thereby prevent replication in T-cell lines challenged with HIV-1 *in vitro* (Dropulic *et al.*, 1992; Ojwang *et al.*, 1992). The potential exists, therefore, to render cells permanently resistant to HIV-1 infection. An expected problem with ribozyme-based HIV-1 inhibition is the development of resistance to the enzyme through sequence variation at the cleavage sites. A means of countering this is to use a number of ribozymes with different sites of action; such 'multitarget' ribozymes have shown enhanced activity, particularly when localised to the same subcellular compartment (Chen *et al.*, 1992a,b, 1994; Menke and Hobom, 1997; Paik *et al.*, 1997).

RNA decoys

Post-integration regulation of HIV-1 gene production can be inhibited using *cis*-acting RNA decoys (Graham and Maio, 1990). The Tat and Rev *trans*-activating proteins have been studied the most thoroughly, and are the specific targets of the TAR and RRE decoys, respectively (Lee *et al.*, 1992, 1994). The decoys prevent replication of laboratory HIV-1 isolates in culture. The TAR decoys provide alternative binding sites for the Tat regulatory proteins, and if present in excess, inhibit Tat-mediated transcriptional activation (Lee *et al.*, 1994). Long RNA TAR decoys have been designed to contain 50 sequence repeats, thereby increasing the degree of Tat 'trapping'. These polymeric sequences have proved active both *in vitro* and *ex vivo* (Lisziewicz *et al.*, 1993; Lori *et al.*, 1994).

The RRE decoys work by the same principle as the TAR decoys, except they target the HIV-1 Rev protein which is involved with mRNA stabilisation and nuclear export. These also regulate viral replication, and inhibition has been shown to prevent viral production *in vitro* (Nakaya *et al.*, 1997).

Dominant-negative proteins

Mutations have been introduced into Gag, Env, Rev and Tat proteins in order to produce *trans*-dominant negative proteins (TNPs) which would inhibit HIV-1 infection (Pearson *et al.*, 1990; Modesti *et al.*, 1991; Bevec *et al.*, 1992; Buchschacher *et al.*, 1995; Lee and Linial, 1995). Mutations within a functionally critical leucine-rich region of Rev produce an inactive peptide that maintains the ability to bind to the RRE ligand, thereby blocking nuclear RNA export and virion assembly. The viral Gag and Env structural proteins form multimers during virion assembly, and these can be disrupted by the introduction of TNPs. Rev TNPs have demonstrated the most significant inhibitory activity; this has been enhanced further with the production of a Tat–Rev fusion protein (TREV), which doubles TNP efficacy (Aguilar-Cordova *et al.*, 1995; Chinen *et al.*, 1997).

Protein sequestration

Single-chain antibodies, or intrabodies, and unique retention signals with the ability to sequester target peptides in the endoplasmic reticulum have shown activity against a number of HIV-1 proteins (Marasco *et al.*, 1999). The principle was used initially with the unique KDEL sequence. This is a tetrapeptide ER retention signal that was incorporated into soluble CD4 (sCD4), resulting in its sequestration within the cell (Buonocore and Rose, 1993; Degar *et al.*, 1996). Viral gp120 synthesised in the same cell would bind to the KDEL–sCD4 complex and, therefore, became trapped and unavailable for particle formation. A drawback was that sufficiently high levels of sCD4 could not be achieved by transfection to allow viral replication at a high MOI. An alternative was to attach the CXC chemokine SDF-1α to KDEL, thereby downregulating the expression of its receptor, CXCR4, on the cell surface (Engel *et al.*, 2000).

Intrabodies have also been used to sequester gp160 in the ER (Chen *et al.*, 1994), but although successful inhibition was achieved using laboratory isolates, primary isolates were poorly affected. Rev (Duan *et al.*, 1994, 1995; Wu *et al.*, 1996), Tat (Mhashilkar *et al.*, 1995, 1997, 1999), integrase (Kitamura *et al.*, 1999) and RT (Maciejewski *et al.*, 1995; Shaheen *et al.*, 1996) have all been sequestered *in vitro* using intrabodies, and results have been encouraging enough to warrant progression to clinical trials.

Immunomodulatory gene therapy directed against HIV-1 infection

The majority of approaches to HIV-1-directed immunotherapy have focused on DNA vaccines and adoptive transfer of autologous effector CTLs (Riddell and Greenberg, 1995; Riddell *et al.*, 2000). Enhancing the host immune responses to HIV-1 peptides may result in the removal of virus or infected cells, thereby reducing further viral replication. Animal studies have demonstrated that both the humoral and cellular immune responses can be enhanced. For example, viral vectors encoding HIV-1 *env* (Wang *et al.*, 1993) and *gag* (Qiu *et al.*, 1999) have been used in mice to induce antibody and cell-mediated responses to infectious HIV-1 isolates. Although the principle can be proved, there is concern that such immune responses may not persist and, therefore, may have limited therapeutic potential. In addition, HIV-1 infection is associated with CD4 cell dysfunction that may accordingly decrease the strength of the response to a genetic vaccine (Pantal *et al.*, 1990; Miedman, 1992).

A more productive approach has been to utilise the patients' own CTLs, and to challenge them *ex vivo* with known HIV-1 epitopes from major proteins such as Gag (Riviere *et al.*, 1989), Pol (Walker *et al.*, 1988) and Env (Riviere *et al.*, 1989; McChesney *et al.*, 1990). CTLs are a major component of the host response to HIV-1 infection, and therefore, their re-introduction in a primed and activated state should enhance HIV-1 clearance by destroying infected cells. Although adoptive transfer of autologous T cells directed against CMV has been demonstrated in mice (Baenziger *et al.*, 1986), further data in humans with HIV-1 infection are required and a number of phase I and II clinical trials have been undertaken.

Clinical trials for the study of gene therapy and HIV-1 infection

The NIH database (National Institutes of Health, 2001) provides an up-to-date account of clinical trials involving gene therapy of HIV-1 infection. At the time of writing a number of such trials are described, of which some are ongoing and others have been completed. The former include a twins study of gene therapy for HIV-1 infection, a study investigating gene therapy, chemotherapy and peripheral stem cell transplantation in treating patients with HIV-1-related non-Hodgkin's lymphoma, a study of stem cell (modified bone marrow) transplantation in HIV-1-infected patients with blood cancer and a pilot study of the patterns of cellular gene expression in HIV-1-infected patients following clinical events which increase plasma virus concentrations.

Those studies that have terminated or are no longer recruiting include another trial of gene therapy in HIV-1-positive patients with non-Hodgkin's lymphoma, a study of the feasibility of setting up a blood bank for gene therapy in HIV-1-infected infants, a phase I trial of APL 400–003 vaccine to determine the safety and immune response evaluations of multiple injections at escalating doses in asymptomatic HIV-1-infected patients, a phase II study of oral Ro24–7429 (Tat antagonist) in patients with HIV-1-related Kaposi's sarcoma, and two studies in HIV-1-infected identical twins: a phase I/II pilot study of the safety of the adoptive transfer of gene-modified cytotoxic syngeneic T lymphocytes and a study of the safety and survival of the adoptive transfer of genetically marked syngeneic lymphocytes. Other trials that have been undertaken include a phase I multicentre trial to evaluate the safety and immunogenicity of the immuno-AG recombinant HIV-1 gp160 in asymptomatic HIV-1-seropositive individuals and a study of the effectiveness of an HIV-1 vaccine (ALVAC vCP205) to boost immune functions in HIV-1-negative volunteers who have already received an HIV-1 vaccine.

Gene therapy is a well-characterised *in vitro* and experimental technique, but it is only through well-designed clinical trials that it will be accepted into a clinical and therapeutic environment. Although there are currently insufficient data, parallels have been drawn with the state of recombinant protein and mononuclear antibody technology in the 1980s (Morgan and Blaese, 1999). These advances have now entered medical practice, having been in a similar position to the one that gene therapy currently occupies.

Gene therapy and other infectious diseases

HIV-1 has been the predominant pathogen targeted for inhibition by gene therapy, however a number of other viruses have also been studied. The major approaches to these are referenced here.

Hepatitis viruses

Gene therapy approaches to controlling hepatitis infections are being evaluated to optimise current antiviral protocols (Zoulim and Trepo, 1999). Antisense DNA successfully inhibited hepatitis B virus (HBV) replication *in vitro* in human hepatocellular carcinoma cells, but the effects were transient (Goodarzi *et al.*, 1990). Animal studies using the naked DNA vaccine have been encouraging (McCluskie *et al.*, 1999), and this approach has entered clinical trials (Tacket *et al.*, 1999). HBV has a double-stranded DNA genome that has been targeted by both antisense RNA and plasmid DNA vaccines. The incidence of both HBV and hepatitis C virus (HCV) infections are increasing without the likelihood of curative medications in the short term, rendering both targets for gene therapy. HCV is, like HIV-1, a positive-stranded RNA virus. Similar approaches have been taken as with HBV, with antisense RNA showing limited results *in vitro*, although encouraging DNA vaccine work is in progress (Forns *et al.*, 1999; Gordon *et al.*, 2000).

Herpesviruses

The herpesviruses represent a large family of double-stranded DNA viruses that include the herpes simplex viruses (HSV-1 and - 2), Epstein–Barr virus (EBV), varicella zoster virus (VZV) and cytomegalovirus (CMV). These can cause a range of clinical conditions, from the minor (e.g. cold sores) to those that are rapidly fatal (e.g. encephalitis), especially in the immunosuppressed patient.

HSV infections may be successfully inhibited with competitive nucleoside analogue inhibitors such as acyclovir or valciclovir, however, as with HIV-1, the emergence of resistant strains is limiting the effectiveness of these drugs. Gene therapy approaches have been explored as an adjunct to chemotherapy. In particular, antisense RNA has shown viral inhibition and prevention of reactivation from latently infected ganglia (Shoji *et al.*, 1998; Aurelian and Smith, 2000).

CMV is a viral infection that is usually cleared by the immune system. In states of immunocompromise, such as AIDS, infection can result in blindness and CNS disease. Although infection can be well-controlled with pharmacological antiviral agents, studies have also demonstrated inhibition using *trans*-dominant negative proteins, antisense constructs and immunotherapy. The latter has been demonstrated *in vivo* using genetically modified CD8+ T cells directed against CMV proteins (Riddell *et al.*, 1991, 1994; Walter *et al.*, 1995). In an immunocompromised host, adoptive transfer of these modified cells demonstrated the induction of a specific host T-cell response to CMV, which was not produced by the unmodified T-cell autologous controls (Riddell *et al.*, 1994; Walter *et al.*, 1995).

Human papillomaviruses

Human papillomavirus (HPV) is a double-stranded DNA virus that can be classified into a number of subtypes known to infect humans, producing conditions such as genital warts (e.g. HPV-2 and - 3) and cervical carcinoma (e.g. HPV-16 and -18) (Tyring, 2000). HPV infections can be treated in the short term, but eradication of the virus is impossible as it persists in a latent episomal form within the basal epithelium. Infection with HPV subtypes 16 and 18 has been associated with malignancy and they have, therefore, been the targets of gene therapy (Shillitoe *et al.*, 1994). Antisense RNA constructs (He *et al.*, 1997; Alvarez-Salas *et al.*, 1999; Venturini *et al.*, 1999) and ribozymes (Chen *et al.*, 1995, 1996; Huang *et al.*, 1996; Alvarez-Salas *et al.*, 1998) have achieved inhibition of HPV replication *in vitro,* and *in vivo* data are awaited.

Conclusions

An enormous amount of research has focused on the gene therapy of infectious diseases, such as HIV-1 infection. Although *in vitro* data have been encouraging and a number of clinical trials initiated, no such therapy has yet entered the arena of clinical practice. This advance is awaited with enthusiasm. As increasing numbers of HIV-infected patients start to fail antiretroviral therapy, other means of viral control will be required and gene therapy may offer an alternative.

Acknowledgement

AJF is funded by the Medical Research Council.

References

Aguilar-Cordova E, Chinen J, Donehower L A, *et al.* (1995) Inhibition of HIV-1 by a double transdominant fusion gene. *Gene Ther* 2: 181–186.

Alvarez-Salas L M, Cullinan A E, Siwkowski A, *et al.* (1998) Inhibition of HPV-16 E6/E7 immortalization of normal keratinocytes by hairpin ribozymes. *Proc Natl Acad Sci USA* 95: 1189–1194.

Alvarez-Salas L M, Arpawong T E, DiPaolo J A (1999) Growth inhibition of cervical tumor cells by antisense oligodeoxynucleotides directed to the human papillomavirus type 16 E6 gene. *Antisense Nucleic Acid Drug Dev* 9: 441–450.

Aurelian L, Smith C C (2000) Herpes simplex virus type 2 growth and latency reactivation by cocultivation are inhibited with antisense oligonucleotides complementary to the translation initiation site of the large subunit of ribonucleotide reductase (RR1). *Antisense Nucleic Acid Drug Dev* 10: 77–85.

Baenziger J, Hengartner H, Zinkernagel R M, Cole G A (1986) Induction or prevention of immunopathological disease by cloned cytotoxic T cell lines specific for lymphocytic choriomeningitis virus. *Eur J Immunol* 16: 387–393.

Baltimore D (1988) Gene therapy. Intracellular immunization [news]. *Nature* 335: 395–396.

Barouch D H, Santra S, Schmitz J E, *et al.* (2000) Control of viremia and prevention of clinical AIDS in rhesus monkeys by cytokine-augmented DNA vaccination. *Science* 290: 486–492.

Bevec D, Dobrovnik M, Hauber J, Bohnlein E (1992) Inhibition of human immunodeficiency virus type 1 replication in human T cells by retroviral-mediated gene transfer of a dominant-negative Rev trans-activator. *Proc Natl Acad Sci USA* 89: 9870–9874.

BHIVA Writing committee on behalf of the BHIVA Executive Committee (2000) British HIV Association Guidelines for the treatment of HIV-1-infected adults with antiretroviral therapy. *HIV Med* 1: 76–101.

Bordier B, Helene C, Barr P J, *et al.* (1992) In vitro effect of antisense oligonucleotides on human immunodeficiency virus type 1 reverse transcription. *Nucleic Acids Res* 20: 5999–6006.

Buchschacher G L J, Freed E O, Panganiban A T (1995) Effects of second-site mutations on dominant interference by a human immunodeficiency virus type 1 envelope glycoprotein mutant. *J Virol* 69: 1344–1348.

Bunnell B A, Morgan R A (1998) Gene therapy for infectious diseases. *Clin Microbiol Rev* 11: 42–56.

Buonocore L, Rose J K (1993) Blockade of human immunodeficiency virus type 1 production in CD4+ T cells by an intracellular CD4 expressed under control of the viral long terminal repeat. *Proc Natl Acad Sci USA* 90: 2695–2699.

Chen C J, Banerjea A C, Haglund K, *et al.* (1992a) Inhibition of HIV-1 replication by novel multitarget ribozymes. *Ann NY Acad Sci* 660: 271–273.

Chen C J, Banerjea A C, Harmison G G, *et al.* (1992b) Multitarget-ribozyme directed to cleave at up to nine highly conserved HIV-1 env RNA regions inhibits HIV-1 replication-potential effectiveness against most presently sequenced HIV-1 isolates. *Nucleic Acids Res* 20: 4581–4589.

Chen S Y, Bagley J, Marasco W A (1994) Intracellular antibodies as a new class of therapeutic molecules for gene therapy. *Hum Gene Ther* 5: 595–601.

Chen Z, Kamath P, Zhang S, *et al.* (1995) Effectiveness of three ribozymes for cleavage of an RNA transcript from human papillomavirus type 18. *Cancer Gene Ther* 2: 263–271.

Chen Z, Kamath P, Zhang S, *et al.* (1996) Effects on tumor cells of ribozymes that cleave the RNA transcripts of human papillomavirus type 18. *Cancer Gene Ther* 3: 18–23.

Chinen J, Aguilar-Cordova E, Ng-Tang D, *et al.* (1997) Protection of primary human T cells from HIV-1 infection by Trev: a transdominant fusion gene. *Hum Gene Ther* 8: 861–868.

Christoffersen R E (1997) Translating genomics information into therapeutics: a key role for oligonucleotides. *Nat Biotechnol* 15: 483–484.

Chun T W, Stuyver L, Mizell S B, *et al.* (1997) Presence of an inducible HIV-1 latent reservoir during highly active antiretroviral therapy. *Proc Natl Acad Sci USA* 94: 13193–13197.

Concorde Coordinating Committee (1994) Concorde: MRC/ANRS randomised double-blind controlled trial of immediate and deferred zidovudine in symptom-free HIV-1 infection. *Lancet* 343: 871–881.

Condra J H, Holder D J, Schleif W A, *et al.* (1996) Genetic correlates of in vivo viral resistance to indinavir, a human immunodeficiency virus type 1 protease inhibitor. *J Virol* 70: 8270–8276.

Degar S, Johnson J E, Boritz E, Rose J K (1996) Replication of primary HIV-1 isolates is inhibited in PM1 cells expressing sCD4-KDEL. *Virology* 226: 424–429.

Delta Coordinating Committee and Virology Group (1999) An evaluation of HIV-1 RNA and CD4 cell count as surrogates for clinical outcome. *AIDS* 13: 565–573.

Dropulic B, Lin N H, Martin M A, Jeang K T (1992) Functional characterization of a U5 ribozyme: intracellular suppression of human immunodeficiency virus type 1 expression. *J Virol* 66: 1432–1441.

Duan L, Bagasra O, Laughlin M A, *et al.* (1994) Potent inhibition of human immunodeficiency virus type 1 replication by an intracellular anti-Rev single-chain antibody. *Proc Natl Acad Sci USA* 91: 5075–5079.

Duan L, Zhu M, Bagasra O, Pomerantz R J (1995) Intracellular immunization against HIV-1 infection of human T lymphocytes: utility of anti-rev single-chain variable fragments. *Hum Gene Ther* 6: 1561–1573.

Engel B C, Bauer G, Pepper K A, *et al.* (2000) Intrakines – evidence for a trans-cellular mechanism of action. *Mol Ther* 1: 165–170.

Finzi D, Hermankova M, Pierson T, *et al.* (1997) Identification of a reservoir for HIV-1 in patients on highly active antiretroviral therapy. *Science* 278: 1295–1300.

Forns X, Emerson S U, Tobin G J, *et al.* (1999) DNA immunization of mice and macaques with plasmids encoding hepatitis C virus envelope E2 protein expressed intracellularly and on the cell surface. *Vaccine* 17: 1992–2002.

Friedman A D, Triezenberg S J, McKnight S L (1988) Expression of a truncated viral trans-activator selectively impedes lytic infection by its cognate virus. *Nature* 335: 452–454.

Gervaix A, Li X, Kraus G, Wong-Staal F (1997) Multigene antiviral vectors inhibit diverse human immunodeficiency virus type 1 clades. *J Virol* 71: 3048–3053.

Goodarzi G, Gross S C, Tewari A, Watabe K (1990) Antisense oligodeoxyribo-nucleotides inhibit the expression of the gene for hepatitis B virus surface antigen. *J Gen Virol* 71: 3021–3025.

Gordon E J, Bhat R, Liu Q, *et al.* (2000) Immune responses to hepatitis C virus structural and nonstructural proteins induced by plasmid DNA immunizations. *J Infect Dis* 181: 42–50.

Graham G J, Maio J J (1990) RNA transcripts of the human immunodeficiency virus transactivation response element can inhibit action of the viral transactivator. *Proc Natl Acad Sci USA* 87: 5817–5821.

Greenberg P D, Reusser P, Goodrich J M, Riddell S R (1991) Development of a treatment regimen for human cytomegalovirus (CMV) infection in bone marrow transplantation recipients by adoptive transfer of donor-derived CMV-specific T cell clones expanded in vitro. *Ann NY Acad Sci* 636: 184–195.

Harrison G S, Long C J, Curiel T J, *et al.* (1992) Inhibition of human immuno-deficiency virus-1 production resulting from transduction with a retrovirus containing an HIV-1-regulated diphtheria toxin A chain gene. *Hum Gene Ther* 3: 461–469.

He Y, Huang L (1997) Growth inhibition of human papillomavirus 16 DNA-positive mouse tumor by antisense RNA transcribed from U6 promoter. *Cancer Res* 57: 3993–3999.

Heidenreich O, Eckstein F (1992) Hammerhead ribozyme-mediated cleavage of the long terminal repeat RNA of human immunodeficiency virus type 1. *J Biol Chem* 267: 1904–1909.

Herskowitz I (1987) Functional inactivation of genes by dominant negative mutations. *Nature* 329: 219–222.

Hervey P S, Perry C M (2000) Abacavir: a review of its clinical potential in patients with HIV-1 infection. *Drugs* 60: 447–479.

Hirsh M S, Conway B, D'Aquila R T, *et al.* (1998) Antiretroviral drug resistance testing in adults with HIV-1 infection. *JAMA* 279: 1984–1991.

Ho D D (1997) Perspectives series: host/pathogen interactions. Dynamics of HIV-1 replication in vivo. *J Clin Invest* 99: 2565–2567.

Ho D D, Neumann A U, Perelson A S, *et al.* (1995) Rapid turnover of plasma virions and CD4 lymphocytes in HIV-1 infection. Nature 373: 123–126.

Hoetelmans R M (1998) Sanctuary sites in HIV-1 infection. *Antivir Ther* 3 (Suppl. 4): 13–17.

Hope T J, Klein N P, Elder M E, Parslow T G (1992) trans-dominant inhibition of human immunodeficiency virus type 1 Rev occurs through formation of inactive protein complexes. *J Virol* 66: 1849–1855.

Huang Y, Kong Y, Wang Y, *et al.* (1996) Stable expression of anti-HPV 16 E7-ribozyme in CV-1 cell lines. *Chin J Biotechnol* 12: 215–220.

Huber B E, Austin E A, Good S S, *et al.* (1993) In vivo antitumor activity of 5-fluorocytosine on human colorectal carcinoma cells genetically modified to express cytosine deaminase. *Cancer Res* 53: 4619–4626.

Kitamura Y, Ishikawa T, Okui N, *et al.* (1999) Inhibition of replication of HIV-1 at both early and late stages of the viral life cycle by single-chain antibody against viral integrase. *J Acquir Immune Defic Syndr Hum Retrovirol* 20: 105–114.

Kuwabara T, Amontov S V, Warashina M, *et al.* (1996) Characterization of several kinds of dimer minizyme: simultaneous cleavage at two sites in HIV-1 tat mRNA by dimer minizymes. *Nucleic Acids Res* 24: 2302–2310.

Ledergerber B, Telenti A, Egger M (1999) Risk of HIV related Kaposi's sarcoma and non-Hodgkin's lymphoma with potent antiretroviral therapy: prospective cohort study. Swiss HIV-1 Cohort Study. *BMJ* 319: 23–24.

Lee P P, Linial M L (1995) Inhibition of wild-type HIV-1 virus production by a matrix deficient Gag mutant. *Virology* 208: 808–811.

Lee S W, Gallardo H F, Gilboa E, Smith C (1994) Inhibition of human immunodeficiency virus type 1 in human T cells by a potent Rev response element decoy consisting of the 13-nucleotide minimal Rev-binding domain. *J Virol* 68: 8254–8264.

Lee T C, Sullenger B A, Gallardo H F, *et al.* (1992) Overexpression of RRE-derived sequences inhibits HIV-1 replication in CEM cells. *New Biol* 4: 66–74.

Levin R, Mhashilkar A M, Dorfman T, *et al.* (1997) Inhibition of early and late events of the HIV-1 replication cycle by cytoplasmic Fab intrabodies against the matrix protein, p17. *Mol Med* 3: 96–110.

Lian Y, De Young M B, Siwkowski A, *et al.* (1999) The sCYMV1 hairpin ribozyme: targeting rules and cleavage of heterologous RNA. *Gene Ther* 6: 1114–1119.

Lisziewicz J, Sun D, Smythe J, *et al.* (1993) Inhibition of human immunodeficiency virus type 1 replication by regulated expression of a polymeric Tat activation response RNA decoy as a strategy for gene therapy in AIDS. *Proc Natl Acad Sci USA* 90: 8000–8004.

Liu J, Woffendin C, Yang Z Y, Nabel G J (1994) Regulated expression of a dominant negative form of Rev improves resistance to HIV-1 replication in T cells. *Gene Ther* 1: 32–37.

Lori F, Lisziewicz J, Smythe J, *et al.* (1994) Rapid protection against human immunodeficiency virus type 1 (HIV-1) replication mediated by high efficiency nonretroviral delivery of genes interfering with HIV-1 tat and gag. *Gene Ther* 1: 27–31.

Maciejewski J P, Weichold F F, Young N S, *et al.* (1995) Intracellular expression of antibody fragments directed against HIV reverse transcriptase prevents HIV infection in vitro. *Nat Med* 1: 667–673.

Mansky L M, Temin H M. Lower in vivo mutation rate of human immunodeficiency virus type 1 than that predicted from the fidelity of purified reverse transcriptase. *J Virol* 69: 5087–5094.

Marasco W A, LaVecchio J, Winkler A (1999) Human anti-HIV-1 tat sFv intrabodies for gene therapy of advanced HIV-1-infection and AIDS. *J Immunol Methods* 231: 223–238.

Mautino M R, Morgan R A (2000) Potent inhibition of human immunodeficiency virus type 1 replication by conditionally replicating human immunodeficiency virus-based lentiviral vectors expressing envelope antisense mRNA. *Hum Gene Ther* 11: 2025–2037.

McChesney M, Tanneau F, Regnault A, *et al.* (1990) Detection of primary cytotoxic T lymphocytes specific for the envelope glycoprotein of HIV-1 by deletion of the env amino-terminal signal sequence. *Eur J Immunol* 20: 215–220.

McCluskie M J, Brazolot M C, Gramzinski R A, *et al.* (1999) Route and method of delivery of DNA vaccine influence immune responses in mice and non-human primates. *Mol Med* 5: 287–300.

Menke A, Hobom G (1997) Antiviral ribozymes. New jobs for ancient molecules. *Mol Biotechnol* 8: 17–33.

Mhashilkar A M, Bagley J, Chen S Y, *et al.* (1995) Inhibition of HIV-1 Tat-mediated LTR transactivation and HIV-1 infection by anti-Tat single chain intrabodies. *EMBO J* 14: 1542–1551.

Mhashilkar A M, Biswas D K, LaVecchio J, *et al.* (1997) Inhibition of human immunodeficiency virus type 1 replication in vitro by a novel combination of anti-Tat single-chain intrabodies and NF-kappa B antagonists. *J Virol* 71: 6486–6494.

Mhashilkar A M, LaVecchio J, Eberhardt B, *et al.* (1999) Inhibition of human immunodeficiency virus type 1 replication in vitro in acutely and persistently infected human CD4+ mononuclear cells expressing murine and humanized anti-human immunodeficiency virus type 1 Tat single-chain variable fragment intrabodies. *Hum Gene Ther* 10: 1453–1467.

Miedema F (1992) Immunological abnormalities in the natural history of HIV infection: mechanisms and clinical relevance. *Immunodefic Rev* 3: 173–193.

Modesti N, Garcia J, Debouck C, *et al.* (1991) Trans-dominant Tat mutants with alterations in the basic domain inhibit HIV-1 gene expression. *New Biol* 3: 759–768.

Morgan R A, Blaese R M (1999) Gene therapy: lessons learnt from the past decade. *BMJ* 319: 1310.

Morvan F, Porumb H, Degols G, *et al.* (1993) Comparative evaluation of seven oligonucleotide analogues as potential antisense agents. *J Med Chem* 36: 280–287.

Mullen C A (1994) Metabolic suicide genes in gene therapy. *Pharmacol Ther* 63: 199–207.

Nakaya T, Iwai S, Fujinaga K, *et al.* (1997) Inhibition of HIV-1 replication by targeting the Rev protein. *Leukemia* 11(Suppl 3): 134–137.

Ojwang J O, Hampel A, Looney D J, *et al.* (1992) Inhibition of human immunodeficiency virus type 1 expression by a hairpin ribozyme. *Proc Natl Acad Sci USA* 89: 10802–10806.

Oldfield E H, Ram Z, Culver K W, *et al.* (1993) Gene therapy for the treatment of brain tumors using intra-tumoral transduction with the thymidine kinase gene and intravenous ganciclovir. *Hum Gene Ther* 4: 39–69.

Paik S Y, Banerjea A, Chen C J, *et al.* (1997) Defective HIV-1 provirus encoding a multitarget-ribozyme inhibits accumulation of spliced and unspliced HIV-1 mRNAs, reduces infectivity of viral progeny, and protects the cells from pathogenesis. *Hum Gene Ther* 8: 1115–1124.

Palella F J J, Delaney K M, Moorman A C, *et al.* (1998) Declining morbidity and mortality among patients with advanced human immunodeficiency virus infection. HIV-1 Outpatient Study Investigators. *N Engl J Med* 338: 853–860.

Pantaleo G, Koenig S, Baseler M, *et al.* (1990) Defective clonogenic potential of CD8+ T lymphocytes in patients with AIDS. Expansion in vivo of a nonclonogenic CD3+CD8+DR+CD25– T cell population. *J Immunol* 144: 1696–1704.

Pearson L, Garcia J, Wu F, *et al.* (1990) A transdominant tat mutant that inhibits tat-induced gene expression from the human immunodeficiency virus long terminal repeat. *Proc Natl Acad Sci USA* 87: 5079–5083.

Perriman R, Delves A, Gerlach W L (1992) Extended target-site specificity for a hammerhead ribozyme. *Gene* 113: 157–163.

Persidis A (1997) Ribozyme therapeutics. *Nat Biotechnol* 15: 921–922.

Pisani E, Schwartlander B, Cherney S, *et al.* (2000) *Report on the Global HIV Epidemic*. UNAIDS/00.44E – WHO/CDS/CSR/EDC/2000.9; 20 avenue Appia, 1211 Geneva 27, Switzerland.

Qiu J T, Song R, Dettenhofer M, *et al.* (1999) Evaluation of novel human immunodeficiency virus type 1 Gag DNA vaccines for protein expression in mammalian cells and induction of immune responses. *J Virol* 73: 9145–9152.

Riddell S R, Greenberg P D (1995) Principles for adoptive T cell therapy of human viral diseases. *Annu Rev Immunol* 13: 545–586.

Riddell S R, Rabin M, Geballe A P, *et al.* (1991) Class I MHC-restricted cytotoxic T lymphocyte recognition of cells infected with human cytomegalovirus does not require endogenous viral gene expression. *J Immunol* 146: 2795–2804.

Riddell S R, Walter B A, Gilbert M J, Greenberg P D (1994) Selective reconstitution of CD8+ cytotoxic T lymphocyte responses in immunodeficient bone marrow transplant recipients by the adoptive transfer of T cell clones. *Bone Marrow Transplant* 14(Suppl. 4): S78–S84.

Riddell S R, Warren E H, Lewinsohn D, *et al.* (2000) Application of T cell immuno-therapy for human viral and malignant diseases. *Ernst Schering Res Found Workshop* 30: 53–73.

Rittner K, Sczakiel G (1991) Identification and analysis of antisense RNA target regions of the human immunodeficiency virus type 1. *Nucleic Acids Res* 19: 1421–1426.

Riviere Y, Tanneau-Salvadori F, Regnault A, *et al.* (1989) Human immunodeficiency virus-specific cytotoxic responses of seropositive individuals: distinct types of effector cells mediate killing of targets expressing gag and env proteins. *J Virol* 63: 2270–2277.

Roberts J D, Bebenek K, Kunkel T A (1988) The accuracy of reverse transcriptase from HIV-1. *Science* 242: 1171–1173.

Roberts J D, Preston B D, Johnston L A, *et al.* (1989) Fidelity of two retroviral reverse transcriptases during DNA-dependent DNA synthesis in vitro. *Mol Cell Biol* 9: 469–476.

Rondon I J, Marasco W A (1997) Intracellular antibodies (intrabodies) for gene therapy of infectious diseases. *Annu Rev Microbiol* 51: 257–283.

Rosenberg S A, Aebersold P, Cornetta K, *et al.* (1990) Gene transfer into humans – immunotherapy of patients with advanced melanoma, using tumor-infiltrating lymphocytes modified by retroviral gene transduction. *N Engl J Med* 323: 570–578.

Rossi J J, Elkins D, Zaia J A, Sullivan S (1992) Ribozymes as anti-HIV-1 therapeutic agents: principles, applications, and problems. *AIDS Res Hum Retroviruses* 8: 183–189.

Sarver N, Cantin E M, Chang P S, *et al.* (1990) Ribozymes as potential anti-HIV-1 therapeutic agents. *Science* 247: 1222–1225.

Shaheen F, Duan L, Zhu M, *et al.* (1996) Targeting human immunodeficiency virus type 1 reverse transcriptase by intracellular expression of single-chain variable fragments to inhibit early stages of the viral life cycle [published erratum appears in *J Virol* 1998 72: 3505–3506]. *J Virol* 70: 3392–3400.

Shillitoe E J, Kamath P, Chen Z (1994) Papillomaviruses as targets for cancer gene therapy. *Cancer Gene Ther* 1: 193–204.

Shoji Y, Ishige H, Tamura N, *et al.* (1998) Enhancement of anti-herpetic activity of antisense phosphorothioate oligonucleotides 5′ end modified with geraniol. *J Drug Target* 5: 261–273.

Smythe J A, Symonds G (1995) Gene therapeutic agents: the use of ribozymes, anti-sense, and RNA decoys for HIV-1 infection. *Inflamm Res* 44: 11–15.

Stein C A, Cheng Y C (1993) Antisense oligonucleotides as therapeutic agents – is the bullet really magical? *Science* 261: 1004–1012.

Sullenger B A, Gallardo H F, Ungers G E, Gilboa E (1990) Overexpression of TAR sequences renders cells resistant to human immunodeficiency virus replication. *Cell* 63: 601–608.

Sullenger BA, Gallardo HF, Ungers GE, Gilboa E (1991) Analysis of trans-acting response decoy RNA-mediated inhibition of human immunodeficiency virus type 1 transactivation. *J Virol* 65: 6811–6816.

Sun L Q, Warrilow D, Wang L, *et al.* (1994) Ribozyme-mediated suppression of Moloney murine leukemia virus and human immunodeficiency virus type I replication in permissive cell lines. *Proc Natl Acad Sci USA* 91: 9715–9719.

Sun L Q, Ely J A, Gerlach W, Symonds G (1997) Anti-HIV-1 ribozymes. *Mol Biotechnol* 7: 241–251.

Tabler M, Homann M, Tzortzakaki S, Sczakiel G (1994) A three-nucleotide helix I is sufficient for full activity of a hammerhead ribozyme: advantages of an asymmetric design. *Nucleic Acids Res* 22: 3958–3965.

Tacket C O, Roy M J, Widera G, *et al.* (1999) Phase 1 safety and immune response studies of a DNA vaccine encoding hepatitis B surface antigen delivered by a gene delivery device. *Vaccine* 17: 2826–2829.

Tyring S K (2000) Human papillomavirus infections: epidemiology, pathogenesis, and host immune response. *J Am Acad Dermatol* 43: S18–S26.

Ulmer J B, Donnelly J J, Parker S E, *et al.* (1993) Heterologous protection against influenza by injection of DNA encoding a viral protein. *Science* 259: 1745–1749.

Venturini F, Braspenning J, Homann M, *et al.* (1999) Kinetic selection of HPV 16 E6/E7-directed antisense nucleic acids: anti-proliferative effects on HPV 16-transformed cells. *Nucleic Acids Res* 27: 1585–1592.

Vickers T, Baker B F, Cook P D, *et al.* (1991) Inhibition of HIV-1-LTR gene expression by oligonucleotides targeted to the TAR element. *Nucleic Acids Res* 19: 3359–3368.

Walker B D, Flexner C, Paradis T J, *et al.* (1988) HIV-1 reverse transcriptase is a target for cytotoxic T lymphocytes in infected individuals. *Science* 240: 64–66.

Walter E A, Greenberg P D, Gilbert M J, *et al.* (1995) Reconstitution of cellular immunity against cytomegalovirus in recipients of allogeneic bone marrow by transfer of T-cell clones from the donor. *N Engl J Med* 333: 1038–1044.

Wang B, Ugen K E, Srikantan V, *et al.* (1993) Gene inoculation generates immune responses against human immunodeficiency virus type 1. *Proc Natl Acad Sci USA* 90: 4156–4160.

Wolff J A, Malone R W, Williams P, *et al.* (1990) Direct gene transfer into mouse muscle in vivo. *Science* 247: 1465–1468.

Wong J K, Hezareh M, Gunthard H F, *et al.* (1997) Recovery of replication-competent HIV-1 despite prolonged suppression of plasma viremia. *Science* 278: 1291–1295.

Wu Y, Duan L, Zhu M, *et al.* (1996) Binding of intracellular anti-Rev single chain variable fragments to different epitopes of human immunodeficiency virus type 1 rev: variations in viral inhibition. *J Virol* 70: 3290–3297.

Zoulim F, Trepo C (1999) New antiviral agents for the therapy of chronic hepatitis B virus infection. *Intervirology* 42: 125–144.

8

Gene therapy approaches for rheumatoid arthritis

Jan Bondeson, Marc Feldmann and Ravinder N Maini

Gene therapy of disease was initially conceived as the delivery of an intact copy of a characterised functional gene into affected cells to correct the physiological defect caused by a gene disorder or deficiency. It was thus a way of treating diseases for which a simple genetic defect was known to be the cause. A good example is the treatment of cystic fibrosis by delivery of the gene for the cystic fibrosis chloride ion transporter protein into the airway epithelial cells of the patients, an approach for which clinical trials are ongoing (Alton *et al.*, 1999; Zuckerman *et al.*, 1999). Another example of a simple monogeneic disease at the forefront of gene therapy clinical trials is severe combined immune deficiency (SCID) caused by adenosine deaminase deficiency (Blaese *et al.*, 1995; Onodera *et al.*, 1998; see also Chapter 4). In recent years, the definition of gene therapy has become much broader. It has been appreciated that in many diseases it may be possible to define therapeutic target genes, and to use various gene therapy strategies to attempt to achieve disease remission, or at least alleviation of the symptoms. Thus gene therapy has been used in multigeneic or even multifactorial diseases. An example is the gene therapy of cancer (see Chapter 5). Thus the *p53* tumour suppressor gene was defined as a therapeutic target, since mutation of this gene is the most frequent abnormality identified in human tumours, and attempts have been made to restore *p53* function by gene replacement therapy (Harris *et al.*, 1996; Roth *et al.*, 1999). Another strategy for cancer in which clinical trials are ongoing aims to facilitate immune destruction of malignant cells by intralesional gene transfer of HLA B7 to increase class I MHC molecule expression (Rini *et al.*, 1999). A third approach is suicide gene therapy, which involves transfer of a gene that renders the tumour cell susceptible to an otherwise non-toxic prodrug. The most successful application of this strategy has used gene transfer of the herpes simplex virus thymidine kinase (HSV *tk*) gene in combination with treatment with the drug ganciclovir, which has the advantage in this context that leakage of toxic metabolites extends the cytotoxic effect to non-transduced tumour cells (Shand *et al.*, 1999).

Rheumatoid arthritis (RA) is a chronic, systemic, inflammatory disease of unknown aetiology, characterised by synovial inflammation and erosion of articular cartilage and subchondral bone. Its prevalence is approximately 1% world-wide. As late as the 1980s, the outlook for RA patients was over-cautionary and pessimistic, because the antirheumatic drugs used at this time lacked efficacy and had significant side effects. For patients with severe RA, the prognosis was particularly poor: many were crippled at an early age, and many suffered severe, chronic pain. At this time, there was also considerable defeatism from the majority of rheumatologists. The 1980s concept of the 'treatment pyramid', commencing with a non-steroidal anti-inflammatory drug (NSAID) alone, and progressing to increasingly potent disease-modifying drugs (DMARDs) if this drug failed to alleviate symptoms, is today perceived as a harmful one. In particular, the notion that only patients with proven disabling and joint destructive disease should receive potent antirheumatic therapy was fallacious, and meant that effective therapy was instituted late, only after permanent damage had occurred.

Our view of the natural history of RA changed dramatically during the 1990s. It became generally accepted that far from being a mild, self-limiting disease, RA is a major source of joint damage, social and functional decline and work disability. Partial control of the inflammation does not appear to prevent the joint damage, and the majority of patients with active disease become clinically disabled within 20 years. For those with aggressive disease or extra-articular manifestations, the mortality is comparable with that of patients with three-vessel coronary arteriosclerosis, or stage IV Hodgkin's disease (Erhardt *et al.*, 1989; Pincus and Callahan, 1993) (Figure 8.1). Many rheumatologists realised that it was important for functional outcome to suppress rheumatoid inflammation early, and to challenge aggressive early RA with the most potent DMARDs available. This coincided with the demonstration in clinical trials that methotrexate, a drug hitherto put on the top of the pyramid and reserved for severe cases, was more efficacious than, and equally just as safe as, the older drugs available (Felson *et al.*, 1990, 1992). Today, methotrexate is the most commonly used DMARD in rheumatoid arthritis.

During the 1990s, knowledge of the molecular basis of rheumatoid inflammation has increased considerably. An important result of this has

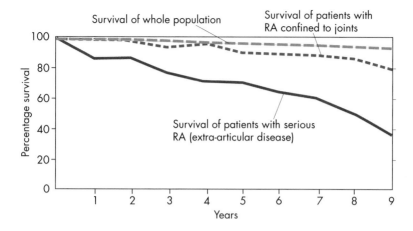

Figure 8.1   The life expectancy of patients with severe rheumatoid arthritis (RA) is reduced. Adapted from Erhardt *et al.* (1989).

been the definition of the proinflammatory cytokine tumour necrosis factor α (TNFα) as a major pathogenic mediator in RA. This has led to the emergence of anti-TNFα therapeutic strategies, which have been proved to be both safe and remarkably efficacious in cases of severe RA that had not responded adequately to DMARD therapy. Both a humanised murine antibody against human TNFα (infliximab) and a p75 TNF receptor–Fc fusion protein (etanercept) are commercially available. The demonstration that inhibition of a single cytokine can have such dramatic effects on rheumatoid inflammation, and that biological therapy with various inhibitors is safe and consistently effective, has led to an upsurge in research interest into developing anti-TNFα strategies further, or defining other therapeutic targets for biological therapy of RA (see review by Maini and Taylor, 2000).

One way of exploiting these advances in the molecular biology and pathology of RA has been to propose gene therapeutic strategies (see reviews by Chernajovsky *et al.*, 1998; Evans and Robbins, 1999; Evans *et al.*, 1999a,b). Many of these aim to deliver gene products to sites of inflammation, where they can specifically block or augment the action of pro- or anti-inflammatory cytokines or other mediators to restore homeostatic balance or re-programme the immune response. TNFα is an obvious therapeutic target, but this review will highlight many others, some of which may have beneficial effects extending those of anti-TNFα strategies. Since RA is a polyarticular disease, systemic gene therapy of RA has been attempted in animal models, but results have not been entirely convincing; in contrast, local (intra-articular) gene therapy has been both safe and effective in animal models of arthritis. The enthusiasm for gene therapy has led to the publication of the results of the first clinical trial of gene therapy of human RA, using *in vitro* retroviral gene transfer into rheumatoid synovial fibroblasts prior to joint surgery (Evans *et al.*, 1999c).

Clinical aspects of rheumatoid arthritis

Epidemiology and genetics of RA

The annual incidence of RA is between 10 and 20 per 100 000 in men and 20–40 per 100 000 in women. Thus there is a female to male excess of between 2 and 4 times, probably due to reproductive and hormonal factors. There is evidence that the incidence of RA is declining (Silman, 1988). The prevalence of RA (0.5–1%) is the same in Europe, North America, South Africa and Asia. It is as high as 5% in certain North American Indian tribes; in contrast, the disease appears to be rare in rural Africa and China.

A recent study of 203 RA patients who had a twin sibling revealed a concordance of 15% in monozygotic twins against 4% in dizygotic twins (Silman *et al.*, 1993). This provides evidence that there is a genetic predisposition for RA, but not a particularly strong one. It has been demonstrated that the major histocompatibility complex (MHC) on chromosome 6 contains genes predisposing to RA. In the United States, United Kingdom and mainland Europe, RA is linked to HLA DR4, but in other parts of the world, like Israel, parts of India and southern Europe, RA is linked to the allele HLA DR1. The third hypervariable region in the HLA DRB1 chain is identical in the HLA DR4 and HLA DR1 molecules, and this 'shared epitope' hypothesis provides evidence that RA appears to be one single disease from an immunogenetical viewpoint. Furthermore, as the only known function of the HLA DR molecules is to bind and present peptides to the T-cell receptor, the shared epitope hypothesis also contributes evidence that T cells are involved in the pathogenesis of RA.

Since identical twins have, by definition, all the genetic risk factors, the low concordance rates for RA in monozygotic twins places a limit on the genetic contribution to this disease. There have been ambitious investigations of possible socioeconomic factors or lifestyle factors that might influence the development of RA, but no definitive answers have been derived. It has long been known that certain viral and bacterial agents can induce a reactive arthritis, and this has been proposed as argument for an external causative agent in RA. But there are no clustering of RA cases in time or space to indicate an infectious spreading of the disease. Nor is there any similarity in the timing of RA outbreak in concordant twins pairs, siblings or spouse pairs. Although there is still research interest in the possible role of Epstein–Barr virus and human parvovirus in triggering RA in genetically susceptible individuals, there is no current epidemiological evidence to implicate a single infectious cause.

The diagnosis of RA

The main characteristic of RA is a chronic, symmetric, inflammatory arthritis affecting many joints, including those of the fingers and hands (see review by Maini and Zvaifler, 1998). The synovitis of the joints is characterised by hyperplasia and inflammation of the synovium, which manifests itself as joint pain and morning stiffness, with swelling and tenderness of joints, and sometimes marked increases in synovial fluid. RA can begin at any age, but onset is highest during and subsequent to the fourth and fifth decades in life. The onset of RA can be acute, subacute or insidious; the latter form is the most common. The American Rheumatism Association criteria (Table 8.1) are useful in standardising the diagnosis of RA, and are widely used. It should be noted that RA is, according to these criteria, a clinical diagnosis: a patient with

Table 8.1   The 1987 American Rheumatism Association (ARA) criteria

1 Morning stiffness	Morning stiffness in and around the joints, lasting at least 1 hour before maximal improvement
2 Arthritis in three or more joint areas	Soft tissue swelling or fluid observed by a physician, present simultaneously for at least six weeks
3 Arthritis of hand joint	Swelling of wrist, metacarpophalangeal joints or proximal interphalangeal joints for at least 6 weeks
4 Symmetric arthritis	Simultaneous involvement of the same joint areas on both sides of the body for at least 6 weeks
5 Rheumatoid nodules	Subcutaneous nodules over bony prominences or close to joints, observed by a physician
6 Rheumatoid factor	Detected by a method positive in less than 5% of normal controls
7 Radiographic changes	Bony decalcification or joint erosions typical of RA seen on hand and wrist radiographs

At least four of these criteria must be met for classification as rheumatoid arthritis.

symmetrical polyarthritis affecting the hands and a history of morning stiffness fulfils the necessary four criteria.

Autoantibodies against a variety of autoantigens occur in the sera of RA patients: in particular, the IgM rheumatoid factor, antibodies to the Fc part of IgG first described by Waaler and Rose, occurs in 70% of patients and is helpful as a diagnostic tool. The presence of the IgM rheumatoid factor in the serum is one of the ARA (or ACR) criteria, but it should be noted that these autoantibodies can also be found in other diseases, in particular Sjögren's syndrome, and low titres may occur in healthy individuals. Rheumatoid nodules, firm subcutaneous swellings that occur on pressure areas, like elbows and finger joints, present in about 20% of patients, are another diagnostic criterium. Histologically, they consist of a central fibrinoid necrosis with surrounding fibroblasts, as a result of small vessel vasculitis. Their distinctive appearance make them a diagnostic aid; yet most patients develop rheumatoid nodules late, and the majority do not have any on presentation. Another characteristic of established RA is the presence of joint erosions on radiographs, but the aim in current practice is to diagnose the disease before structural joint damage is present.

Almost every joint in the body can be affected in RA. In particular, the proximal interphalangeal joints and metacarpophalangeal joints (knuckles) are commonly affected early in the disease, as are the wrist and elbow joints. Similarly, both ankle joints and metatarsophalangeal joints often show early synovitis. Large joint involvement, usually in shoulders and knees, may occur early, but the hip is usually spared until late in disease. Tendon sheaths are often affected, and persistent flexor or extensor tenosynovitis of the wrist can be characteristic in early RA, and sometimes gives rise to complications. Flexor tenosynovitis can give rise to a 'trigger finger' phenomenon, and also to carpal tunnel syndrome; extensor tenosynovitis may lead to tendon rupture.

The clinical course of RA

The clinical course of RA has been subdivided into three alternatives. In the monocyclic form of the disease, affecting 20% of patients, there is just one flare of synovitis, and the disease is self-limiting. More common is the polycyclic variety, consisting of a series of flares of variable severity; this affects approximately 70% of patients. Some of these patients may experience remission, but it is rare. Most patients with established disease experience chronic, smouldering disease activity, punctuated by flares. The most severe form of RA is the steadily progressive, aggressive disease, which consists of one long, steady flare of persistent inflammation. Patients with progressive disabling disease often have negative prognostic factors, like positivity for HLA DR4 and the IgM rheumatoid factor, and an insidious onset of disease. They quickly develop irreversible joint damage.

Although the synovial inflammation is the most obvious clinical feature of RA, there is also clear evidence of a systemic disease. Patients with active RA have an elevated erythrocyte sedimentation rate and high levels of C-reactive protein and other acute phase reactants, as well as mild to moderate anaemia, granulocytosis and thrombocytosis. About one quarter of patients have extra-articular manifestations of disease, of which rheumatoid nodules are the most common manifestation. More uncommon are lung and kidney fibrosis, the Felty syndrome of hypersplenism and increased turnover of leukocytes and platelets, and the so-called malignant rheumatoid arthritis, characterised by aggressive vasculitis and neuropathy.

Pathophysiology and treatment of rheumatoid arthritis

The inflammatory process of RA

A normal joint has a lining layer 1–3 cells thick, consisting of fibroblastoid and macrophage-type cells without a basement membrane, resting on an interstitium of connective tissue with a few blood vessels. In contrast, the RA synovium has a much thicker lining layer, and a markedly hypercellular deeper layer. The lining layer can be 6–10 cells thick. There is perivascular accumulation of cells, a marked increase in the number of small vessels, and cells infiltrating in between the vessels (Figure 8.2). The most abundant cells are macrophages, activated fibroblasts and T lymphocytes, with plasma cells, dendritic cells, B cells and endothelium contributing to the rest of the synovial cell mass. Thus, the majority of cells in the RA synovium are blood-borne, indicating the importance of cell trafficking and recruitment in the pathogenesis of the disease. The fibroblast-like synoviocytes proliferate and possess some phenotypic characteristics of transformed cells. There is extensive formation of new blood vessels in the synovial tissue, dense perivascular infiltrates of macrophages and T cells, and occasional formation of follicles with germinal centres indicative of an ongoing immune response. The large number of capillaries supporting the

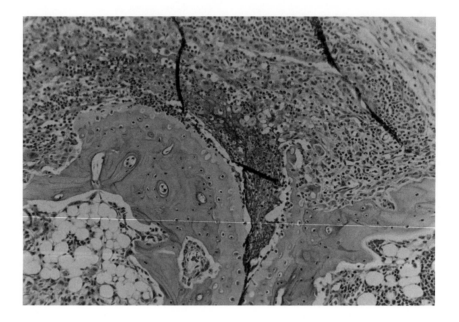

Figure 8.2 The rheumatoid synovium: erosion of bone and cartilage by pannus tissue arising from adjacent synovium in inflammatory arthritis.

hypercellular, proliferative tissue suggests that angiogenesis contributes to the disease process.

In later stages of the rheumatoid inflammation, erosion of cartilage and bone takes place, usually at the site where the fibrous capsule of the joint lined by synovium abuts the cartilage and bone. This tissue over-lying and invading cartilage and bone is referred to as pannus. This destructive process is seen as joint space narrowing and subchondral defects (erosions) of bone on joint radiographs.

The limitations of current pharmacotherapy of RA

The old-fashioned paradigm for the pharmacological treatment of RA used the concept of the treatment pyramid. In patients with early RA, treatment commenced with a non-steroidal anti-inflammatory drug (NSAID), such as diclofenac or indometacin, and if treatment response was insufficient, a mild disease-modifying drug (DMARD) like hydroxy-chloroquine or the lipophilic gold compound auranofin was added. The more potent disease-modifying compounds, like sulfasalazine and methotrexate, were reserved for severe, therapy-resistant cases, and usually administered several years after the diagnosis had initially been made. But the view of the natural history of RA and its management has changed dramatically during the 1990s. It has become generally accepted that far from being a mild, self-limiting disease, RA is a major source of joint damage, functional decline and work disability. The life expectancy of patients with severe RA is considerably reduced. Partial control of the inflammation does not appear to prevent joint damage, and the majority of patients with active disease show progressive disability. With the modern knowledge of the pathological process in RA, and a more realistic view of the long-term prognosis of the disease, it has become increasingly clear that treatment with potent DMARDs should be instituted as early as possible after diagnosis, and prior to functional deterioration. The main obstacle for achieving the target of controlling the rheumatoid inflammation leading to progressive joint destruction has been the inadequacy of the drugs available. Most of the older drugs used to treat arthritis have entered rheumatology in a serendipitous manner rather than a rational one: the gold compounds were originally used as tuberculostatics, the chloroquine derivatives as antimalarials, and methotrexate as an antiproliferative agent used in the treatment of malignancies.

Gold compounds like aurothiomalate and auranofin are still used in antirheumatic therapy: both have been shown to be superior to placebo in controlled trials (see review by Champion et al., 1990). These compounds probably have multiple mechanisms of action: both compounds inhibit neutrophil functions like phagocytosis and superoxide release, and auranofin also inhibits the formation of 5-lipoxygenase products (Bondeson, 1997). It is of interest that auranofin, but not hydrophilic gold compounds like aurothiomalate, inhibit lipopolysaccharide (LPS)-induced TNFα and IL-1β in macrophages (Bondeson and Sundler, 1995), possibly through an effect on the transcription factor NF-κB (Bratt et al., 2000). But in a meta-analysis of antirheumatic compounds, auranofin proved to be less effective than aurothiomalate and other more potent antirheumatic compounds (Felson et al., 1990, 1992), and in another study (Pincus et al., 1992), it was tolerated for a significantly shorter time than any other antirheumatic drug. In contrast, aurothiomalate was one of the most potent DMARDs in the same meta-analysis (Felson et al., 1990, 1992), but also more toxic than any other compound. The use of antirheumatic gold compounds today is decreasing, and this is true also for other older drugs, like D-penicillamine and the cytotoxic compound azathioprine.

Antimalarial drugs, like chloroquine and hydroxychloroquine, are superior to placebo in RA (Clark *et al.*, 1993; HERA study group, 1995). They are still used to some extent, since although they are less effective than the more potent drugs (van der Heijde *et al.*, 1989; Felson *et al.*, 1990, 1992), their low toxicity make them an attractive therapeutic option. Antimalarial compounds are also likely to have multiple mechanisms of action, including inhibition of neutrophil function, inhibition of phospholipase A_2, and inhibition of macrophage-derived, proinflammatory cytokines (Bondeson, 1997).

Sulfasalazine was synthesised in the 1930s as a combination between an (antibacterial) sulfonamide moiety and an (anti-inflammatory) salicylic acid derivative, since it was at that time believed that RA was an infectious disease. It is still used in RA, and has been shown to be superior to hydroxychloroquine and auranofin (van der Heijde *et al.*, 1989; Felson *et al.*, 1990, 1992). Its mechanisms of action have been proposed to include inhibition of neutrophil functions, including the formation of 5-lipoxygenase products, and a potentiation of the production of the anti-inflammatory autocoid adenosine, thereby reducing leukocyte trafficking (Cronstein, 1995); it is unlikely that physiological concentrations of sulfasalazine or its metabolites have any effect on the production of TNFα and IL-1β in macrophages (Bondeson, 1997).

In the 1990s, methotrexate has emerged as the leading DMARD on the market. There are various suggestions about its mechanism of action in RA: an attractive hypothesis with a good deal of experimental support is that it promotes the production of adenosine and thus reduces leukocyte trafficking (Cronstein, 1996). Methotrexate does not appear to influence the induction of TNFα or IL-1β in macrophages (Bondeson and Sundler, 1995), but it does inhibit the induction of TNFα and interferon γ from T cells. Clinical studies have provided evidence that methotrexate is at least as efficacious as the most potent other DMARDs and that it has a more rapid onset of effect, that it is often effective when other DMARDs have failed, and that it is generally tolerated over long periods of time (Felson *et al.*, 1990, 1992; Pincus *et al.*, 1992; Bannwarth *et al.*, 1994). However, although methotrexate may be the most effective DMARD currently available, it fails to induce disease remission in most patients.

The most recent DMARD on the market is leflunomide, an isoxazol derivative whose active metabolite blocks the clonal expansion of T cells by preventing *de novo* synthesis of pyrimidines (Fox *et al.*, 1999). Clinical studies have shown that leflunomide is more effective than placebo in rheumatoid arthritis, and similar to sulfasalazine or methotrexate (Smolen *et al.*, 1999).

Another concept that has gained prominence in the 1990s is combination therapy with two or more DMARDs. Combination therapy with methotrexate and ciclosporin has given some encouraging results, but the occurrence of renal and hypertensive side effects is a major concern. Hydroxychloroquine–methotrexate or sulfasalazine–methotrexate combination therapy is not infrequently used (Calguneri *et al.*, 1999; Hawley *et al.*, 1999). Recent studies of triple therapy with methotrexate, sulfasalazine and hydroxychloroquine in RA have shown impressive benefits from this combination, without increased toxicity during long-term follow-up (O'Dell, 1999).

T cells, macrophages, interleukin 1 and tumour necrosis factor α as therapeutic targets in RA

In the 1980s and early 1990s, there was much enthusiasm about the T cell as a therapeutic target in RA. The T lymphocyte was considered as the prime mover in rheumatoid inflammation, directing the activity of other synovial cells. There is no controversy about the importance of the T cell in the initiation of RA, but in the 1990s, there has been considerable opposition to the concept of the T cell as the central player in established, chronic rheumatoid synovitis (Firestein and Zvaifler, 1990). If the T cells were actively supporting the rheumatoid inflammation, they would be expected to proliferate, express surface activation markers and produce cytokines. But it has been pointed out that rheumatoid T cell mitotic figures and surface activation markers are low (Firestein and Zvaifler, 1990), proliferation responses when stimulated with recall antigens or mitogens suboptimal (Cope *et al.*, 1994) and lymphokine levels in synovial tissue and exudates very low (Firestein *et al.*, 1988, 1990). In a study of synovial biopsies, no correlation was found between synovial lymphocyte infiltration and the development of radiological articular destruction (Mulherin *et al.*, 1996). An argument in favour of the T cell as a therapeutic target in RA is that ciclosporin, a potent inhibitor of T-cell proliferation and cytokine induction, has been shown to be moderately effective in RA, but this drug also acts on other cell types, including macrophages (Nguyen *et al.*, 1990; Svensson *et al.*, 1995). Much work has been put into the development of anti-CD4 antibodies for use in RA as a specific therapy against T cells. These antibodies have been demonstrated to reduce levels of circulating T cells within hours of infusion, and after 5 days of treatment, some T-cell depletion was seen in the synovial tissue. Some early, uncontrolled studies of lytic anti-CD4 monoclonal antibody therapy in RA gave promising results, but later, placebo-controlled studies failed to show any significant benefit (Choy *et al.*, 1992; Moreland *et al.*, 1995; van der Lubbe *et al.*, 1995).

In contrast, a steadily growing body of evidence has pointed out the macrophage as a therapeutic target cell in RA. Macrophages are numerous in the inflamed rheumatoid synovium, and there is no doubt, from studies of cell morphology, expression of surface activation markers, and proinflammatory cytokine production, that these cells are highly activated (Chu *et al.*, 1992; Cutolo *et al.*, 1993). There is a clear correlation between macrophage activation markers and the general inflammatory activity in synovial biopsy specimens (Sack *et al.*, 1994). Another synovial biopsy study (Mulherin *et al.*, 1996) observed a correlation between macrophage numbers in the lining and sublining layers of the rheumatoid synovium and the subsequent development of articular erosions. In marked contrast to the T-cell cytokines, macrophage-produced cytokines, such as TNFα, IL-1 and IL-6, are abundant in the rheumatoid synovium. In particular, activated macrophages expressing IL-1α and TNFα are prominent near the cartilage–pannus junction (Chu *et al.*, 1992; Wood *et al.*, 1992). In contrast to the brief cytokine response to immune stimulation or infection, the cytokine production in the rheumatoid synovium is prolonged and chronic (Feldmann *et al.*, 1996). Although anti-inflammatory mediators, such as IL-10, the IL-1 receptor antagonist and the soluble TNF receptors, were also upregulated in RA tissue, their levels were not sufficient to antagonise the actions of the proinflammatory macrophage cytokines (Figure 8.3).

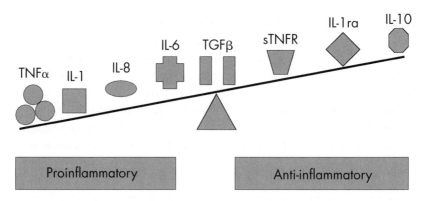

Figure 8.3 Disequilibrium of proinflammatory cytokines and their inhibitors in active rheumatoid arthritis (RA). This concept explains why both pro- and anti-inflammatory pathways are upregulated in RA.

After the macrophage had gained prominence as a major player in disease perpetuation in established RA, the debate turned to concentrate on which of its cytokines is the most promising therapeutic target. In particular, the proinflammatory cytokines TNFα and IL-1 have attracted much interest, as both are highly proinflammatory and expressed in the rheumatoid joint. TNFα is produced as a 26-kDa active precursor molecule, which is membrane bound. It can be proteolytically cleaved by a specific enzyme, known as TACE or ADAM-17, to yield the 17-kDa soluble TNFα molecule. This readily forms an active, 52-kDa TNFα trimer, which is the main extracellular form of TNFα. Two different TNF receptors are known: the non-inducible p55 receptor and the inducible p75 receptor, both of which can be cleaved to yield soluble TNF receptors. TNFα has many proinflammatory effects in various cell types (reviewed by Aggarwal *et al.*, 2001). It is a potent activator of macrophages and inducer of IL-1 (Turner *et al.*, 1989), an activator of IL-8 production and adhesion molecule expression by endothelial cells (Nawroth *et al.*, 1986), an inhibitor of proteoglycan synthesis (Saklatvala, 1986), and an inducer of prostaglandin E_2 and matrix metalloproteinase production from synovial cells (Dayer *et al.*, 1985).

IL-1 occurs in two forms, IL-1α and IL-1β, which are the products of separate genes, both of which are situated on chromosome 2 (see review by Dinarello, 2001). They have different amino acid sequences but are structurally similar on the three-dimensional level and act through the same receptors. IL-1α is synthesised in a biologically active 31-kDa precursor, which may remain intracellular or become expressed on the cell surface, where it may be cleaved into the mature 17.5-kDa IL-1α molecule by extracellular proteases. IL-1β is proteolytically processed by the so-called IL-1β-converting enzyme (caspase 1) to yield mature IL-1β, which can then freely leave the cell. Two types of IL-1 receptors exist: the type I receptor, which has a longer cytoplasmic segment and a higher affinity for IL-1α, and the type II receptor, which has a shorter cytoplasmic segment and a higher affinity for IL-1β. Both receptors bind both IL-1 and the so-called IL-1 receptor accessory protein. The type II receptor is a non-signalling 'decoy' that is present in large excess on the target cells over both the type I receptor and the IL-1 receptor accessory protein; this makes shedding of the type II receptor extracellular domain an important critical event in IL-1 signalling. Furthermore, proteolytic cleavage of the type II IL-1 receptor yields the so-called soluble IL-1 receptor, which can inhibit the action of IL-1β. In addition, a molecule known as the IL-1 receptor antagonist, which has structural similarity to IL-1, can bind to IL-1 receptors without activating the target cell. But less than 5%

of IL-1 receptors need to be engaged by IL-1 to induce a biological response, and it is estimated that a 10- to 100-fold excess of the IL-1 receptor antagonist is needed to achieve a 50% inhibition of the IL-1 response (Arend *et al.*, 1990). Thus, although the IL-1 receptor antagonist is also upregulated in the RA synovium, it is inadequate to affect the IL-1-induced inflammatory response.

IL-1 is well known as a potent mediator of bone and cartilage breakdown. It induces proteoglycan degradation and inhibition of synthesis, including aggrecan, biglycan and decorin (Page *et al.*, 1991; von den Hoff *et al.*, 1995). It acts on fibroblasts, chondrocytes and synovial cells to induce the formation of prostaglandin E_2 and large amounts of collagenase 1, stromelysin 1 and other matrix metalloproteinases (MacNaul *et al.*, 1992). Indeed, some animal studies spoke in favour of IL-1 being a more powerful inducer of cartilage destruction than TNFα (O'Byrne *et al.*, 1990; van Lent *et al.*, 1995; Kuiper *et al.*, 1998), and this led to a hypothesis that although TNFα was the main cytokine regulating synovitis in RA (Brennan *et al.*, 1992), IL-1 was the dominant mediator of cartilage destruction (e.g. van den Berg, 1998).

Biological therapy of RA

In 1988, it was observed that in cell cultures from dissociated rheumatoid synovial tissue, proinflammatory cytokine production continued over several days in the absence of extrinsic stimulation (Buchan *et al.*, 1988). This suggested the presence of some intrinsic signal driving cytokine production in these cultures, which consist of a heterogeneous population of cells producing multiple cytokines. A key observation was that after incubation of these rheumatoid synovial tissue cultures with neutralising anti-TNF antibodies, the production of IL-1 virtually ceased (Brennan *et al.*, 1989). Later, it was demonstrated that the production of other proinflammatory cytokines, such as IL-6, IL-8 and GM-CSF, from RA synovial cultures was strikingly reduced by treatment with neutralising anti-TNF antibodies (Haworth *et al.*, 1991; Butler *et al.*, 1995; Feldmann *et al.*, 1996). This formulated the concept of TNFα as the dominant proinflammatory mediator in rheumatoid inflammation, occupying a key position at the apex of the cytokine cascade (Figure 8.4). These observations defined TNFα as a potential therapeutic target in RA. This hypothesis was tested by treating mice with collagen-induced arthritis with either specific anti-TNF monoclonal antibodies or a soluble TNF receptor (sTNFR) fused to the immunoglobulin Fc fragment. Both these strategies potently ameliorated clinical symptoms and prevented joint destruction (Williams *et al.*, 1992; Piguet *et al.*, 1992). Another important observation was that mice with a high level of expression of a human TNFα transgene developed a disease resembling RA 4–6 weeks after birth, and that this arthritis could be prevented by administration of anti-TNF monoclonal antibody (Keffer *et al.*, 1991). Blocking IL-1 action with an anti-IL-1 receptor (type I) monoclonal antibody also led to effective prevention of arthritis, thus confirming that the proinflammatory effects of TNFα overexpression involve IL-1 (Probert *et al.*, 1995).

These observations set the stage for clinical trials of anti-TNF strategies in RA. Early short term trials of infliximab, a humanised murine antibody against human TNFα, performed in 1992 and 1993, showed that infusions of this antibody were both safe and efficacious. Patients exhibited a marked reduction (over 60%) in pain, stiffness, swelling and joint tenderness within 24 hours. Maximum benefit was observed at around 2–4 weeks and was sustained for the entire eight-week duration of the trial in most patients (Elliott *et al.*, 1993). These findings prompted a multicentre, placebo-controlled, randomised, double-blind study in 73 patients, conducted in 1993–1994 (Elliott *et al.*, 1994). Infliximab was administered as a single intravenous infusion of either 1 or 10 mg/kg and was compared with a placebo infusion. According to the Paulus criteria for 20% improvement in RA (Paulus *et al.*, 1990), 79% and 44% of patients had responded to the high- and low-dose infusions of infliximab, but only 8% of patients receiving placebo infusions

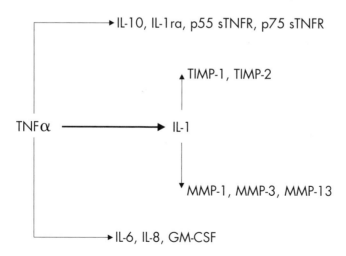

Figure 8.4   The cytokine cascade in rheumatoid arthritis (RA).

responded after four weeks. In patients receiving the higher dose of 10 mg/kg, response duration lasted eight weeks. There were impressive decreases in IL-6, C-reactive protein (CRP) and erythrocyte sedimentation rate (ESR). The mechanism of action of infliximab has been shown to involve not only diminution of other cytokines, such as IL-1 and IL-6, but also inhibition of angiogenesis and downregulation of vascular endothelial growth factor, and blocking of neutrophil recruitment into joints (Paleolog *et al.*, 1996; Tak *et al.*, 1996; Taylor *et al.*, 2000; Lorenz *et al.*, 2000).

The success of infliximab in these short-term clinical trials resulted in a longer term European multicentre, placebo-controlled, randomised, double-blind study in 101 RA patients who had active disease despite receiving methotrexate. Patients received infliximab infusions at entry and at weeks 2, 6, 10 and 14, in combination with either placebo or low-dose methotrexate. Again, patients receiving 3 mg/kg or 10 mg/kg of infliximab had a >60% Paulus 20% response, which was sustained during the 14 weeks of treatment. There was a clear synergy between infliximab and methotrexate, particularly with regard to duration of response (Maini *et al.*, 1998). These data provided the rationale for a randomised phase III study involving 428 patients, all receiving methotrexate. Again, benefit from infliximab was both pronounced and sustained over a long period of time; patients were receiving maintenance therapy every four or eight weeks (Maini *et al.*, 1999). Infliximab was well tolerated throughout the 54 weeks of the study.

The establishment of TNFα as the major therapeutic target in RA also led to a search for the mechanisms by which this cytokine exerts its effects. Many symptoms in RA patients, including pain, stiffness and joint swelling, respond well to anti-TNFα therapy, and are likely to be directly dependent on proinflammatory cytokines (Feldmann *et al.*, 1996, 1997; Maini and Feldmann, 2000). An important problem, however, is the regulation of the process of joint destruction. In mice with collagen-induced arthritis (Williams *et al.*, 1992) or in transgenic mice with a disregulated TNFα transgene (Keffer *et al.*, 1991), joint destruction can be abolished by blocking TNFα. Whether this is also the case in human RA has been intensely debated, one school of thought suggesting that while TNFα is the major cytokine regulating synovitis in RA, IL-1 is the dominant cytokine implicated in cartilage destruction (van Lent *et al.*, 1995). It is of high interest that in spite of the animal data suggesting that IL-1 and not TNFα was the central cytokine for joint destruction, a radiological monitoring of joint erosions in the phase III study discussed earlier showed that joint damage was arrested in patients treated with infliximab (Lipsky *et al.*, 1999). Thus, control of inflammation with anti-TNFα therapy also appears to control the development of joint erosions in human RA.

The second major anti-TNF therapeutic strategy in RA has been to use a p75 TNF receptor–Ig fusion protein (etanercept). The development of etanercept has been rapid, clinical trials commencing in 1994 and phase III studies being completed in 1998. Whereas monoclonal anti-TNFα antibodies like infliximab are specific strategies against TNFα, the related cytokine lymphotoxin (TNFβ) also binds to etanercept and other soluble TNF receptor dimers. Another difference is that infliximab, but not etanercept, can mediate complement-dependent lysis of TNFα-expressing cells *in vitro* (Barone *et al.*, 1999); whether this also happens *in vivo* is not clear. The clinical effects of etanercept are also quite impressive, however, with benefit similar to that observed with infliximab in a multicentre, randomised, placebo-controlled trial (Moreland *et al.*, 1997), and a second trial involving patients with persistent disease despite taking methotrexate (Weinblatt *et al.*, 1999). There was no comparison of combination therapy with etanercept alone, and it is thus not clear whether there is any synergy between etanercept and methotrexate, as was the case with infliximab.

Both etanercept and infliximab have been approved for the treatment of rheumatoid arthritis, among other inflammatory diseases, and are commercially available. In contrast to many of the old antirheumatic drugs, they have proved remarkably safe, and are widely used, particularly in the United States. Many pharmaceutical companies are in the process of developing alternative anti-TNFα strategies, including other anti-TNF antibodies (Kempeni, 1999) and TNF receptor–Ig fusion proteins (Edwards, 1999) as well as small molecule inhibitors of TNFα synthesis.

Some important therapeutic target genes in rheumatoid arthritis

Inhibitors of proinflammatory cytokines

In the early 1990s, inhibition of IL-1 was seen as being of great importance for the treatment of RA. This concept was supported by data from experimental SCID mouse models (Muller-Ladner *et al.*, 1997) and animal arthritis models (reviewed by van den Berg, 1997) indicating a major role for IL-1 in the development of perichondrocytic matrix degradation leading to joint damage, and also an impressive effect of anti-IL-1 therapy in animal models of arthritis (van Lent *et al.*, 1995; Joosten *et al.*, 1996; Kuiper *et al.*, 1998). In animal studies, recombinant soluble type I IL-1 receptor and recombinant IL-1 receptor antagonist were both effective (Joosten *et al.*, 1996), but an early human study of recombinant human soluble type I IL-1 receptor was disappointing, and later studies have concentrated on recombinant human IL-1 receptor antagonist. After an initial study (Campion *et al.*, 1996) had established the safety of this form of treatment, and suitable dosage schedules for daily subcutaneous injections of the IL-1 receptor antagonist, a 24-week, double-blind, placebo-controlled, multicentre study compared placebo injections with either 30, 75 or 150 mg daily injections of the IL-1 receptor antagonist in a total of 472 patients. A modest clinical benefit, without dose dependence, was observed, and also a modest decrease in ESR and CRP levels (20–35% reduction as compared with 60–70% with infliximab or etanercept). Interestingly, there was also some anti-erosive effect of the IL-1 receptor antagonist in this study, statistically significant only in the two lower dose regimens (Bresnihan *et al.*, 1998); reduction of radiological progression of RA in patients treated with the IL-1 receptor antagonist was also observed after 48 weeks (Jiang *et al.*, 2000).

The emergence of TNFα as the major therapeutic target in RA also has implications for gene therapy approaches, since an obvious course of action would be to transfer genes that inhibit TNFα. In particular, a construct encoding a soluble TNF receptor–Ig fusion protein would be of interest, as both p75 (Weinblatt *et al.*, 1999) and p55 (Edwards, 1999) TNF receptor–Ig fusion proteins have been shown to be effective in RA. The recent demonstration that the infliximab anti-TNFα antibody has a potent anti-erosive effect in RA patients has disproved the concept that TNF controls inflammation and IL-1 joint destruction: it instead appears that these processes are more tightly linked than presumed earlier, and that TNFα is a key mediator of them both. Indeed, a comparison between recent clinical studies of long-term trials of anti-IL-1 (Bresnihan *et al.*, 1998) and anti-TNF (Lipsky *et al.*, 1999; Maini *et al.*, 1999) strategies in RA would favour the latter concept both with regard to regulation of inflammation and prevention of joint erosions.

IL-6 is a cytokine with mainly proinflammatory effects, including the induction of acute phase proteins from hepatocytes and activation of osteoclasts to absorb bone. It has been shown to play a role in murine collagen-induced arthritis (Takagi *et al.*, 1998; Sasai *et al.*, 1999), and early uncontrolled studies of intravenous infusions of a murine anti-IL-6 monoclonal antibody has been shown to have beneficial effects in two preliminary, uncontrolled studies in patients with active RA (Wendling *et al.*, 1993; Yoshizaki *et al.*, 1998).

The Th1 cytokine IL-12 has also attracted interest as a therapeutic target in arthritis, as neutralisation of this cytokine might have beneficial effects on the Th1/Th2 cytokine balance. In murine collagen-induced arthritis, administration of antibodies against IL-12 prior to disease onset attenuated disease severity (Joosten *et al.*, 1997a; Malfait *et al.*, 1998), and there was a synergistic effect with anti-TNF antibodies (Butler *et al.*, 1999). Clinical trials of anti-IL-12 strategies in RA are being planned.

Anti-inflammatory cytokines

The anti-inflammatory cytokine that has attracted most notice as a potential therapeutic in RA is IL-10. Produced mainly by mononuclear cells and T cells, this anti-inflammatory cytokine inhibits the production of TNFα, IL-1 and IL-6 by activated monocytes and macrophages, upregulates the production of soluble TNF receptors and the IL-1 receptor antagonist, and downregulates MHC class II expression on antigen-presenting cells (Moore *et al.*, 1993; St Clair, 1999). This would point towards an anti-inflammatory effect of IL-10, and has prompted trials of systemic administration of this cytokine in the murine collagen-induced arthritis model. IL-10 treatment suppressed the clinical manifestations of both early and established murine collagen-induced arthritis, and reduced histological signs of joint inflammation, synovial tissue expression of TNFα and IL-1 mRNA, and the destruction of articular bone and cartilage (Walmsley *et al.*, 1996; Joosten *et al.*, 1997b). These encouraging findings have prompted clinical studies of IL-10 administration in humans. A dose-escalating, double-blind, placebo-controlled phase I trial of daily subcutaneously administered IL-10 (1.0–20 μg/kg) in 72 patients with active RA showed no major side effects and an increase in serum levels of soluble TNF receptors and the IL-1 receptor antagonist. Although it was not possible to draw any conclusions concerning clinical efficacy, there was a trend toward improvement in disease activity compared with placebo recipients. Treatment was well tolerated (Maini *et al.*, 1997).

Another possible therapeutic cytokine in RA is IL-4, a product mainly of Th2 cells that suppresses Th1 function. IL-4 also inhibits the expression of TNFα, IL-1, IL-6 and other proinflammatory cytokines, as well as prostaglandin E_2, in activated macrophages and monocytes, and facilitates the expression and release of soluble IL-1 and TNF receptors (Chomarat *et al.*, 1995; Woods *et al.*, 1999). There is also experimental evidence in favour of IL-4 inhibiting growth factor-induced proliferation of RA synoviocytes (Dechanet *et al.*, 1993), and having a beneficial effect both on cartilage degradation (van Roon *et al.*, 1996) and on bone resorption (Miossec *et al.*, 1994). IL-4 levels are normally extremely low in the RA joint. A study of overexpressing IL-4 in RA synovial cell cultures by means of adenoviral gene transfer showed an impressive reduction in proinflammatory cytokines like TNFα and IL-1, in prostaglandin E_2 and in chemokines like IL-8 and MCP-1, and also in growth-related fibroblast gene products (Woods *et al.*, 1999). Treatment of experimental arthritis with IL-4 had to be administered by daily injections or by constant infusion due to the short half-life of the injected molecule. Both in streptococcal cell wall arthritis and murine collagen-induced arthritis, this strategy induced significant suppression of disease (Allen *et al.*, 1993; Horsfall *et al.*, 1997; Joosten *et al.*, 1997b). Interestingly, treatment of established murine collagen-induced arthritis with combined IL-4 and IL-10 markedly augments the improvement noted with IL-10 alone (Joosten *et al.*, 1997b). In contrast, a phase I dose-escalating study of recombinant human IL-4 administered three times a week for six weeks in patients with active RA failed to demonstrate significant clinical benefit compared with placebo (van den Bosch *et al.*, 1998).

A third anti-inflammatory cytokine in RA is IL-11, a pleiotropic cytokine that acts in synergy with IL-10 to suppress the induction of proinflammatory cytokines in macrophages or RA cells (Hermann *et al.*, 1998). In murine collagen-induced arthritis, treatment with recombinant human IL-11 in established disease significantly attenuates clinical severity and affords some protection against joint destruction (Walmsley *et al.*, 1998). IL-11 is also particularly effective in a model of HLA B27 transgenic rats that spontaneously develop arthritis and inflammatory bowel disease (Peterson *et al.*, 1998). In a phase I dose-escalating study of weekly subcutaneous injections of recombinant human IL-11 in RA, treatment was well tolerated except for injection site reactions, and there was a modest trend toward improvement for those patients receiving the highest dose (15 μg/kg once weekly) (Moreland *et al.*, 1999).

Transforming growth factor β (TGFβ) is a potent immunomodulatory cytokine with both pro- and anti-inflammatory properties. Its effects on many macrophage and T-cell functions in inflammation are mainly inhibitory, and it stimulates repair and regeneration of connective tissue, but is an inducer of leukocyte recruitment to sites with inflammatory activity (Prud'homme and Piccirillo, 2000). Data with regard to the role of TGFβ in arthritis are contradictory: one study found that TGFβ administration antagonised the development of streptococcal cell wall arthritis in rats (Brandes *et al.*, 1991), another that antibodies against TGFβ inhibited tissue pathology and inflammatory cell recruitment in a similar model of experimental polyarthritis (Wahl *et al.*, 1993).

While interferon γ therapy is not superior to placebo in RA (Veys *et al.*, 1997), there has been some interest in interferon β, which is used in multiple sclerosis and has been shown to have beneficial effects on the production of both proinflammatory cytokines and metalloproteinases in RA synovial cell cultures (Smeets *et al.*, 2000). A study of subcutaneous injections of recombinant interferon β in rhesus monkeys with collagen-induced arthritis had markedly beneficial effects, but results from an early, uncontrolled study in RA patients showed more modest benefits, and no clear-cut dose–response relationship (Tak *et al.*, 1999a).

The transcription factor NF-κB as a therapeutic target

The definition of TNFα as a therapeutic target in RA has led to increased interest in the mechanisms controlling TNFα production, the blockade of which might mimic the clinical benefit of anti-TNFα therapy. In RA joints, macrophages are the cells producing the majority of TNFα (Chu *et al.*, 1992). In particular, the role of the transcription factor NF-κB in TNFα regulation has been considered of interest. In the mouse macrophage cell line RAW 264 (Shakhov *et al.*, 1990), in the human monocytic cell line THP-1 (Makarov *et al.*, 1997) and in mouse bone marrow-derived macrophages (Han and Beutler, 1990), NF-κB is essential for TNFα production, but this is not the case in human lymphoid cell lines (Goldfeld *et al.*, 1991). This prompted us to investigate, using a novel adenoviral technique to infect in excess of 95% of normal human macrophages, whether an adenovirus (Wrighton *et al.*, 1996) transferring the endogenous NF-κB inhibitor IκBα was able to inhibit TNFα production (Figure 8.5). Using Northern analysis of TNFα mRNA and ELISA studies of TNFα production, 80% inhibition of this cytokine was observed (Foxwell *et al.*, 1998). There are both NF-κB-dependent and -independent pathways to induce NF-κB and other proinflammatory cytokines: while LPS- and phorbol myristate acetate (PMA)-induced TNFα is NF-κB-dependent, zymosan-induced TNFα is not. Another finding of interest was that the proinflammatory cytokines IL-1, IL-6 and

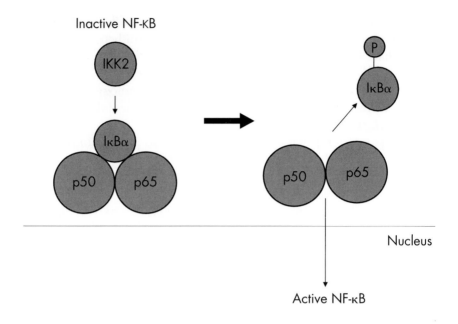

Figure 8.5 Schematic view of the activation of NF-κB.

IL-8 were NF-κB-dependent in human macrophages, but that IL-10 and the IL-1 receptor antagonist were not (Bondeson *et al.*, 1999a).

We used the same adenoviral technique to study the effect of NF-κB blockade on the key destructive enzymes matrix metalloproteinases (MMP)-1, MMP-3 and MMP-13, and their inhibitor TIMP-1, in human fibroblasts and chondrosarcoma cells (Bondeson *et al.*, 2000). MMP-1 and MMP-3 have been shown to be upregulated in the RA synovial membrane, and have been implicated in the development of joint damage. While there was some prior evidence that MMP-1 was NF-κB-dependent (Tewari *et al.*, 1996; Vincenti *et al.*, 1998), little was known about the regulation of MMP-3 and MMP-13, except that some studies (reviewed by Fini *et al.*, 1998) indicated that the transcription factor AP-1 played a major role. The results were that both MMP-1, MMP-3 and MMP-13 were inhibited by NF-κB blockade, irrespective of stimulus (IL-1, TNF, PMA), but that TIMP-1 was unaffected (Bondeson *et al.*, 2000). Further evidence for the NF-κB-dependence of MMP-1 in rabbit synovial fibroblasts (Barchowsky *et al.*, 1999) and human fibroblast-like synoviocytes (Aupperle *et al.*, 1999) has been obtained.

It was possible to extend this technique of adenoviral gene transfer also to a mixed culture of rheumatoid synovial cells. After it had been ascertained that more than 90% of all cell types (macrophages, T cells and fibroblasts) in the joint cultures could be infected with adenovirus, and that the IκBα adenovirus was functional with regard to IκBα over-expression, it was possible to analyse the spontaneous production of a variety of cytokines and destructive enzymes (Bondeson *et al.*, 1999b). Thus it was possible to study the effect of IκBα overexpression on not only the balance between pro- and anti-inflammatory cytokines in the inflamed joint tissue, but also the balance between destructive metallo-proteases and their inhibitors. While the spontaneous production of TNFα, IL-1β, IL-6 and IL-8 was inhibited, there was no effect on IL-10, IL-11 and the IL-1 receptor antagonist. MMP-1, MMP-3 and MMP-13 were also inhibited, but the spontaneous production of TIMP-1 instead somewhat potentiated (Figure 8.6).

There is also evidence that the combined inhibition of NF-κB and TNFα treatment induced apoptosis in cell lines, but not in primary macrophages (Foxwell *et al.*, 1998). In a recent study, adenoviral over-expression of IκBα in primary RA synovial fibroblast cell lines did not promote apoptosis *per se*, but facilitated TNFα-induced apoptosis (Zhang *et al.*, 2000). This may well add another desirable characteristic to anti-NF-κB targeted strategies in RA, since lack of control of apop-tosis in the proliferating synovial fibroblasts is of importance for the ability of these cells to invade the surrounding tissues, leading to joint destruction.

These results clearly point out NF-κB as a key target for therapeutic intervention. As NF-κB blockade resulted in a significant reduction of proinflammatory cytokines and destructive enzymes, while not directly affecting anti-inflammatory mechanisms and the tissue inhibitor of MMPs, these results, along with the finding of nuclear NF-κB in active RA joints (Marok *et al.*, 1996; Sioud *et al.*, 1998), suggest that selective blockade of NF-κB in the diseased tissue would be of considerable benefit in rheumatoid arthritis.

Gene delivery systems suitable for rheumatoid arthritis

Non-viral strategies

Among the key components of a successful gene therapy protocol for rheumatoid arthritis is an effective gene delivery system, which requires a vector capable of efficiently delivering the gene of interest to the target cells in the diseased synovium. Non-viral vectors are usually simple and

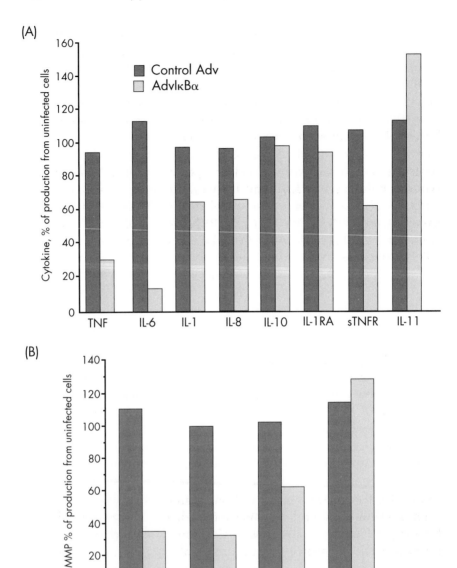

Figure 8.6   Proinflammatory and destructive mediators (e.g. TNFα, IL-1 and MMP-1) are inhibited, but anti-inflammatory and anti-destructive mediators (e.g. IL-11, IL-1RA and TIMP-1) are spared in rheumatoid synovial cultures infected by an adenovirus transferring IκBα, the inhibitory subunit of NF-κB. Adapted from Bondeson *et al.* (1999b, 2000).

inexpensive. They are non-antigenic and have not been derived from pathogens. The simplest vector imaginable is just a string of naked plasmid DNA. To aid uptake, one technique is to coat naked DNA onto small inert particles, which are projected into cells using a 'gene gun', but this is cumbersome and requires specialised equipment. Another strategy to enhance gene transfer is to use cationic liposome-encapsulated DNA, or DNA–carrier complexes that utilise ligands designed to facilitate receptor-mediated uptake. The major drawback of all these strategies is their inefficiency: cellular uptake is generally low, also in synovial fibroblasts *in vitro* and in synovial cells after intra-articular injection (Nita *et al.*, 1996). Nevertheless, there are some examples of naked plasmid DNA (Ragno *et al.*, 1997; Song *et al.*, 1998) or linear DNA 'decoy' oligonucleotides (Miagkov *et al.*, 1998; Tomita *et al.*, 1999) being used with some success in animal models of arthritis, although the significance of this is unclear.

Viral strategies

Viruses are the obvious choice for gene delivery; over millions of years they have perfected their ability to infect cells and to introduce their own genes into the genome of their host. For use as gene therapy vectors, viruses have to be genetically disabled to minimise their pathogenicity while retaining their capacity to infect cells; once the genes have been delivered, the virus must not replicate and harm the patient or experimental animal. Several types of viruses have been modified in this way.

Retroviruses are RNA viruses that replicate through a double-stranded DNA intermediate, which integrates into the host DNA and expresses viral RNA for the lifetime of the cell. Established methods exist for the production of infectious, replication- incompetent retroviruses through deletion of some viral genes essential for replication, and the use of a packaging cell line expressing these genes. Such retroviruses have been extensively used in gene therapy protocols, particularly as *ex vivo* gene delivery vehicles, and much is known about their biology and safe handling. It is well known that retroviruses integrate their genetic material into the cells they infect, which increases their potential for long-term gene expression, a useful characteristic in the gene therapy of chronic disease. Another advantage of retroviruses is that they do not express viral genes in the cells they infect, since viral proteins are often antigenic and lead to immune reactions against infected cells. Most retroviral vectors currently in use are based on the Moloney murine leukaemia virus (MoMLV), an extensively characterised, non-pathogenic virus that has no homology with human retroviruses. MoMLV-based vectors are unable to infect non-dividing cells, and are thus often used in *ex vivo* gene therapy protocols, in which the target cells are removed, infected outside the body, and then re-implanted in the organ system in question. This also allows for screening the cells for replication-competent retrovirus before they are re-introduced into the patient or experimental animal. A second safety concern with retroviruses is the risk of insertional mutagenesis leading to malignant transformation of cells, which has been shown to occur in mice infected with replication-competent retrovirus, but never with replication-incompetent retrovirus. Direct retroviral gene transfer *in vivo* into rheumatoid synovium is not possible, due to the lack of infectivity, but strategies have been devised to get around this problem. High-titre MoMLV-based retroviruses can infect synovial cells *in vivo*, if these cells have been challenged with mitotic stimuli or with the polycationic molecule polybrene; this has been demonstrated in rabbit knees (Ghivizzani *et al.*, 1997) and in SCID mice engrafted with human rheumatoid synovial tissue (Jorgensen *et al.*, 1997). A second approach has used retroviral vectors based on lentiviruses, which are able to infect non-dividing cells (Naldini *et al.*, 1996), but this technique has yet to be shown to work safely and reliably in synovial tissue.

Adeno-associated viruses are non-pathogenic, stable parvoviruses that can transduce both dividing and non-dividing cells, and do not make viral proteins. Like retroviruses, they integrate their genetic material into the cells they infect, which increases their potential for long-term gene expression. They efficiently infect a variety of cells, including human skeletal myocytes (Kessler *et al.*, 1996) and human chondrocytes (Arai *et al.*, 2000). The use of adeno-associated viruses in gene therapy has been limited by the fact that they are relatively difficult to produce, and have a small packaging capacity, but the protocols for their effective production have improved in recent years. In a study of acute LPS-induced arthritis in rats, using local injection of a recombinant adeno-associated virus expressing β-galactosidase, there was a striking correlation between vector transgene expression and disease severity in injected joints. The inflammatory reaction peaked after 3–7 days, and at that time, 95% of synovial cells had high level transgene expression. Even more interesting, the diminished transgene expression could effectively be reactivated by a repeated challenge with LPS after 30 days (Pan *et al.*, 1999). This observation of inflammation-regulated transgene expression was later reproduced using an adeno-associated virus containing an IL-1 receptor antagonist transgene (Pan *et al.*, 2000). Another study evaluated the use of adeno-associated viruses for *in vivo* intra-articular use, either in normal mice or in mice with arthritis induced by overexpression of TNFα. Interestingly, transduction levels were much higher in arthritic knees, and both synovial fibroblasts and chondrocytes were infected (Goater *et al.*, 2000).

Adenoviruses are double-stranded DNA viruses that are known to cause mild respiratory and eye infections in a number of species, including humans. They have four early genes, E1–E4, encoding various proteins that are essential for the viral life cycle. The proteins encoded by the E1 region are essential to activate transcription of the E2–E4 genes, and this has been utilised to make E1-deleted, so-called first-generation adenoviruses, which are replication deficient. They still express a low level of viral proteins, leading to a stimulation of the immune response against infected cells and cessation of gene expression (Yang *et al.*, 1994). This might be desirable in some contexts, such as 'suicide gene' therapy of malignant disease, but is definitely not desirable in arthritis, since prolonged expression is required for therapy. One way around this problem has been to use E4-deleted, second-generation adenoviruses, which are less immunogenic, but also exhibit a decrease in transgene expression. A good deal of work has gone into the production of 'gutted' or 'gutless' adenoviruses, with deletion of large parts, or even all, the viral genome, leading to a further decrease in viral immunogenicity, but retaining their infectivity (Hartigan-O'Connor *et al.*, 1999; Morral *et al.*, 1999).

Adenoviruses have many advantages as vectors in gene therapy. They are easy to produce in high titres, have a large transgene packaging capacity, and infect with high efficiency a wide variety of both dividing and non-dividing cells, such as endothelial cells (Wrighton *et al.*, 1996), mature macrophages (Foxwell *et al.*, 1998) and fibroblasts and fibroblast-like cells (Bondeson *et al.*, 2000). Adenoviral infection of cells occurs in two steps. The viral fibre protein binds to a receptor on the surface of the target cell known as the coxsackie-adenoviral receptor (CAR), or possibly class II MHC, and virus internalisation is then accomplished through interaction between an RGD motif in the viral penton base and $\alpha_v\beta_3$ and $\alpha_v\beta_5$ integrins on the cell surface (Figure 8.7). It is an interesting observation that rheumatoid joint T cells, but not peripheral blood T cells, can be infected with a modest titre of adenovirus (Bondeson *et al.*, 1999b). Similarly, sarcoid lung T cells and macrophages harvested by bronchoalveolar lavage are readily infectible with adenovirus, but not peripheral blood monocytes or T cells from the same patients, or normal macrophages and T cells from bronchoalveolar lavages performed on normal volunteers. This difference is explained by increased expression of both CAR and $\alpha_v\beta_3$ and $\alpha_v\beta_5$ integrins on the surface of the cells coming from an inflammatory milieu (Conron *et al.*, 2001).

The fact that the three major varieties of rheumatoid joint cells – macrophages, T cells and synoviocytes – have all been proven to be readily infectible with adenovirus (Bondeson *et al.*, 1999b) implies that these viruses would be very useful for local gene delivery to the inflamed synovium in various animal models of arthritis. This had also been shown to be the case: in rhesus monkey (Goossens *et al.*, 1999), rabbit (Roessler *et al.*, 1993; Ghivizzani *et al.*, 1998), rat (Le *et al.*, 1997), guinea pig (Ikeda *et al.*, 1998) and mouse (Apparailly *et al.*, 1998; Ma *et al.*, 1998) models of arthritis, local adenoviral gene delivery has been proven to be very efficient, as judged either by staining of infected synovium after infection with an adenovirus transferring the β-galactosidase gene, or analysis of the expression of various transgenes. Systemic, intravenous administration of adenovirus in animal models of arthritis is also a feasible strategy, although problems with immunogenicity have been noted (Quattrocchi *et al.*, 1999), and safety concerns of course preclude this form of gene therapy in human RA.

Herpes simplex viruses are large, linear DNA viruses that can infect a variety of dividing and non-dividing cells. Replication-incompetent

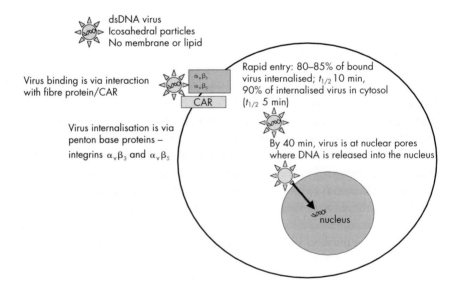

Figure 8.7 Schematic view of the mechanisms involved in adenovirus infection CAR, Coxsackie-adenoviral receptor.

herpes simplex viruses, constructed by the deletion of certain early viral genes that are essential for virus morphogenesis, can be grown in packaging cells that express these particular viral genes. Second-generation herpes simplex viruses have further deletions of the viral genome, and consequent advantages with regard to viral toxicity. Herpes simplex viruses have a large packaging capacity, but because they are cytotoxic, and cumbersome to produce, have been less widely used in gene therapy. A recent study (Oligino *et al.*, 1999) showed that while both first- and second-generation herpes simplex viruses could infect rabbit synovial fibroblasts, only the second-generation vector was capable of inducing transgene expression in an animal model of arthritis.

Gene therapy in animal models of arthritis

Neutralisation of proinflammatory cytokines

Many studies of gene therapy in animal models of arthritis have used anti-IL-1 antibodies or the IL-1 receptor antagonist, on the strength of the excellent results with direct administration of these molecules in animal models of arthritis (Joosten *et al.*, 1996; Kuiper *et al.*, 1998). However, recombinant IL-1 receptor antagonist protein injections do not achieve sufficient excess of this molecule to neutralise IL-1 in RA, due to its short half-life. Gene therapy with the IL-1 receptor antagonist has been seen as a means to improve on this. An early study (Makarov *et al.*, 1996) used *ex vivo* retroviral gene transfer of cDNA for the IL-1 receptor antagonist molecule, and observed local suppression of rat bacterial cell wall-induced arthritis. Other studies reported anti-arthritic and anti-invasive properties of re-implanted fibroblasts transfected with the IL-1 receptor antagonist in murine collagen-induced arthritis (Bakker *et al.*, 1997) or similar co-implantation of human cartilage and transduced (but not untransduced) synovial fibroblasts in SCID mice (Muller-Ladner *et al.*, 1997). *In vivo* local adenoviral gene therapy with a soluble IL-1 receptor–IgG fusion protein was associated with an anti-arthritic effect in rabbit antigen-induced arthritis; interestingly, not only the injected knee but also the contralateral one showed reduction of synovitis (Ghivizzani *et al.*, 1998). Local gene therapy using the IL-1 receptor antagonist gene was shown to be effective using a herpes simplex virus vector in rabbit antigen-induced arthritis (Oligino *et al.*, 1999), as was an adeno-associated virus vector in rat lipopolysaccharide-induced arthritis (Pan *et al.*, 2000).

An early study (Kolls *et al.*, 1994) demonstrated that intravenous injection of mice with an adenovirus transferring a chimaeric soluble p55 TNF receptor–IgG fusion protein resulted in high (1 mg/ml) plasma levels of TNF inhibitor for four weeks. These animals, but not mice injected with a control adenovirus, also showed susceptibility to infection with *Listeria monocytogenes*. Another study (Le *et al.*, 1997) indicated that this over-expression of the chimaeric soluble TNF receptor was sufficient to suppress the severity of rat collagen-induced arthritis when the adenovirus was administered systemically, either before or after onset of disease. In contrast, systemic gene therapy with the same chimaeric soluble TNF receptor in murine collagen-induced arthritis led to some initial amelioration of disease, but there was gradual loss of benefit and rebound to greater inflammatory activity, probably at least in part due to the development of agonistic antibodies against the construct, which activate TNF receptor-mediated signals (Quattrocchi *et al.*, 1999). In an early study in rat collagen-induced arthritis, local intra-articular gene transfer of the same chimaeric soluble p55 TNF receptor–IgG was limited by adenoviral synovitis (Le *et al.*, 1997), but the same construct was successfully used in local adenoviral gene therapy of rabbit adjuvant-induced arthritis (Ghivizzani *et al.*, 1998). Interestingly, comparison between this chimaeric soluble TNF receptor construct and a soluble IL-1 receptor–IgG fusion protein was in favour of the latter: it was equally potent in suppressing synovitis, and significantly better in reducing white cell infiltration into the joint space and cartilage matrix destruction (Ghivizzani *et al.*, 1998). These observations should not be taken as evidence that anti-IL-1 gene therapy strategies are superior to anti-TNF approaches in human RA, since the initial promise of anti-IL-1 biological therapy in animal models of biological therapy has not been fulfilled in clinical studies in RA patients, whereas anti-TNF therapy has been very efficacious.

There are no studies on the use of anti-IL-6 gene therapy. One group has used intraperitoneal adenoviral transfer of the IL-12 molecule in the murine collagen-induced arthritis model, and observed that the systemic transient overexpression of IL-12 that resulted led to accelerated disease progression and augmentation of arthritis severity. Conversely, neutralisation of endogenous IL-12 using a monoclonal antibody led to delay in disease onset and attenuation of severity (Parks *et al.*, 1998).

Overexpression of anti-inflammatory cytokines

There have also been successful animal trials of gene therapy using IL-10; all have used adenoviruses as vectors. All these studies have used a variant of the IL-10 molecule known as viral IL-10. Murine and human IL-10 cDNA sequences have a strong homology to an open reading frame in the Epstein–Barr virus genome called viral IL-10. The viral IL-10 molecule, which has 84% homology with human IL-10, shares many of its anti-inflammatory and immunosuppressive properties, but does not induce MHC class II expression on B cells or act as a co-stimulatory molecule in T-cell activation. Most studies have thus focused on gene transfer of the viral IL-10 molecule as an anti-arthritic strategy, as it might not only serve as a superior anti-inflammatory agent, but also act as a 'stealth molecule' that reduces the body's immune reaction to the adenoviral vector.

An early study (Apparailly *et al.*, 1998) used systemic administration of an adenovirus expressing viral IL-10 on day 30 of murine collagen-induced arthritis, when clinical signs of arthritis start. The transgene delayed the onset of arthritis, decreased severity and suppressed joint pathology. Viral IL-10 could be detected in the serum of the mice for 7 days. A second study (Ma *et al.*, 1998) of systemic administration of an adenovirus expressing viral IL-10 reproduced these findings, but found that treatment of established disease was ineffective. These authors also used intra-articular injection of the same virus into knee joints; when performed prior to the onset of arthritis, this strategy inhibited the development of arthritis in the injected paw, but it did not reduce established arthritis. An important observation, also using intra-articular adenoviral transfer of viral IL-10 in the murine collagen-induced arthritis model, was that development of arthritis was suppressed in both injected and uninjected paws (Whalen *et al.*, 1999). This also held true in rabbit antigen-induced arthritis: disease was ameliorated in both injected and contralateral control knees. The mechanism for this protection of distal joints after a single intra-articular injection is being debated. It is possible that transduced cells, including immature dendritic cells, may travel from one joint to another, and thus lead to immunoregulation in peripheral joints, or that adenovirus leakage might occur, leading to infection of a proportion of cells also in joints other than the one injected. A recent study (Watanabe *et al.*, 2000) found that protection of non-injected paws in murine collagen-induced arthritis occurred only upon systemic or intra-articular, but not peri-articular, adenoviral transfer of viral IL-10; it was suggested that circulating viral IL-10 protein was a major mediator of distal protection.

Similarly, there is impressive evidence in favour of a chondroprotective effect of intra-articular gene therapy using IL-4. One study has used adenoviral transfer of IL-4 in murine collagen-induced arthritis, injections being administered to the knee joints just before the expected onset of arthritis. Although considerable overexpression of IL-4 was achieved in injected joints, there was no effect on the course of arthritis. In contrast, joint erosion was markedly reduced, as evidenced by radiographic and histologic analysis. This was proposed to be secondary to reductions in IL-1β and IL-6 protein which stimulate osteoclasts, as well as a decrease in granulocyte influx, and inhibition of MMP-3 and other destructive enzymes (Lubberts *et al.*, 1999). In addition, the expression of the Th1 activator IL-12, and the chondrodestructive, T cell-derived cytokine IL-17 was suppressed. The synovial level of the osteoclast-activating mediator osteoprotegerin ligand was also significantly reduced in the animals receiving the IL-4 adenovirus, while its antagonist osteoprotegerin was unaffected. Another study used intra-articular retroviral transfer of IL-4 in rat adjuvant-induced arthritis, finding a significant reduction in both paw swelling and radiographic joint damage in animals injected with the IL-4 retrovirus on day 12 of arthritis (Boyle *et al.*, 1999). Interestingly, this group found an increase in IL-4 production also in the uninjected, contralateral paw of animals injected with the IL-4 retrovirus, which was suspected to be secondary to trafficking of naïve T cells from the injected joint.

There is only one study of local adenoviral transfer of TGFβ, in normal guinea pigs; it was observed that TGFβ was produced in the synovial tissue, and that levels persisted in the joint fluid for two weeks (Ikeda *et al.*, 1998). However, its therapeutic effect was not evaluated in animal models of arthritis. In another study of gene therapy of rat streptococcal cell wall arthritis, the administration of naked plasmid DNA encoding TGFβ1, had strikingly beneficial effects on the development of chronic erosive disease when administered at the peak of the acute phase of disease (Song *et al.*, 1998).

One study has used *ex vivo* retroviral gene therapy with murine interferon β, with intraperitoneal implantation of infected fibroblasts in mice with collagen-induced arthritis. Suppression of TNFα, IL-12 and interferon γ levels, and amelioration of disease, was observed (Triantaphyllopoulos *et al.*, 1999).

NF-κB as a therapeutic target

Experimental data from human synovial cell cultures has identified NF-κB as a key regulator of synovial inflammation, and probably also destruction, in RA (Bondeson *et al.*, 1999b). In a study of intra-articular injections of a modified adenovirus transferring a non-degradable

IκBα mutant in rats with streptococcal cell wall-induced arthritis, the severity of the arthritis was significantly inhibited in both the injected joint and in the untreated, contralateral one (Miagkov *et al.*, 1998). The authors proposed a mechanism of increased apoptosis for this effect, but this is unlikely to be the main mechanism, since the effects of NF-κB are more complex than envisaged.

Another recent animal study (Tak *et al.*, 1999b) used local adeno-viral transfer of wild-type or dominant-negative versions of IKK-2, the enzyme responsible for cleaving the inhibitory subunit IκB to activate NF-κB. Thus transfer of wild-type IKK-2 should result in NF-κB activation, and transfer of dominant-negative IKK-2 in NF-κB inhibition. In a model of rat adjuvant arthritis local injection of the adenovirus transferring dominant-negative IKK-2 resulted in quite potent suppression of arthritis in the injected paw, and also some anti-arthritic effect in the contralateral paw. In contrast, injection of wild-type IKK-2 into a normal rat paw caused significant arthritis. This study adds valuable evidence in support of the central role of NF-κB and IKK-2 in arthritis, and strengthens the concept of NF-κB as a therapeutic target.

Other approaches

Since it is known that the abnormal proliferation of synovial fibroblasts plays a role in the process of cartilage destruction in RA, various approaches to induce apoptosis of synoviocytes have been attempted in the gene therapy of experimental arthritis. The simplest approaches have used suicide gene therapy: gene transfer of the herpes simplex virus promoter driving the thymidine kinase gene in combination with treatment with the drug ganciclovir. In rhesus monkey collagen-induced arthritis, transfer of the thymidine kinase gene followed by ganciclovir treatment resulted in increased apoptotic cell death, and ablation of the lining layer, in knees injected with the thymidine kinase adenovirus (Goossens *et al.*, 1999). Apoptosis is normally mediated by the Fas/Fas ligand system, but in the RA synovium there is clearly a defect in the regulation of apoptosis, resulting in synovial hyperplasia and infiltration. Another approach has used transfer of the Fas ligand gene to synovium to induce apoptosis of synoviocytes in mice with collagen-induced arthritis (Zhang *et al.*, 1997).

One interesting study used adenoviral transfer of the Fas-associated death domain protein (FADD), which plays an important role in Fas-mediated apoptosis. This caused upregulation of FADD expression, and apoptosis, in cultured RA synoviocytes. Local injection of the FADD adenovirus into engrafted human synovial tissue in SCID mice also induced apoptosis of synovial cells, but not chondrocytes (Kobayashi *et al.*, 2000). Another target for interfering with the cell cycle turnover of synovial fibroblasts are cyclin-dependent kinases, in particular the INK4 family. It has been demonstrated that synovial cells derived from rheumatoid hyperplastic synovial tissue express the p16^{INK4a} gene when they were growth inhibited, and that adenoviral transfer of this gene was capable of inducing growth inhibition of cultured synovial fibroblasts. Using local adenoviral transfer of the p16^{INK4a} gene to knee joints of rats with adjuvant arthritis inhibited joint swelling, synovial tissue hyperplasia and histological joint destruction (Taniguchi *et al.*, 1999).

Tyrosine kinases of the Src family are involved in various intracellular signalling pathways, including mitogenic responses to growth factors in fibroblasts and osteoclastic bone resorption. Infecting cultured rheumatoid synoviocytes with an adenovirus transferring the *csk* gene, which negatively regulates Src family tyrosine kinases, it was observed that Src kinase activity, IL-6 production and proliferative responses were all inhibited, as was the bone-resorbing activity of osteoclasts infected with the same virus. Local injection of this adenovirus into the ankle joints of rats with adjuvant arthritis suppressed both inflammation and bone destruction (Takayanagi *et al.*, 1999).

What is the mechanism for the 'contralateral effect'?

A finding of considerable interest in animal studies of local adenoviral gene therapy of arthritis is the 'contralateral effect': that not only the injected joint, but other non-injected joints as well, show improvement after injection of adenovirus. This is a highly encouraging observation, indicating that intra-articular gene therapy of RA, using local injection of adenovirus into the knee joint, may well have a polyarticular effect. The mechanism for the 'contralateral effect' has been debated, and several hypotheses brought forward. One study using adenoviral transfer of IL-1 or TNF soluble receptors found no systemic transgene expression in non-injected joints, but there was evidence of leukocyte trafficking from the treated joint to other, non-treated ones (Ghivizzani *et al.*, 1998). These migrating cells were likely to be transduced antigen-presenting cells, which could generate Th2 lymphocytes (Evans *et al.*, 1999b). Another study, using an adenovirus transferring the IL-4 gene suggested that IL-4 overexpression in the treated joint generates Th2 lymphocytes locally, and that these cells then traffic to other joints (Boyle *et al.*, 1999).

One study of adenoviral transfer of viral IL-10 in rabbit antigen-induced arthritis found high levels of viral IL-10 protein in the injected joint and in draining lymph nodes, but very low levels of viral IL-10 in serum and contralateral joints, and suggested that transduced antigen-presenting cells could migrate and generate Th2 lymphocytes (Lechman *et al.*, 1999). In contrast, a very similar study in murine collagen-induced arthritis found that after intravenous or intra-articular injection of the adenovirus transferring the viral IL-10 gene, viral IL-10 cDNA could be found not only in distal joints, but also in the liver. There was a correlation between serum levels of viral IL-10 and the degree of protection of distal joints, suggesting that circulating viral IL-10 protein is the major mediator of distal protection. According to this model, the finding of a small number of transduced cells in distal joints could be explained by the entry of adenovirus virions into the systemic circulation (Watanabe *et al.*, 2000).

The 'contralateral effect' has to date been observed with many different constructs: not only with IL-1 and TNF soluble receptors, IL-4 and IL-10, but also with adenoviral transfer of the IKK2 dominant negative (Tak *et al.*, 1999b) and even in a study of Fas ligand gene transfer (Zhang *et al.*, 1997). It is thus not transgene-dependent, and this would render it less likely that the systemic production of any one cytokine, or the immunomodulatory effects induced by local overexpression of any particular molecule, could be the explanation. It is known (Yoshimura *et al.*, 2001) that both mature and immature dendritic cells can be infected with adenovirus, and it may well be that transduced immature dendritic cells may travel to peripheral joints, where they can exert immunomodulatory effects. This question could be resolved by investigating the presence of mature and immature dendritic cells expressing the transgene in injected and non-injected joints.

Combination constructs and inducible promoters

The prospect of using combination therapy with two therapeutic genes has been investigated in rabbit antigen-induced arthritis, where combination therapy with adenoviruses transferring both IL-1 and TNF soluble receptors had a greater effect than either of these viruses on its own (Ghivizzani *et al.*, 1998). Similarly, a combination of adenoviruses transferring viral IL-10 and a soluble TNF receptor had a greater effect in murine collagen-induced arthritis than either of these vectors on its own (Kim *et al.*, 2000), both with regard to incidence and severity of arthritis. In adenoviral gene therapy, it is possible to make constructs that express more than one therapeutic gene, and this could be used to achieve higher efficiency: for example, an adenovirus transferring the genes for both IL-10 (anti-inflammatory) and IL-4 (anti-erosive) would probably be of considerable therapeutic value.

Normally, viruses used for gene therapy have promoters that are constitutionally active. This may not be optimal in a disease like RA, which has periods of exacerbation and remission. The optimal system would be to have a promoter that is spontaneously turned on by an increase in inflammatory activity. One study (reviewed by Evans *et al.*, 1999b) used an inducible promoter based on elements taken from the C3 HIV promoter, since C3 is upregulated as part of the acute phase response by inflammatory stimuli. An adenovirus with IL-10 as the therapeutic gene under control of this promoter was injected into the ankle joints of rats. Induction of arthritis led to IL-10 levels that were equal to those obtained in animals injected with an adenovirus with a constitutive cytomegalovirus promoter. IL-10 expression inhibited arthritis, and this led to diminuation of IL-10 production in animals injected with the adenovirus with the inducible promoter. One drawback with this technique would be that a joint infection would also turn on this promoter, which could have disastrous consequences since the host defence mechanisms would be compromised. A good inducible promoter for use in gene therapy of RA should thus be optimally regulated by a mediator unique for this disease. Another option would be to use an inducible promoter construct that responds to a specific activator molecule that can be taken orally, like tetracycline.

Current clinical trials of gene therapy in rheumatoid arthritis

The only clinical trial of gene therapy of RA upon record was begun in 1996 and completed three years later (Evans *et al.*, 1999c). The criteria were strict: in all, nine female RA patients were recruited, who were scheduled to have both metacarpophalangeal (MCP) joint arthroplasty on at least one hand, along with some other form of joint surgery on another site. Autologous synovial tissue was removed when the patients had joint surgery, and the synovial fibroblasts were then expanded *in vitro*. These cells were divided into two batches, one of which was then infected with a retrovirus carrying IL-1 receptor antagonist cDNA.

These cells were carefully tested for adventitious agents before being re-introduced into the MCP joints by means of injection: two joints were injected with modified cells and two with uninfected cells. No patient had any adverse reaction to this procedure.

One week later, the MCP joint arthroplasty was performed and the synovial tissue was removed for analysis. All joints receiving transfected cells showed evidence of IL-1 receptor antagonist expression at both the mRNA and protein levels. Interestingly, some joints receiving uninfected cells also showed evidence of transgene expression. This may be due to inter-articular trafficking of cells. The first clinical study of local *ex vivo* retroviral gene therapy of RA thus showed that safe and effective transgene expression could be achieved (Evans *et al.* 1999c). A German trial along the same lines, except that a period of one month, instead of one week, is scheduled between the injection of control or modified autologous synovial fibroblasts and the MCP joint surgery, was begun in 1997 and had treated two patients by 1999 (Evans and Robbins, 1999).

Discussion

While there is no denying that RA is a serious disease with significant morbidity and mortality, it is no longer correct to describe it, as some reviewers of gene therapy approaches in this disease have done (Evans and Robbins, 1999; Evans *et al.*, 1999b), as incurable and virtually untreatable. In fact, DMARD therapy is effective in a proportion of patients, and anti-TNF strategies in combination with methotrexate has emerged as the new 'gold standard' for antirheumatic therapy: it is more efficacious, with regard to both control of inflammation and prevention of joint erosions, than any other strategy. Another great advantage is that anti-TNF therapy is safe, and virtually devoid of serious side effects. Gene therapy approaches may well find it difficult to improve on anti-TNF therapy for RA.

Nevertheless, it should be remembered that a significant percentage (30–40%) of RA patients do not respond to anti-TNF therapy, and that the relatively high cost of the drugs available today will necessitate strict selection of which patients to treat. Gene therapy approaches may well offer a cost-effective alternative or complement to anti-TNF therapy. The optimal gene therapy strategy for RA should offer site-specific, preferably long-lasting and controllable delivery of a therapeutic protein that targets a significant disease process that is characteristic and unique for RA. For reasons of both efficacy and practicality, *in vivo* gene therapy of arthritis is superior to *ex vivo* approaches. A systematic study of various vectors for gene transfer to synovium has pointed out that non-viral strategies are insufficient to achieve high-level gene transfer, that retroviruses are not suitable for *in vivo* use due to their inability to infect non-dividing cells, and that herpes simplex virus vectors are limited by their cytotoxicity (Nita *et al.*, 1996). In contrast, adenoviruses are very well suited for local gene transfer to synovium *in vivo*, and have been successfully used in many animal models of arthritis, including non-human primates (Goossens *et al.*, 1999); there is no reason to suppose that this strategy would not work in human RA patients. The 'contralateral effect' observed in many animal studies of local adenoviral gene transfer, which appears to be transgene-independent, is of high interest, since it holds out a promise that local adenoviral gene transfer to one or two large joints would have widespread beneficial effects in other inflamed joints. Adeno-associated viruses may have additional advantages as gene therapy vectors, due to their propensity to infect inflammatory cells, but are not yet sufficiently well studied for use in human clinical trials.

In the early and mid-1990s, several studies pointed out IL-1 as an important therapeutic target in animal arthritis, particularly with regard to the development of joint erosions. The later demonstration that anti-TNF strategies were superior to treatment with the IL-1 receptor antagonist, both with regard to control of inflammation and prevention of erosions, has disproved this assumption of the superiority of anti-IL-1 strategies, either for biological therapy or gene therapy of RA. Thus, there are no convincing data to support the possibility that gene therapy with the IL-1 receptor antagonist would have any advantages over gene therapy with a TNF receptor–Ig fusion protein. Both viral IL-10 and IL-4 also have potential as therapeutic genes: in particular, a combination of these two would combine a potent anti-inflammatory effect with anti-erosive properties. Also of great potential is the IκBα inhibitor of NF-κB, which combines an upstream inhibitory effect on TNFα with beneficial effects on other proinflammatory cytokines, while sparing anti-inflammatory mediators. In addition, NF-κB inhibition would bring about inhibition of several metalloproteinases, without reducing the activity of their endogenous inhibitor. The pro-apoptotic effect of inhibiting NF-κB might provide additional benefit in the rheumatoid synovium.

It is possible to speculate that the first *in vivo* human clinical trial of gene therapy of RA might employ local adenoviral transfer of either a soluble TNF receptor, viral IL-10 (and/or IL-4), or an NF-κB inhibitor. Although concerns have recently been raised about the safety of adenoviral gene therapy after the death of a participant in a clinical trial in circumstances suggestive of adenoviral inflammation (see Greenberg, 2000), it is important to stress that the adenoviral gene therapy of arthritis will be local, not systemic, it will not use high viral doses, and the viruses used will contain potent anti-inflammatory constructs that will also serve to alleviate viral toxicity. Furthermore, modern gutted adenoviruses have reduced immunogenicity, due to reduced expression of adenoviral proteins. A human trial of *in vivo* adenoviral gene therapy could consist of intra-articular injection of either an empty gutted adenovirus or a gutted adenovirus containing one of the constructs discussed above into the knee joint of RA patients. First, it will be necessary to demonstrate the safety of the procedure, and secondly to measure transgene expression through using an adenovirus transferring the β-galactosidase gene, in both the injected knee and the contralateral one, preferentially through arthroscopic joint biopsies, and also monitoring of viral spread. The duration of the expression of the construct, and its effects on cellular infiltration, cytokine and matrix metalloproteinase production, could be performed by immunohistochemistry techniques as well as analysis of joint fluid, and effects on joint swelling and synovial proliferation could be performed by means of ultrasound and magnetic resonance imaging (MRI). Clinical scoring of the injected and contralateral knees, and also other affected joints, should be performed at regular intervals. Such a study would thus determine the safety, and potentially the efficacy, of local adenoviral gene transfer in RA, with regard to both biochemical, histological, clinical and radiographic parameters, in the injected knee as well as in other joints.

References

Aggarwal B B, Samanta A, Feldmann M (2001) TNFα. In: Oppenheim J J, Feldmann M, eds. *The Cytokine Reference*. London: Academic Press, pp. 413–434.

Allen J B, Wong H L, Costa G L, et al (1993) Suppression of monocyte function and differential regulation of IL-1 and IL-1ra by IL-4 contribute to resolution of experimental arthritis. *J Immunol* 151: 4344–4351.

Alton E W, Stern M, Farley R, *et al.* (1999) Cationic lipid-mediated CFTR gene transfer to the lungs and nose of patients with cystic fibrosis: a double-blind placebo-controlled trial. *Lancet* 353: 947–953.

Apparailly F, Vervaerde C, Jacquet C, *et al.* (1998) Adenovirus-mediated transfer of viral IL-10 gene inhibits murine collagen-induced arthritis. *J Immunol* 160: 5213–5220.

Arai Y, Kubo T, Fushiki S, *et al.* (2000) Gene delivery to human chondrocytes by an adeno associated virus vector. *J Rheumatol* 27: 979–982.

Arend W P, Welgus H G, Thompson R C, Eisenberg S P (1990) Biological properties of recombinant human monocyte-derived interleukin-1 receptor antagonist. *J Clin Invest* 85: 1694–1697.

Aupperle K R, Bennett B L, Boyle D L, *et al.* (1999) NF-kappa B regulation by I kappa B kinase in primary fibroblast-like synoviocytes. *J Immunol* 163: 427–433.

Bakker A C, Joosten L A, Arntz O J, *et al.* (1997) Prevention of murine collagen-induced arthritis in the knee and ipsilateral paw by local expression of human interleukin-1 receptor antagonist protein in the knee. *Arthritis Rheum* 40: 893–900.

Bannwarth B, Labat L, Moride Y, Schaeverbeke T (1994) Methotrexate in rheumatoid arthritis. An update. *Drugs* 47: 25–50.

Barchowsky A, Brinckerhoff C E, Vincenti M (1999) Activation of MMP-1 transcription through the NF-κB and MAPK/AP-1 pathways in primary synovial fibroblasts. *Arthritis Rheum* 42 (Suppl. 9): S198.

Barone D, Krantz C, Lambert D, *et al.* (1999) Comparative analysis of the ability of Etanercept and Infliximab to lyse TNF-expressing cells in a complement dependent fashion. *Arthritis Rheum* 42 (Suppl. 9): S90.

Blaese R M, Culver K W, Miller A D (1995) T lymphocyte-directed gene therapy for ADA-SCID: initial trial results after 4 years. *Science* 270: 475–480.

Bondeson J (1997) The mechanisms of action of disease-modifying antirheumatic drugs. A review with emphasis on macrophage signal transduction and the induction of proinflammatory cytokines. *Gen Pharmacol* 29: 127–150.

Bondeson J, Sundler R (1995) Auranofin inhibits the induction of interleukin 1β and tumor necrosis factor α mRNA in macrophages. *Biochem Pharmacol* 50: 1753–1759.

Bondeson J, Browne K A, Brennan F M, *et al.* (1999a) Selective regulation of cytokine induction by adenoviral gene transfer of IκBα into human macrophages: LPS- but not zymosan-induced proinflammatory cytokines are inhibited, but IL-10 is inhibited. *J Immunol* 162: 2939–2945.

Bondeson J, Foxwell B M J, Brennan F M, Feldmann M (1999b) A new approach to defining therapeutic targets: blocking NF-κB inhibits both inflammatory and destructive mechanisms in rheumatoid synovium, but spares anti-inflammatory mediators. *Proc Natl Acad Sci USA* 96: 5668–5673.

Bondeson J, Brennan F M, Foxwell B M J, Feldmann M (2000) Effective adenoviral transfer of IκBα into human fibroblasts and chondrosarcoma cells reveals that the induction of matrix metalloproteases and proinflammatory cytokines is NF-κB dependent. *J Rheumatol* 27: 2078–2089.

Boyle D L, Nguyen K H Y, Zhang S, *et al.* (1999) Intra-articular IL-4 gene therapy in arthritis: anti-inflammatory effect and enhanced Th2 activity. *Gene Ther* 6: 1911–1918.

Brandes M E, Allen J B, Ogawa Y, Wahl S M (1991) Transforming growth factor beta 1 suppresses acute and chronic arthritis in experimental animals. *J Clin Invest* 87: 1108–1113.

Bratt J, Belcher J, Vercellotti G M, Palmblad J (2000) Effects of anti-rheumatic gold salts on NF-kappa-B mobilization and tumour necrosis factor α-induced neutrophil-dependent cytotoxicity for human endothelial cells. *Clin Exp Immunol* 120: 79–84.

Brennan F M, Chantry D, Jackson A, *et al.* (1989) Inhibitory effect of TNFα antibodies on synovial cell interleukin-1 production in rheumatoid arthritis. *Lancet* ii: 244–247.

Brennan F M, Maini R N, Feldmann M (1992) TNFα – A pivotal role in rheumatoid arthritis? *Br J Rheumatol* 31: 293–298.

Bresnihan B, Alvaro-Garcia J M, Cobby M, *et al.* (1998) Treatment of rheumatoid arthritis with recombinant human interleukin-1 receptor antagonist. *Arthritis Rheum* 41: 2196–2204.

Buchan G, Barrett K, Turner M, *et al.* (1988) Interleukin-1 and tumour necrosis factor mRNA expression in rheumatoid arthritis: prolonged production of IL-1 alpha. *Clin Exp Immunol* 73: 449–455.

Butler D M, Maini R N, Feldmann M, Brennan FM (1995) Modulation of proinflammatory cytokine release in rheumatoid synovial membrane cultures. Comparison of monoclonal anti TNF-α antibody with the interleukin-1 receptor antagonist. *Eur Cytokine Netw* 6: 225–230.

Butler D M, Malfait A-M, Maini R N, *et al.* (1999) Anti-IL-12 and anti-TNF antibodies synergistically suppress the progression of murine collagen-induced arthritis. *Eur J Immunol* 29: 2205–2212.

Calguneri M, Pay S, Caliskander Z, *et al.* (1999) Combination therapy versus monotherapy for the treatment of patients with rheumatoid arthritis. *Clin Exp Rheumatol* 17: 699–704.

Campion G V, Lebsack M E, Lookabaugh J, *et al.* (1996) Dose-range and dose-frequency study of recombinant human interleukin-1 receptor antagonist in patients with rheumatoid arthritis. *Arthritis Rheum* 39: 1092–1101.

Champion G D, Graham G G, Ziegler JB (1990) The gold complexes. *Baillière's Clin Rheumatol* 4: 491–534.

Chernajovsky Y, Annenkov A, Herman C, *et al.* (1998) Gene therapy for rheumatoid arthritis. Theoretical considerations. *Drugs Aging* 12: 29–41.

Chomarat P, Vannier E, Dechanet J, *et al.* (1995) Balance of IL-1 receptor antagonist/IL-1 beta in rheumatoid synovium and its regulation by IL-4 and IL-10. *J Immunol* 154: 1432–1439.

Choy E H S, Chikanza I C, Kingsley G H, *et al.* (1992) Treatment of rheumatoid arthritis with single dose or weekly pulses of chimeric anti-CD4 monoclonal antibody. *Scand J Immunol* 36: 291–298.

Chu C Q, Field M, Allard S, *et al.* (1992) Detection of cytokines at the cartilage/pannus junction in patients with rheumatoid arthritis: implications of the role of cytokines in cartilage destruction and repair. *Br J Rheumatol* 31: 653–661.

Clark P, Casas E, Tugwell P, *et al.* (1993) Hydroxychloroquine compared with placebo in rheumatoid arthritis. A randomized controlled trial. *Ann Intern Med* 119: 1067–1071.

Conron M, Bondeson J, Foxwell B M J, *et al.* (2001) High-efficiency adenoviral gene transfer to sarcoid lung cell cultures reveals that both macrophage-produced and T lymphocyte produced proinflammatory cytokines are NF-κB dependent. *J Immunol*, submitted *Am J Resp Cell Mol Biol* (in press).

Cope A P, Londei M, Chu R, *et al.* (1994) Chronic exposure to tumor necrosis factor (TNF) in vitro impairs the activation of T cells through the T cell receptor/CD3 complex; reversal *in vivo* by anti-TNF antibodies in patients with rheumatoid arthritis. *J Clin Invest* 94: 749–760.

Cronstein B N (1995) The antirheumatic agents sulphasalazine and methotrexate share an anti-inflammatory mechanism. *Br J Rheumatol* 34 (Suppl. 2): 30–32.

Cronstein B N (1996) Molecular therapeutics. Methotrexate and its mechanism of action. *Arthritis Rheum* 39: 1951–1960.

Cutolo M, Sulli A, Barone A, *et al.* (1993) Macrophages, synovial tissue and rheumatoid arthritis. *Clin Exp Rheumatol* 11: 331–339.

Dayer J-M, Beutler B, Cerami A (1985) Cachectin/tumor necrosis factor stimulates collagenase and prostaglandin E2 production by human synovial cells and dermal fibroblasts. *J Exp Med* 162: 2163–2168.

Dechanet J, Briolay J, Rissoan M C, *et al.* (1993) IL-4 inhibits growth factor-stimulated rheumatoid synoviocyte proliferation by blocking the early phases of the cell cycle. *J Immunol* 151: 4908–4917.

Dinarello C A (2001) Interleukin-1. In: Oppenheim J J, Feldmann M, eds. *The Cytokine Reference*. London: Academic Press, pp. 351–374.

Edwards C K III (1999) PEGylated recombinant human soluble tumour necrosis factor receptor type I (r-Hu-sTNF-RI): novel high affinity TNF receptor designed for chronic inflammatory diseases. *Ann Rheum Dis* 58 (Suppl. 1): I73–I81.

Elliott M J, Maini R N, Feldmann M, *et al.* (1993) Treatment of rheumatoid arthritis with chimeric monoclonal antibodies to tumour necrosis factor α. *Arthritis Rheum* 36: 1681–1690.

Elliott M J, Maini R N, Feldmann M, *et al.* (1994) Randomised double-blind comparison of chimeric monoclonal antibody to tumour necrosis factor α. *Lancet* 344: 1105–1110.

Erhardt C C, Mumford P A, Venables P J, Maini R N (1989) Factors predicting a poor life prognosis in rheumatoid arthritis: an eight year prospective study. *Ann Rheum Dis* 48: 7–13.

Evans C H, Robbins P D (1999) Gene therapy of arthritis. *Intern Med* 38: 233–239.

Evans C H, Ghivizzani S C, Kang R, *et al.* (1999a) Gene therapy for rheumatoid arthritis. *Arthritis Rheum* 42: 1–16.

Evans C H, Rediske J J, Abramson S B, Robbins P D (1999b) Joint efforts: tackling arthritis using gene therapy. *Mol Med Today* 5: 148–151.

Evans C H, Robbins P D, Ghivizzani S C, *et al.* (1999c) Results from the first human clinical trial of gene therapy for arthritis. *Arthritis Rheum* 42 (Suppl. 9): S170.

Feldmann M, Brennan F M, Maini R N (1996) Role of cytokines in rheumatoid arthritis. *Annu Rev Immunol* 14: 397–440.

Feldmann M, Elliott M J, Woody J N, Maini RN (1997) Anti-tumor necrosis factor α therapy of rheumatoid arthritis. *Adv Immunol* 64: 283–350.

Felson D T, Anderson J J, Meenan R F (1990) The comparative efficacy and toxicity of second-line drugs in rheumatoid arthritis. *Arthritis Rheum* 33: 1449–1461.

Felson D T, Anderson J J, Meenan R F (1992) Use of short-term efficacy/toxicity tradeoffs to select second-line drugs in rheumatoid arthritis. *Arthritis Rheum* 35, 1117–1125.

Fini M E, Cook J R, Mohan R, Brinckerhoff C E (1998) Regulation of matrix metalloproteinase expression. In: Parks W C, Mecham W C, eds. *Matrix Metalloproteinases*. San Diego: Academic Press, 299–356.

Firestein G S, Zvaifler N J (1990) How important are T cells in chronic rheumatoid synovitis? *Arthritis Rheum* 33: 769–773.

Firestein G S, Xu W-D, Townsend K, *et al.* (1988) Cytokines in chronic inflammatory arthritis I. *J Exp Med* 168: 1573–1586.

Firestein G S, Alvaro-Garcia J M, Maki R (1990) Quantitative analysis of cytokine gene expression in rheumatoid arthritis. *J Immunol* 144: 3342–3353.

Fox R I, Herrmann M L, Frangou C G, *et al.* (1999) Mechanism of action for leflunomide in rheumatoid arthritis. *Clin Immunol* 93: 198–208.

Foxwell B M J, Browne K A, Bondeson J, *et al.* (1998) Efficient adenoviral infection with IκBα reveals that macrophage TNFα production in rheumatoid arthritis is NF-κB dependent. *Proc Natl Acad Sci USA* 95: 8211–8215.

Ghivizzani S C, Lechman E R, Tio C, *et al.* (1997) Direct retrovirus-mediated gene transfer to the synovium of the rabbit knee: implications for arthritis gene therapy. *Gene Ther* 4: 977–982.

Ghivizzani S C, Lechman E R, Kang R, *et al.* (1998) Direct adenovirus-mediated gene transfer of interleukin 1 and tumor necrosis factor α soluble receptors to rabbit knees with experimental arthritis has local and distal effects. *Proc Natl Acad Sci USA* 95: 4613–4618.

Goater J, Muller H, Kollias G, *et al.* (2000) Empirical advantages of adeno associated viral vectors *in vivo* gene therapy for arthritis. *J Rheumatol* 27: 983–989.

Goldfeld A E, Strominger J L, Doyle C (1991) Human tumor necrosis factor alpha gene regulation in phorbol ester stimulated T and B cell lines. *J Exp Med* 174: 73–81.

Goossens P H, Schouten G J, 't Hart B A, *et al.* (1999) Feasibility of adenovirus-mediated nonsurgical synovectomy in collagen-induced arthritis-affected rhesus monkeys. *Hum Gene Ther* 10: 1139–1149.

Greenberg D S (2000) Stricter regulation proposed for US gene therapy trials. *Lancet* 355: 1977.

Han J, Beutler B (1990) The essential role of the UA-rich sequence in endotoxin-induced cachectin/TNF synthesis. *Eur Cytokine Netw* 1: 71–75.

Harris M P, Sutjipto S, Wills K N, *et al.* (1996) Adenovirus-mediated p53 gene transfer inhibits growth of human tumor cells expressing mutant p53 protein. *Cancer Gene Ther* 3: 121–130.

Hartigan-O'Connor D, Amalfitano A, Chamberlain J S (1999) Improved production of gutted adenovirus in cells expressing adenovirus preterminal protein and DNA polymerase. *J Virol* 73: 7835–7841.

Hawley D J, Wolfe F, Pincus T (1999) Use of combination therapy in the routine care of patients with rheumatoid arthritis: physician and patient surveys. *Clin Exp Rheumatol* 17 (6 Suppl. 18): S78–82.

Haworth C, Brennan F M, Chantry D, *et al.* (1991) Expression of granulocyte-macrophage colony-stimulating factor (GM-CSF) in rheumatoid arthritis: regulation by tumour necrosis factor α. *Eur J Immunol* 21: 2575–2579.

HERA Study Group (1995) A randomized trial of hydroxychloroquine in early rheumatoid arthritis. The HERA study. *Am J Med* 98: 156–168.

Hermann J A, Hall M A, Maini R N, *et al.* (1998) Important immunoregulatory role of interleukin-11 in the inflammatory process in rheumatoid arthritis. *Arthritis Rheum* 41: 1388–1397.

Horsfall A C, Butler D M, Marinova L, *et al.* (1997) Suppression of collagen-induced arthritis by continuous administration of IL-4. *J Immunol* 159: 5687–5696.

Ikeda T, Kubo T, Arai Y, *et al*. (1998) Adenovirus mediated gene delivery to the joints of guinea pigs. *J Rheumatol* 25: 1666–1673.

Jiang Y, Genant H K, Watt I, *et al*. (2000) A multicenter, double-blind, dose-ranging, randomized, placebo-controlled study of recombinant human interleukin-1 receptor antagonist in patients with rheumatoid arthritis: radiologic progression and correlation of Genant and Larsen scores. *Arthritis Rheum* 43: 1001–1009.

Joosten L A, Helsen M M, van de Loo F A, van den Berg W B (1996) Anticytokine treatment of established type II collagen-induced arthritis in DBA/1 mice. A comparative study using anti-TNF alpha, anti-IL-1 alpha/beta, and IL-1 Ra. *Arthritis Rheum* 39: 797–809.

Joosten L A, Lubberts E, Helsen M M A, van den Berg W B (1997a) Dual role of IL-12 in early and late stages of murine collagen type II arthritis. *J Immunol* 159: 4094–4102.

Joosten L A, Lubberts E, Durez P, *et al*. (1997b) Role of interleukin-4 and interleukin-10 in murine collagen-induced arthritis. Protective effect of interleukin-4 and interleukin-10 treatment on cartilage destruction. *Arthritis Rheum* 40: 249–260.

Jorgensen C, Demoly P, Noel D, *et al*. (1997) Gene transfer to human rheumatoid synovial cells engrafted in SCID mice. *J Rheumatol* 24: 2076–2079.

Keffer J, Probert L, Cazlaris H, *et al*. (1991) Transgenic mice expressing human tumour necrosis factor: a predictive genetic model of arthritis. *EMBO J* 10: 4025–4031.

Kempeni J (1999) Preliminary results of early clinical trials with the fully human anti-TNFα monoclonal antibody D2E7. *Ann Rheum Dis* 58 (Suppl. 1): I70–I72.

Kessler P D, Podsakoff G M, Chen X, *et al*. (1996) Gene delivery to skeletal muscle results in sustained expression and systemic delivery of a therapeutic protein. *Proc Natl Acad Sci USA* 93: 14082–14087.

Kim K-N, Watanabe S, Ma Y, *et al*. (2000) Viral IL-10 and soluble TNF receptor act synergistically to inhibit collagen-induced arthritis following adenovirus-mediated gene transfer. *J Immunol* 164: 1576–1581.

Kobayashi T, Okamoto K, Kobata T, *et al*. (2000) Novel gene therapy for rheumatoid arthritis by FADD gene transfer: induction of apoptosis of rheumatoid synoviocytes but not chondrocytes. *Gene Ther* 7: 527–533.

Kolls J, Peppel K, Silva M, Beutler B (1994) Prolonged and effective blockade of tumor necrosis factor activity through adenovirus-mediated gene transfer. *Proc Natl Acad Sci USA* 91: 215–219.

Kuiper S, Joosten L A, Bendele A M, *et al*. (1998) Different roles of tumour necrosis factor alpha and interleukin 1 in murine streptococcal cell wall arthritis. *Cytokine* 10: 690–702.

Le C H, Nicolson A G, Morales A, Sewell K J (1997) Suppression of collagen-induced arthritis through adenovirus-mediated transfer of a modified tumor necrosis factor alpha receptor gene. *Arthritis Rheum* 40: 1662–1669.

Lechman E R, Jaffurs D, Ghivizzani S C, *et al*. (1999) Direct adenoviral gene transfer of viral IL-10 to rabbit knees with experimental arthritis ameliorates disease in both injected and contralateral control knees. *J Immunol* 163: 2202–2208.

Lipsky P, St Clair W, Furst D, *et al.* (1999) 54-week clinical and radiographic results from the Attract trial: a phase III study of Infliximab (Remicade) in patients with active RA despite methotrexate. *Arthritis Rheum* 42 (Suppl. 9): S401.

Lorenz H M, Grunke M, Hieronymus T, *et al.* (2000) *In vivo* blockade of tumor necrosis factor-α in patients with rheumatoid arthritis: longterm effects after repeated infusions of chimeric monoclonal antibody cA2. *J Rheumatol* 27: 304–310.

Lubberts E, Joosten L A B, van den Bersselaar L, *et al.* (1999) Adenoviral vector-mediated overexpression of IL-4 in the knee joint of mice with collagen-induced arthritis prevents cartilage destruction. *J Immunol* 163: 4564–4556.

Ma Y, Thornton S, Duwel L E, *et al.* (1998) Inhibition of collagen-induced arthritis in mice by viral IL-10 gene transfer. *J Immunol* 161: 1516–1524.

MacNaul K L, Chartrain N, Lark M, *et al.* (1992) Differential effects of IL-1 and TNF alpha on the expression of stromelysin, collagenase and their natural inhibitor, TIMP, in rheumatoid human synovial fibroblasts. *Matrix* Suppl. 1: 198–199.

Maini R N, Feldmann M (2000) *Pocket Reference to TNFα Antagonism and Rheumatoid Arthritis.* London: Science Press.

Maini R N, Taylor P C (2000) Anti-cytokine therapy for rheumatoid arthritis. *Annu Rev Med* 51: 207–229.

Maini R N, Zvaifler N J (1998) Rheumatoid arthritis and other synovial disorders. In: Klippel J H, Dieppe P D, eds. *Rheumatology*, 2nd edn. London: Mosby Publishers, Section 5.

Maini R N, Paulus H, Breedveld F C, *et al.* (1997) rHuIL-10 in subjects with active rheumatoid arthritis (RA): a phase I and cytokine receptor study. *Arthritis Rheum* 40 (Suppl. 9): S224.

Maini R N, Breedveld F C, Kalden J R, *et al.* (1998) Therapeutic efficacy of multiple intravenous infusions of anti-tumor necrosis factor α monoclonal antibody combined with low-dose weekly methotrexate in rheumatoid arthritis. *Arthritis Rheum* 41: 1552–1563.

Maini R N, St Clair E, Breedveld F C, *et al.* (1999) Infliximab (chimeric anti-tumour necrosis factor α monoclonal antibody) versus placebo in rheumatoid arthritis patients receiving concomitant methotrexate: a randomised phase III trial. *Lancet* 354: 1932–1939.

Makarov S S, Olsen J C, Johnston W N, *et al.* (1996) Suppression of experimental arthritis by gene transfer of interleukin 1 receptor antagonist cDNA. *Proc Natl Acad Sci USA* 93: 402–406.

Makarov S S, Johnston W N, Olsen J C, *et al.* (1997) NF-kappa B as a target for anti-inflammatory gene therapy: suppression of inflammatory responses in monocytic and stromal cells by stable gene transfer of I kappa B alpha. *Gene Ther* 4: 846–852.

Malfait A-M, Butler D M, Presky D H, *et al.* (1998) Blockade of interleukin 12 during the induction of collagen-induced arthritis markedly attenuates the severity of the arthritis. *Clin Exp Immunol* 111: 377–383.

Marok R, Winyard PG, Coumbe A, *et al.* (1996) Activation of the transcription factor nuclear factor-kappaB in human inflamed joint tissue. *Arthritis Rheum* 39: 583–591.

Miagkov A V, Kovalenko D V, Brown C E, *et al.* (1998) NF-kappaB activation provides the potential link between inflammation and hyperplasia in the arthritic joint. *Proc Natl Acad Sci USA* 95: 13859–13864.

Miossec P, Chomarat P, Dechanet J, *et al.* (1994) Interleukin-4 inhibits bone resorption through an effect on osteoclasts and proinflammatory cytokines in an *ex vivo* model of bone resorption in rheumatoid arthritis. *Arthritis Rheum* 37: 1715–1722.

Moore K W, O'Garra A, de Waal Malefyt R, Vieira P, Mosmann T R (1993) Interleukin-10. *Annu Rev Immunol* 11: 165–190.

Moreland L W, Pratt P, Mayes M D, *et al.* (1995) Double-blind, placebo-controlled multicenter trial using chimeric monoclonal anti-CD4 antibody, cM-T412, in rheumatoid arthritis patients receiving methotrexate. *Arthritis Rheum* 38: 1581–1588.

Moreland L W, Baumgartner S W, Schiff M H, *et al.* (1997) Treatment of rheumatoid arthritis with a recombinant human tumor necrosis factor receptor (p75)-Fc fusion protein. *N Engl J Med* 337: 141–147.

Moreland L, Chase W, Fife R, *et al.* (1999) Phase I/II study evaluating the safety and potential efficacy of recombinant interlukin-11 in patients with refractory rheumatoid arthritis. *Arthritis Rheum* 41 (Suppl. 9): S171.

Morral N, O'Neal W, Rice K, *et al.* (1999) Administration of helper-dependent adenoviral vectors and sequential delivery of different vector serotype for long-term liver-directed gene transfer in baboons. *Proc Natl Acad Sci USA* 96: 12816–12821.

Mulherin D, Fitzgerald O, Bresnihan B (1996) Synovial tissue macrophage populations and articular damage in rheumatoid arthritis. *Arthritis Rheum* 39: 115–124.

Muller-Ladner U, Roberts C R, Franklin B N, *et al.* (1997) Human IL-1Ra gene transfer into human synovial fibroblasts is chondroprotective. *J Immunol* 158: 3492–3498.

Naldini L, Blomer U, Gallay P, *et al.* (1996) *In vivo* delivery and stable transduction of non-dividing cells by lentiviral vector. *Science* 272: 263–267.

Nawroth P, Bank I, Handley D, *et al.* (1986) Tumor necrosis factor interacts with endothelial cells to induce release of IL-1. *J Exp Med* 163: 1363–1375.

Nguyen D T, Eskandal M K, DeForge L E, *et al.* (1990) Cyclosporin A modulation of tumor necrosis factor gene expression and effects in vitro and *in vivo*. *J Immunol* 144: 3822–3828.

Nita I, Ghivizzani S C, Galea-Lauri J, *et al.* (1996) Direct gene delivery to synovium. An evaluation of potential vectors *in vitro* and *in vivo*. *Arthritis Rheum* 39: 820–828.

O'Byrne E M, Blancuzzi V, Wilson D E, *et al.* (1990) Elevated substance P and accelerated cartilage degradation in rabbit knees injected with interleukin-1 and tumor necrosis factor. *Arthritis Rheum* 33: 1023–1028.

O'Dell J R (1999) Combination DMARD therapy with hydroxychloroquine, sulfasalazine, and methotrexate. *Clin Exp Rheumatol* 17 (6 Suppl. 18): S53–58.

Oligino T, Ghivizzani S C, Wolfe D, *et al.* (1999) Intra-articular delivery of a herpes simplex virus IL-1Ra gene vector reduces inflammation in a rabbit model of arthritis. *Gene Ther* 6: 1713–1720.

Onodera M, Ariga T, Kawamura N, *et al.* (1998) Successful peripheral T-lympho-cyte-directed gene transfer for a patient with severe combined immune deficiency caused by adenosine deficiency. *Blood* 91: 30–36.

Page T D P, King B, Stephens T, Dingle J T (1991) *In vivo* studies of cartilage regeneration after damage induced by catabolin/interleukin-1. *Ann Rheum Dis* 50: 75–80.

Paleolog E M, Hunt M, Elliott M J, *et al.* (1996) Monoclonal anti-tumour necrosis factor α deactivates vascular endothelium in rheumatoid arthritis. *Arthritis Rheum* 39: 1082–1091.

Pan R Y, Xiao X, Chen C L, *et al.* (1999) Disease-inducible transgene expression from a recombinant adeno-associated virus vector in a rat arthritis model. *J Virol* 73: 3410–3417.

Pan R Y, Chen S-L, Xiao X, *et al.* (2000) Therapy and prevention of arthritis by recombinant adeno-associated virus vector with delivery of interleukin-1 receptor antagonist. *Arthritis Rheum* 43: 289–297.

Parks E, Strieter R M, Lukacs N W, *et al.* (1998) Transient gene transfer of IL-12 regulates chemokine expression and disease severity in experimental arthritis. *J Immunol* 160: 4615–4619.

Paulus H E, Egger M J, Ward J R, *et al.* (1990) Analysis of improvement in individual rheumatoid arthritis patients treated with disease-modifying drugs, based on the findings in patients treated with placebo. *Arthritis Rheum* 33: 477–484.

Peterson R L, Wang L, Albert L, *et al.* (1998) Molecular effects of recombinant human interleukin-11 in the HLA-B27 rat model of inflammatory bowel disease. *Lab Invest* 78: 1503–1512.

Piguet P F, Grau G E, Vesin C, *et al.* (1992) Evolution of collagen arthritis in mice is arrested by treatment with anti-tumour necrosis factor (TNF) antibody or a recombinant soluble TNF receptor. *Immunology* 77: 510–514.

Pincus T, Callahan L F (1993) What is the natural history of rheumatoid arthritis? *Rheum Dis Clin North Am* 19: 123–151.

Pincus T, Marcum S B, Callahan L F (1992) Longterm drug therapy for rheumatoid arthritis in seven rheumatology private practices: II. second line drugs and prednisone. *J Rheumatol* 19: 1885–1894.

Probert L, Plows D, Kontogeorgos G, Kollias G (1995) The type I interleukin-1 receptor acts in series with tumor necrosis factor (TNF) to induce arthritis in TNF-transgenic mice. *Eur J Immunol* 25: 1794–1797.

Prud'homme G J, Piccirillo C A (2000) The inhibitory effects of transforming growth factor-beta1 (TGF-beta1) in autoimmune diseases. *J Autoimmun* 14: 23–42.

Quattrocchi E, Walmsley M, Browne K, *et al.* (1999) Paradoxical effects of adenovirus-mediated blockade of TNF activity in murine collagen-induced arthritis. *J Immunol* 163: 1000–1009.

Ragno S, Colston M J, Lowrie D B, *et al.* (1997) Protection of rats from adjuvant arthritis by immunization with naked DNA encoding for mycobacterial heat shock protein 65. *Arthritis Rheum* 40: 277–283.

Rini B I, Selk L M, Vogelzang N J (1999) Phase I study of direct intralesional gene transfer of HLA-B7 into metastatic renal carcinoma lesions. *Clin Cancer Res* 5: 2766–2772.

Roessler B J, Allen E D, Wilson J M, *et al.* (1993) Adenoviral gene transfer to rabbit synovium *in vivo. J Clin Invest* 92: 1085–1092.

Roth J A, Swisher S G, Meyn R E (1999) p53 suppressor gene therapy for cancer. *Oncology* 13 (10 Suppl. 5): 148–154.

Sack U, Stiehl P, Geiler G (1994) Distribution of macrophages in rheumatoid synovial membrane and its association with basic activity. *Rheumatol Int* 13: 181–186.

St Clair E W (1999) Interleukin 10 treatment for rheumatoid arthritis. *Ann Rheum Dis* 58 (Suppl. 1): I99–I102.

Saklatvala J (1986) Tumour necrosis factor-α stimulates resorption and inhibits synthesis of proteoglycan in cartilage. *Nature* 322: 547–549.

Sasai M, Saeki Y, Ohshima S, *et al.* (1999) Delayed onset and reduced severity of collagen-induced arthritis in interleukin-6-deficient mice. *Arthritis Rheum* 42: 1635–1643.

Shakhov AN, Collart MA, Vassalli P, *et al.* (1990) κB-type enhancers are involved in lipopolysaccharide-mediated transcriptional activation of the tumor necrosis factor α gene in primary macrophages. *J Exp Med* 171: 35–47.

Shand N, Weber F, Mariani L, *et al.* (1999) A phase I-II clinical trial of gene therapy for recurrent glioblastoma multiforme by tumor transduction with the herpes simplex thymidine kinase gene followed by ganciclovir. *Hum Gene Ther* 10: 2325–2335.

Silman A J (1988) Has the incidence of rheumatoid arthritis declined in the United Kingdom? *Br J Rheumatol* 27: 77–79.

Silman A J, MacGregor A J, Thomson W, *et al.* (1993) Twin concordance rates for rheumatoid arthritis: results from a nationwide study. *Br J Rheumatol* 32: 903–907.

Sioud M, Mellbye O, Forre O (1998) Analysis of the NF-κB p65 subunit, Fas antigen, fas ligand and Bcl-2-related proteins in the synovium of RA and polyarticular JRA. *Clin Exp Rheumatol* 16: 125–134.

Smeets T J, Dayer J M, Kraan M C, *et al.* (2000) The effects of interferon-beta treatment of synovial inflammation and expression of metalloproteinases in patients with rheumatoid arthritis. *Arthritis Rheum* 43: 270–274.

Smolen J S, Kalden J R, Scott D L, *et al.* (1999) Efficacy and safety of leflunomide compared with placebo and sulphasalazine in active rheumatoid arthritis: a double-blind, randomised, multicentre study. *Lancet* 353: 259–266.

Song X Y, Gu M, Jin W W, *et al.* (1998) Plasmid DNA encoding transforming growth factor-beta1 suppresses chronic disease in a streptococcal cell wall-induced arthritis model. *J Clin Invest* 101: 2615–2621.

Svensson U, Holst E, Sundler R (1995) Cyclosporin-sensitive expression of cytokine mRNA in mouse macrophages responding to bacteria. *Mol Immunol* 32: 157–165.

Tak P P, Taylor P C, Breedveld F C, *et al.* (1996) Decrease in cellularity and expression of adhesion molecules by anti-tumor necrosis factor alpha monoclonal antibody treatment in patients with rheumatoid arthritis. *Arthritis Rheum* 39: 1077–1081.

Tak P P, 't Hart B A, Kraan M C, *et al.* (1999a) The effects of interferon beta treatment on arthritis. *Rheumatology (Oxford)* 38: 362–369.

Tak P P, Gerlag D M, Aupperle K R, *et al.* (1999b) IkB kinase (IKK2) is a key regulator of synovial inflammation. *Arthritis Rheum* 42 (Suppl. 9): S400.

Takagi N, Mihara M, Moriya Y, *et al.* (1998) Blockage of interleukin-6 receptor ameliorates joint disease in murine collagen-induced arthritis. *Arthritis Rheum* 41: 2117–2121.

Takayanagi H, Juji T, Miyazaki T, *et al.* (1999) Suppression of arthritic bone destruction by adenovirus-mediated csk gene transfer to synoviocytes and osteoclasts. *J Clin Invest* 104: 137–146.

Taniguchi K, Kohsaka H, Inoue N, *et al.* (1999) Induction of the p16^{INK4a} senescence gene as a new therapeutic strategy for the treatment of rheumatoid arthritis. *Nat Med* 5: 760–767.

Taylor P C, Peters A M, Paleolog E, *et al.* (2000) Reduction of chemokine levels and leukocyte traffic to joints by tumor necrosis factor alpha blockade in patients with rheumatoid arthritis. *Arthritis Rheum* 43: 38–47.

Tewari M, Tuncay O C, Milchman A, *et al.* (1996) Association of interleukin-1-induced, NFκB DNA binding activity with collagenase gene expression in human gingival fibroblasts. *Arch Oral Biol* 41: 461–468.

Tomita T, Takeuchi E, Tomita N, *et al.* (1999) Suppressed severity of collagen-induced arthritis by *in vivo* transfection of nuclear factor κB decoy oligodeoxynucleotides as a gene therapy. *Arthritis Rheum* 42: 2532–2542.

Triantaphyllopoulos K A, Williams R O, Tailor H, Chernajovsky Y (1999) Amelioration of collagen-induced arthritis and suppression of interferon-gamma, interleukin-12, and tumor necrosis factor alpha production by interferon-beta gene therapy. *Arthritis Rheum* 42: 90–99.

Turner M, Chantry D, Buchan G, *et al.* (1989) Regulation of expression of human IL-1α and IL-1β genes. *J Immunol* 143, 3556–3561.

Van den Berg W B (1997) Lessons for joint destruction from animal models. *Curr Opin Rheumatol* 9: 221–228.

Van den Berg W B (1998) Joint inflammation and cartilage destruction may occur uncoupled. *Springer Semin Immunopathol* 20: 149–164.

Van den Bosch F, Russell A, Keystone E C, *et al.* (1998) rHuIL-4 in subjects with active rheumatoid arthritis (RA): a phase I dose escalating safety study. *Arthritis Rheum* 41 (Suppl. 9): S56.

Van der Heijde D M, van Riel P L, Nuwer-Swart I H, *et al.* (1989) Effects of hydroxychloroquine and sulphasalazine on progression of joint damage in rheumatoid arthritis. *Lancet* i, 1036–1038.

Van der Lubbe P A, Dijkmans B A C, Markusse H M, *et al.* (1995) A randomized, double-blind, placebo-controlled study of CD4 monoclonal antibody therapy in early rheumatoid arthritis. *Arthritis Rheum* 38: 1079–1106.

Van Lent P L E M, Fons A J, Van de Loo A E M, *et al.* (1995) Major role for interleukin 1 but not for tumor necrosis factor in early cartilage damage in immune complex arthritis in mice. *J Rheumatol* 22: 2250–2258.

Van Roon J A, van Roy J L, Gmelig-Meyling F H, *et al.* (1996) Prevention and reversal of cartilage degradation in rheumatoid arthritis by interleukin-10 and interleukin-4. *Arthritis Rheum* 39: 829–835.

Veys E M, Menkes C J, Emery P (1997) A randomised double-blind study comparing treatment with recombinant interferon gamma versus placebo in the treatment of RA. *Arthritis Rheum* 40: 62–68.

Vincenti M P, Coon C I, Brinckerhoff C E (1998) Nuclear factor κB/p50 activates an element in the distal matrix metalloprotease I promoter in interleukin-1β-stimulated synovial fibroblasts. *Arthritis Rheum* 41: 1987–1994.

Von den Hoff H, De Koenig M, Van Kampen J, Van der Korst J (1995) Interleukin-1 reversibly inhibits the synthesis of biglycan and decorin in intact articular cartilage in culture. *J Rheumatol* 22, 1520–1526.

Wahl S M, Allen J B, Costa G L, *et al.* (1993) Reversal of acute and chronic synovial inflammation by anti-transforming growth factor beta. *J Exp Med* 177: 225–230.

Walmsley M, Katsikis P D, Abney E, *et al.* (1996) IL-10 inhibits progression of established collagen-induced arthritis. *Arthritis Rheum* 39: 495–503.

Walmsley M, Marinova-Mustafchieva L, Butler D M, Feldmann M (1998) An anti-inflammatory role for interleukin-11 in established murine collagen-induced arthritis. *Immunology* 94: 31–37.

Watanabe S, Kim K-N, Imagawa T, *et al.* (2000) On the mechanism of protection of distal joints after local gene transfer in collagen-induced arthritis. *Hum Gene Ther* 11: 751–758.

Weinblatt M E, Kremer J M, Bankhurst A D, *et al.* (1999) A trial of etanercept, a recombinant tumor necrosis factor receptor: Fc fusion protein, in patients with rheumatoid arthritis receiving methotrexate. *N Engl J Med* 340: 253–259.

Wendling D, Racadot E, Wildenes J (1993) Treatment of severe rheumatoid arthritis by anti-interleukin-6 monoclonal antibody. *J Rheumatol* 20: 259–262.

Whalen J D, Lechman E L, Carlos C A, *et al.* (1999) Adenoviral transfer of the viral IL-10 protein periarticularly to mouse paws suppresses development of collagen-induced arthritis in both injected and uninjected paws. *J Immunol* 162: 3625–3632.

Williams RO, Feldmann M, Maini RN (1992) Anti-tumor necrosis factor ameliorates joint disease in murine collagen-induced arthritis. *Proc Natl Acad Sci USA* 89: 9784–9788.

Wood NC, Dickens E, Symons JA, Duff GW (1992) In situ hybridization of interleukin-1 in CD14-positive cells in rheumatoid arthritis. *Clin Immunol Immunopathol* 62: 295–300.

Woods J M, Tokuhira M, Berry J C, *et al.* (1999) Interleukin-4 adenoviral gene therapy reduces production of inflammatory cytokines and prostaglandin E2 by rheumatoid arthritis synovium *ex vivo. J Invest Med* 47: 285–292.

Wrighton C J, Hofer-Warbinek R, Moll T, *et al.* (1996) Inhibition of endothelial cell activation by adenovirus-mediated expression of IκBα, an inhibitor of the transcription factor NF-κB. *J Exp Med* 183: 1013–1022.

Yang Y, Nunes F A, Berencsi K, *et al.* (1994) Cellular immunity to viral antigens limits E1-deleted adenoviruses for gene therapy. *Proc Natl Acad Sci USA* 91: 4407–4411.

Yoshimura S, Bondeson J, Foxwell BMJ, *et al.* (2001) Antigen presenting capacity in dendritic cells is NF-κB dependent. *Int Immunol* 13: 675–683.

Yoshizaki K, Nishimoto N, Mihara M, Kishimoto T (1998) Therapy of rheumatoid arthritis by blocking IL-6 signal transduction with a humanized anti-IL-6 receptor antibody. *Springer Semin Immunopathol* 20: 247–259.

Zhang H, Yang Y, Horton J L, *et al.* (1997) Amelioration of collagen-induced arthritis by CD95 (Apo-1/Fas)-ligand gene transfer. *J Clin Invest* 100: 1951–1957.

Zhang H G, Huang N, Liu D, *et al.* (2000) Gene therapy that inhibits nuclear translocation of nuclear factor kappaB results in tumor necrosis factor alpha-induced apoptosis of human synovial fibroblasts. *Arthritis Rheum* 43: 1094–1105.

Zuckerman J B, Robinson C B, McCoy K S, *et al.* (1999) A phase I study of adenovirus-mediated transfer of the human cystic fibrosis transmembrane conductance regulator gene to a lung segment of individuals with cystic fibrosis. *Hum Gene Ther* 10: 2973–2985.

9

The use of gene therapy in neurological diseases

*Paul A Smith, Graham J Wallace
and Sandra Amor*

Advances in the molecular basis of neurological diseases coupled with improvements in gene transfer systems has allowed the development of novel therapeutic strategies with which to treat otherwise 'incurable' neurological diseases. While the correction of genetic neurological abnormalities and the cure of progressive chronic neurological disorders are the ultimate goals of such therapy, many steps have yet to be taken. In this chapter we will outline some of the probable pathogenic mechanisms operating in several major neurological disorders and the possible therapeutic approaches taken to limit such diseases. Although important advances in gene delivery systems make the use of gene therapy an attractive possibility, neurological disorders present major problems due to the introduction of 'therapeutic genes' into post-mitotic neurons and the relative inaccessibility of the central nervous system. This chapter reviews the experimental and clinical data on gene therapy as a therapeutic strategy for human neurodegenerative disorders such as multiple sclerosis, Parkinson's disease and motor neuron disease and discusses the inherent problems associated with targeting gene therapies to the central nervous system.

The nervous system

The nervous system is composed of the peripheral nervous system (PNS) and the central nervous system (CNS). For the purpose of this review the major cell types of the CNS and PNS will be outlined and, where appropriate, those involved in neurological diseases mentioned.

Neurons, glia and myelin

The CNS receives information from the sensory organs via the PNS: the impulses are transmitted along axons many of which are protected by myelin. Damage to neurons and/or myelin or myelin-producing cells leads to a loss in the conductivity, resulting in neurological deficit. In Alzheimer's disease, atrophy, degeneration and the presence of neurofibrillary changes of nerve cells give rise to dementia, whereas in multiple sclerosis (MS) demyelination and/or axonal damage leads to paralysis. While the exact mechanism of myelin damage in MS and Guillain–Barré syndrome is unknown, alterations in the function of or damage to the myelin-producing cells (oligodendrocytes in the CNS and Schwann cells in the PNS) are thought to play an important role in the development of these diseases. Neurological defect results from neuronal damage and/or damage to the axons. Since neurons are post-mitotic cells they do not regenerate; axonal damage, on the other hand, may be repaired, but this regeneration is a very slow process. Axonal and neuronal dysfunction may also occur as a result of inflammation; oedema, for example, may compress the axon, blocking impulses. In this case when the inflammation subsides, neurological deficit is restored.

Neuroimmunology

The introduction of foreign antigens into the nervous system is probably far more likely to cause problems than systemic administration. The possibility that vector systems are themselves immunogenic, coupled with the fact that some therapies for neurological disorders are designed to modulate the immune response, makes it pertinent to discuss several aspects of immunology.

Activation of T cells

The clonal expansion and differentiation of naïve T cells entails a two-signal process (Figure 9.1). Signal 1 is antigen-specific and involves the recognition of the 'foreign' antigenic peptide bound to the major histocompatibility complex (MHC) of the antigen-presenting cell (APC). Signal 2 is the interaction of an accessory receptor on the T cell with its ligand on the APC. This is termed co-stimulation. Failure of co-stimulation during T-cell receptor (TCR) engagement results in anergy or non-responsiveness and provides an important mechanism of peripheral tolerance *in vivo*. There are several co-stimulation interactions possible between the T cell and APC, however the major co-stimulation signal is via the CD28 receptor on the T cell binding to the CD80 (B7) or CD86 ligand on the APC. A counter-receptor for the ligands CD80 and CD86 exists that delivers a negative signal to the naïve T cell. Cytotoxic T lymphocyte-associated molecule 4 (CTLA-4) is a homologue of CD28 and probably arose due to gene duplication. CTLA-4 down-regulates peripheral T-cell responses by causing death in activated CD4+ T cells via a Fas-independent mechanism, whereas in naïve T cells cross-linking inhibits interleukin 2 (IL-2) production and arrests cell cycle G_0/G_1 progression without apoptosis (programmed cell death). CTLA-4 may also initiate an inhibitory signal transduction pathway effecting T-cell activation (Saito, 1998).

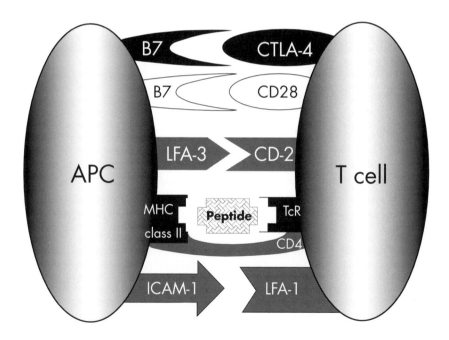

Figure 9.1   Activation of T cells following interaction with antigen-presenting cells. Clonal expansion and differentiation of naïve T cells requires a two-signal process. Signal 1 involves the recognition of the 'foreign' antigenic peptide bound to the major histocompatibility complex (MHC) of the antigen-presenting cell (APC) while signal 2 is provided by the interaction of an accessory receptor on the T cell with its ligand on the APC (i.e. co-stimulation).

Cytokines

Once activated, T cells perform a number of effector and signalling functions, including the activation of other effector cells such as cytotoxic T cells, macrophages and B cells via direct cell-to-cell contact or by secretion of signalling molecules such as cytokines, which are critically involved in determining the type of effector phase. It is generally accepted that activated T cells are classified into two major groups, depending on the type of cytokines they produce. Type 1 helper cells (Th1 cells) promote the inflammatory processes, cell-mediated immune responses and weak antibody formation. The major cytokines secreted by Th1 cells are interferon γ (IFNγ), tumour necrosis factor α (TNFα) and lymphotoxin. The other group, referred to as type 2 (Th2) cells, is associated with marked antibody production including IgG2b, IgE and IgA, less inflammation and secretion of IL-4, IL-5 and IL-10 (Singh *et al.*, 1999). Why particular T cells are selected to be Th1 or Th2 type is unknown, but the quality and affinity of the TCR interaction with the peptide in the context of the MHC may be an important factor.

Mechanisms of damage and repair in the CNS

Mechanisms leading to damage

Damage within the nervous system may result from infection, inflammation and degeneration. Obviously the causes of some diseases are unknown and novel mechanisms may be involved. Viruses may directly infect the neuron or glia cell and result in cell lysis or, alternatively, may stimulate cell death via a cytotoxic immune response. Another mechanism of virus-induced cell death is via apoptosis, in which case the virus infection switches on the programmed cell death pathway. Alternatively, viruses may cause mild damage and induce the release of CNS proteins, which are themselves immunogenic, thus inducing an autoreactive response. Yet further is the phenomenon of molecular mimicry, whereby a protein sequence of an infectious agent shares peptide sequences with neural and/or myelin antigens, thus stimulating a specific immunological response to the agent which also recognises and damages the normal host tissue.

Pathogenic immune responses are also heterogeneous. Activation of macrophages stimulates the release of proinflammatory cytokines, such as TNFα, reactive oxygen species and proteases, which all induce cell damage. Identification of the mechanisms operating in the induction of CNS/PNS diseases allows these to be targeted for therapeutic regimens.

Repair strategies

In addition to controlling the pathogenic processes, strategies aimed at repairing damaged tissues using tropic factors to stimulate the growth of glia and neurons (Figure 9.2), may also make use of gene therapeutic approaches. A group of compounds that have recently progressed from preclinical to clinical studies are the neurotrophic factors; these occur naturally and function to support the development and survival of neurons. Neurotrophic factors have been put forward as a strategy for the prevention, slowing or reversal of a number of neurological diseases (Doering, 1994).

Gene transfer into the nervous system

The two important considerations in the use of gene therapeutic strategies in neurological disease are the delivery of the vector systems to the CNS, i.e. delivery of agents across the blood–brain barrier, and the expression of the therapeutic gene in the cells of the CNS such as the terminally differentiated neurons.

Blood–brain barrier

The blood–brain barrier (BBB) was first identified following systemic injection of dyes which 'stained' all the organs except for the brain and spinal cord. While oxygen, small molecules and some viruses are able to cross the semi-permeable BBB, other compounds, including therapeutic agents, are excluded. The exclusion is due mainly to the structure of the endothelial cell tight junctions. In addition astrocytic foot-processes and specialised macrophage-like cells called pericytes, as well as the basement membrane of the endothelial cells are thought to play a role in this barrier. While intrathecal and intracranial administration can be used to avoid the BBB, such treatments have obvious drawbacks. To aid the passage of therapeutic agents to the brain, BBB disruption techniques have been applied in experimental systems. For example, mannitol

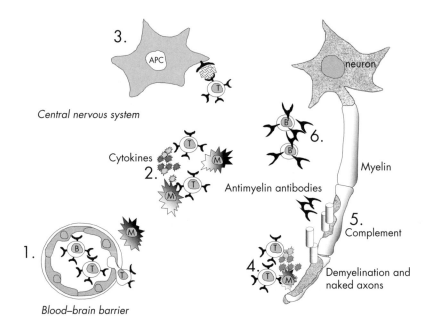

Figure 9.2 Pathogenic mechanism leading to central nervous system (CNS) damage. Activated lymphoctyes and monocytes cross the blood–brain barrier and enter the CNS (1). Further activation occurs following recognition of specific antigen presented by antigen-presenting cells (APCs) – either macrophages (2) or resident microglia cells (3). Such activation leads to production of cytokines to exacerbate the recruitment and proliferation of potentially pathogenic cells. Activated macrophages (M) and lymphocytes (T, B) produce damaging soluble components – free radicals and cytokines (4), complement (5), antibodies (6) – leading to myelin and/or axonal damage.

induces temporary shrinkage in the endothelial cells to allow a cancer drug to enter the CNS (Siegal *et al.*, 2000). More recently, the use of modified neurotropic viruses which carry the transgene of interest has been studied; these may prove to be the best method of targeting the brain.

Delivery systems

The four main methods used to introduce DNA into organisms are liposomes, naked DNA, viral vectors and *ex vivo* transfer of genetically transformed cells.

Viral vectors

Many different viruses, including adenoviruses, vaccinia viruses, herpesviruses and retroviruses, have been used as vectors to introduce foreign genes. Ideally, a viral vector should have the following five properties: long-term expression, no pathogenicity, able to contain a large insert, non-immunogenic, and expressed at therapeutic levels, and the treatment should be reversible (Bankiewicz *et al.*, 1997; Hermens and Verhaagen, 1998). Every system studied so far has been found to have fundamental strengths and weaknesses, and none fulfil all of the criteria. A problem encountered by all vector systems is that serial inoculations or long-term expression may induce an immune response that prevents the full beneficial effects of the system becoming apparent (Byrnes *et al.*, 1995). Delivery of genes directly into the brain, which guarantees expression where it needs to be for neurological disorders, is problematic at best but should reduce any systemic response. There are some areas that need to be addressed before inoculation can occur directly into the brain, such as ensuring that critical neurological functions are not interrupted following intrathecal administration and over-coming limited access to the brain that would prevent repeated injection of the therapeutic genes (Constantini *et al.*, 2000). At the present time, the majority of studies in mice have involved stereotactic inoculations of viral vectors resulting in focal transduction with limited spread by retrograde or anterograde axonal transport (Constantini *et al.*, 2000).

Adenovirus vectors   Adenoviruses have several properties that make them good candidates for use as vectors. The advantages include a wide host range, ability to accommodate large inserts, high titres, ability to grow in non-dividing cells and the genome exists as an episome which decreases the probability of integration (Le Gal La Salle *et al.*, 1993). Genes of interest are generally cloned into the vector under the control of a Rous sarcoma virus long terminal repeat or a cytomegalovirus promoter. Adenoviral vectors infect neurons, astrocytes and microglia after intracranial inoculation and can travel by retrograde axonal transport (Byrnes *et al.*, 1995; Wood *et al.*, 1996; Peltékian *et al.*, 1997). The major disadvantages of so-called first-generation adenovirus vectors for use in neurological disorders are their inflammatory potential, cytotoxicity and low level of transgene expression. Although the vectors sustain prolonged transgene expression in the brains of naïve animals, expression is rapidly eliminated by a severe inflammatory infiltration in animals primed against adenovirus by peripheral infection. In contrast, the new generation high-capacity vectors persist in the CNS and induce high levels of transgene expression. Intracerebral inoculation evades an anti-adenoviral T-cell response elicited through peripheral immune priming (Simonato *et al.*, 2000).

Retroviral/lentiviral vectors   Retrovirus vectors, although very widely used in gene therapy, are of limited use in neuroscience as they are unable to replicate in post-mitotic neurons. However, they may be useful for targeting neural precursors and tumour cells as well as in *ex vivo* transplantation strategies using fibroblasts, astrocytes, endothelial cells and neural progenitor cells. Several studies have engineered cells to secrete trophic factors, neurotransmitters and metabolic enzymes by transfection via retroviral vectors or plasmids. While these systems are efficacious in experimental models the use of human fetal tissue for therapy in humans poses major ethical questions. The most commonly used retroviral vector is murine leukaemia virus but this is unable to infect and transduce quiescent cells, rendering it of limited value to brain disorders (Hermens and Verhaagen, 1998).

Vectors based on lentiviruses with the ability to integrate into quiescent neural cells are showing more potential for treatment of neurodegenerative disorders (Hermens and Verhaagen, 1998). These vectors are an obvious choice since inserts of up to 9 kb can be accommodated and they are not very immunogenic because of their integration and gene expression mechanisms (Federco, 1999). Intrastriatal inoculation of exogenous genes using a lentiviral vector transduces a higher number of cells than the use of adeno-associated virus vectors at all times post inoculation and more cells than adenoviral vectors at late time points (Constantini *et al.*, 2000). The vectors are also expressed at areas far away from the inoculation site due to retrograde axonal transport; expression has been found up to 24 weeks post inoculation, probably as a result of integration, with only a small immune response produced (Blömer *et al.*, 1997).

Herpes simplex virus 1 vectors   The herpes simplex virus 1 (HSV-1) system is advantageous because the virus naturally infects neurons, wherein it becomes latent for the life of the host, large inserts can be accommodated because half of the genome is non-essential and can be deleted (Simonato *et al.*, 2000) and the inserted gene may be expressed over an extended period of time (Maidment *et al.*, 1996). The virus can also travel by retrograde axonal transport, allowing it to move easily through the brain (Byrnes *et al.*, 1995) and express antigen in areas far from the inoculation site. This means that an extraneural delivery of herpes simplex is sufficient for intraneural gene expression. Disadvantages of the vector include induction of a T-cell and macrophage response (Byrnes *et al.*, 1995) and the difficulty of finding a promoter that is active in the latent state. HSV-1 is able to induce a latent infection within neurons, but prolonged expression of a transgene in latently infected neurons has proven difficult due to transcriptional silencing of exogenous promoters. Ongoing studies are currently looking at using the HSV latency-associated promoter to drive the expression of therapeutic genes (Lachmann and Efstathiou, 1999). In addition to immune responses to the selected gene, the vector itself may also provoke an immune response leading to rapid 'clearance' and decreased effectivity of the vector by the immune system.

Alphaviral vectors   The alphavirus Semliki Forest virus (SFV) is neurotropic and has been used to express antigens within the CNS. SFV has a wide host range, allowing replication and gene expression in a large number of cells, which may be problematic for gene therapy, when expression needs to be limited. SFV vectors are non-replicating since the structural genes are replaced with an exogenous antigen, making the vector relatively safe, as there is no method of spreading to other cells. Two types of vector are used: layered DNA/RNA and infectious particles, both of which induce apoptosis late in infection, curtailing expression of viral and exogenous genes (Glasgow *et al.*, 1998).

The layered DNA/RNA system involves promoter control at both the DNA and RNA levels. Typically, the vector is inoculated as DNA and, under the control of a eukaryotic promoter, transcription to RNA occurs. Following this, the subgenomic viral promoter is responsible for production of the foreign gene. This method of expression provided a 10- to 200-fold increase when compared with standard DNA vectors expressing the same antigen (Lundstrom, 1997).

The infectious particle vaccine requires a recombinant genome expressing the exogenous antigen and the structural proteins (known as the vector replicon) as well as a helper virus, which provides the missing non-structural genes. Before inoculation, the helper virus and the vector replicon are co-transfected into cells, leading to the production of virus particles containing the vector replicon. This is purified to remove the helper virus then inoculated. Infectious particles are very efficient at infecting cells because they have a viral envelope that induces receptor-mediated endocytosis. To date the SFV vector system has concentrated on extraneural effects. Influenza nucleoprotein has been engineered into the SFV vector and promotes both CD4+ and CD8+ T-cell responses (Zhou *et al.*, 1995). SFV infectious particles have also been shown to promote responses to Simian immunodeficiency virus (SIV) *env* gene products (Mossman *et al.*, 1996). It remains a possibility that SFV vectors may be used for expression in the CNS in the future.

Non-viral gene delivery systems

Gene delivery systems that do not use viral vectors include naked DNA, cationic lipids and polycationic polymers while the *ex vivo* approach relies on genetically transduced cells.

Naked DNA   Naked DNA is composed of plasmid DNA, which expresses an exogenous antigen after direct inoculation into a tissue. The DNA is taken up and enters the cellular cytoplasm, followed by the nucleus (Constantini *et al.*, 2000). DNA is not used widely for treating neurodegenerative disorders because vehicles based on viruses are inherently more efficient at entering cells and expressing antigen, even though the same inoculation problems occur with both.

Liposomes   If the naked DNA is coupled to specific polypeptides and ligands, it is possible to restrict transfection to specific cell types (Constantini *et al.*, 2000). The DNA is enclosed in positively charged particles (liposomes) that are taken up by receptor-mediated endocytosis. Compared to whole virus vector, DNA and liposomes do not contain as much 'foreign' material and are therefore less immunogenic. Liposomes are not a favoured method of gene therapy in the brain because although they can enter the CNS after an intraperitoneal delivery, the precise level of expression following this has not been determined (Princen *et al.*, 2000). Furthermore, liposomes aggregate when added to saline solution, leading to low levels of exogenous antigen in the brain following intravenous inoculation (Shi and Pardridge, 2000). Liposomes still require some development before they can be exploited to treat neurodegenerative disorders.

Ex vivo *transfer of modified cells*   A foreign gene or antigen that is inserted into a vector to allow expression in any cell is referred to as 'transduced' or 'transfected'. In neurological disease to date such approaches have used fibroblasts, astrocytes, endothelial cells, progenitor cells and, in one case, myelin-reactive T cells. This technique involves the infection of neurons *in vivo* followed by implantation into the brain to replace lost cells. The isolation of stem cells from the CNS in recent years has expanded the possibilities of *ex vivo* therapy; their use allows cell differentiation to occur within the host. The stem cells are immortalised, allowing infinite passages and manipulations in culture (Martínez-Serrano and Björklund, 1997). Unfortunately, it was found that some implanted cells caused tumours or promoted an immune response. Subsequent studies now use fibroblasts, myoblasts, glial cells or fetal and embryonic cells (Raymon *et al.*, 1997). Retroviral vectors expressing cDNA for reporter genes, neurotrophic factors and metabolic enzymes have been used to infect the cell lines prior to *ex vivo* transfer (Martínez-Serrano and Björklund, 1997). The main advantage of the *ex vivo* technique is that production of the exogenous antigen can be assayed *in vitro* prior to implantation. Studies have shown that nerve growth factor (NGF)-expressing cells, after *ex vivo* transfer into the rat, can prevent neurological deficits from becoming apparent up to nine months post inoculation (Martínez-Serrano and Björklund, 1997).

Ex vivo gene transfer can be used for the treatment of metabolic defects. In the disease mucopolysaccharidosis type VII (MPS VII) there is an inherited deletion of the β-glucuronidase (GUSB) gene, resulting in mental retardation and neuronal and glial degeneration. A retroviral vector was used to transduce a cell line with human GUSB. After implantation of these cells into mice suffering from MPS VII, the disease was corrected by the GUSB produced from the cells (Martínez-Serrano and Björklund, 1997).

Gene therapy for neurological diseases

Gene therapeutic approaches for neurological disease may be used to protect against neurological disease, to slow the progression of disease or to assist in the repair of damaged tissues. In addition, downregulation of active disease-promoting gene products may be targeted using antisense genes or used to replace proteins lost due to gene malfunction. Such approaches are discussed below in several major neurological disorders.

Multiple sclerosis

Aetiology

Multiple sclerosis (MS) is the most prevalent demyelinating disease of the CNS with around 1 in 1000 affected in northern Europe and the USA. The first clinical signs of MS generally begin between the ages of

20 and 40 with a female/male ratio of approximately 2 : 1. While the aetiology of the disease is unknown, genetic and environmental factors are thought to play a major role in predisposition to the disease. Clinically, several forms of MS are observed, the most common being relapsing–remitting MS, which is manifested over many years by episodes of relapse followed by remission. Clinical symptoms are inextricably linked to the pathology of the CNS, with motor disturbances affecting the ability to walk and use of hands; disturbances in visual acuity, double vision; incoordination; bowel and bladder incontinence; spasticity; and sensory disturbances including loss of touch, pain and temperature perception. Multiple sclerosis and its animal model experimental allergic encephalomyelitis (EAE) are generally accepted to be mediated by an autoimmune attack on the myelin surrounding the neurons of the CNS. Such damage within the CNS is observed as lesions of myelin damage or demyelination with varying degrees of axonal involvement.

Pathology

While the aetiology and the exact mechanism(s) leading to myelin damage in MS are unknown, it is generally thought that a virus may be implicated in the onset of disease. However, once initiated, the disease is probably (auto)immune-mediated. A major step in the development of CNS disease is influx of inflammatory cells into the CNS. Naïve T cells do not enter the CNS, but activated T cells, irrespective of the antigen-specificity, can cross the BBB. Therefore, by inhibiting the priming and activation of T cells it may be possible to alleviate the CNS infiltration by encephalitogenic T cells. Thus the steps to T-cell activation and/or migration into the CNS may be targeted in therapeutic intervention. Once inflammatory cells have entered the CNS, a cascade of events occurs, as described above and depicted in Figure 9.2. The points numbered 1 to 6 in Figure 9.2 represent possible points at which the inflammatory response may be targeted.

The myelin-reactive T cells may be further activated by myelin components in the context of antigen-presenting cells and myelin peptides, while macrophages may become activated following phagocytosis of myelin debris. Under experimental conditions, such activation gives rise to the production of many potentially myelin-damaging soluble mediators, including reactive oxygen species, nitric oxide and proteases.

Current therapies

While some new therapies are currently in clinical trials, several have recently entered the clinic. These include the interferons, such as interferon β1a and interferon β1b. Interferons are compounds produced by the body to fight viral infections and are immunomodulatory. Although their exact therapeutic mechanism in MS remains unclear, interferon β1b has been shown to slow the progression of secondary progressive MS and interferon β1a reduces the number of relapses in relapsing–remitting MS. Another therapeutic regimen is glatiramer acetate or co-polymer 1, a synthetic amino acid co-polymer of L-alanine, L-glutamic acid, L-lysine and L-tyrosine that cross-reacts with the myelin protein MBP. Intradermal injection of co-polymer 1 prevents EAE in the guinea pig prior to the onset of disease and at the time of clinical onset. The mode of action is thought to be the generation of suppressor T cells and inhibition of MBP-reactive T cells. In MS, co-polymer 1 reduces the frequency of attacks in patients suffering from relapsing–remitting MS. Other anti-inflammatory drugs include mitroxantrone and cladribine, which may reduce relapses and slow disease progression in relapsing–remitting and secondary progressive MS. More specifically, antibodies directed to the adhesion molecule VLA-4, a molecule expressed on cells crossing the BBB, blocks the entry of pathogenic immune cells into the brain and spinal cord. In clinical trials the use of these antibodies (LeukArrest by ICOS Corporation and Antegren by Athena Neurosciences) was shown to reduce the severity and duration of MS relapses.

Another form of therapy uses intravenous immunoglobulins (i.v. Ig). A reduction in relapse rate and decreased MRI activity has been reported following i.v. Ig treatment in relapsing–remitting MS, and there is evidence to support its use in secondary progressive or primary progressive MS (Lisak, 1998).

Gene therapy

To date, gene therapy has not been used in MS itself, however many approaches have used the experimental model of MS, EAE, to examine potential mechanisms of administering immune-modulating regimes in order to suppress disease. These include gene delivery of antibodies directed to cytokines, CTLA-4, catalase in viral vectors and liposomes and local delivery of interleukin 4 by retrovirus-transduced T lymphocytes. While such therapies have been shown to modulate the disease in

EAE, the effect is more pronounced when the genes are administered intracranially.

Altering the balance of the cytokine milieu in favour of Th2 cytokines with gene insertion or reducing Th1 cytokine levels via gene knockout are currently being evaluated as gene therapy in animal models of Th1-mediated diseases such as EAE. For example, Martino *et al.* (2000) demonstrated that the use of non-replicative HSV-1-derived viral vectors engineered with heterologous cytokine genes was effective in modulating EAE. A single direct CNS injection of a DNA–cationic liposome complex encoding anti-inflammatory cytokines such as IL-4, IL-10, IFNα and TGFβ has also been reported to inhibit EAE (Croxford *et al.*, 1998). Other soluble mediators such as free radicals may also be involved in myelin damage in MS and EAE and thus therapies aimed at controlling such mediator may be useful in controlling the disease. Superoxide anions are converted to hydrogen peroxide by the enzyme superoxide dismutase (SOD) by interaction with transition metals. SOD consists of four classes, containing either a dinuclear (Cu, Zn) or a mononuclear (Fe, Mn or Ni) co-factor. Hydrogen peroxide is in turn converted to water and oxygen by catalase. Hydrogen peroxide is relatively unreactive to organic molecules, however it has been reported to induce apoptosis at high concentrations. Catalase is a tetrameric haemin enzyme consisting of four identical tetra-arranged subunits of 60 kDa, which scavenges hydrogen peroxide via the 'peroxidative reaction' in order to oxidise a variety of other substrates, including phenols, formic acid and alcohol. Suppression of oxidative injury by adenoviral-mediated transfer of the human catalase gene has been found to increase catalase activity 2-fold in the endothelia, oligodendroglia, astrocytes and axons of the optic nerve. Catalase gene insertion has been reported to reduce demyelination, disruption of the BBB, cellular infiltration and *in vivo* levels of hydrogen peroxide (Guy *et al.*, 1998).

In addition to reducing pathogenic processes, therapeutic strategies aimed at repairing damaged tissues are under development, including gene therapeutic approaches. In MS and EAE, it has been reported that nerve growth factor (NGF) levels increase in the cerebrospinal fluid (CSF) and closely follow the acute phase of the disease. It has been hypothesised that the enhanced production of NGF by glial cells is necessary to compensate for the effect of axonal and/or neuronal cell body injury occurring in EAE (Mincera *et al.*, 1998). Alternatively, that oligodendrocytes are damaged or destroyed in MS suggests that therapies aimed at increasing oligodendrocyte numbers to induce remyelination may be beneficial. Thus, repopulating damaged areas with oligodendrocytes by inducing migration of oligodendrocyte progenitors into the area and/or introducing glial cell growth factors by gene therapy to stimulate maturation of myelin-forming oligodendrocytes may be feasible in MS. Figure 9.3 depicts the development and maturation steps of oligodendrocytes and the associated growth factors which may be targets for gene therapy.

One neurotrophic factor that has stimulatory effects on oligodendrocytes and Schwann cells is glial growth factor 2 (GGF2). This is a secreted isoform of neuregulin, a family of soluble and transmembrane proteins belonging to the epidermal growth factor superfamily. Because oligodendrocytes are targeted for destruction during MS progression, with subsequent remyelination during remission it has been suggested that increasing levels of GGF might ameliorate the disease. Treatment with rhGGF2 during the course of EAE has been reported to delay clinical signs, decrease their severity and to result in significant reductions in relapse rate. CNS lesions also showed more remyelination than controls (Cannela *et al.*, 1998).

The beneficial effects seen with rhGGF2 are attributable to increased proliferation and survival of the oligodendrocytes and an associated increase in the expression of Th2 cytokines. It remains to be seen whether administration of neural/glia cell growth factors via gene therapy is able to promote oligodendrocyte repair.

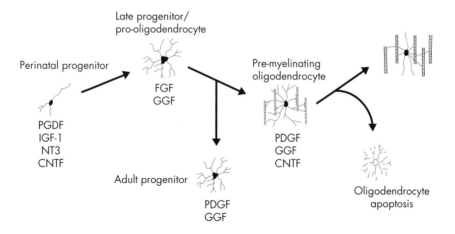

Figure 9.3 Development of the oligodendrocyte lineage. The cell types seen during oligodendrocyte development together with the growth factors involved in the differentiation steps. PDGF, platelet-derived growth factor; FGF, fibroblast growth factor; GGF, glial growth factor; IGF-1, insulin-like growth factor 1; NT3, neurotrophin 3; CNTF, ciliary neurotrophic factor. Apoptosis of oligodendrocytes only occurs if a pre-myelinating oligodendrocyte does not contact with enough axons.

Guillain–Barré syndrome

Aetiology

Guillain–Barré syndrome (GBS) or acute inflammatory demyelinating polyradiculoneuropathy (AIDP) is a self-limiting autoimmune disease of the peripheral nervous system. Estimations of the incidence rate of GBS range from 1.3 to 1.9 per 100 000 annually in the under 40 years of age group, however there are two peaks – one in late adolescence and young adulthood and a second in the elderly. There is no bias in incidence towards either sex. Clinically, GBS results in rapidly evolving symmetrical limb weakness, loss of tendon reflexes, autonomic dysfunctions and absent or mild sensory signs (Hahn, 1998). GBS is a post-infectious illness that is initially triggered by a respiratory tract (cytomegalovirus) or gastrointestinal tract infection (*Campylobactor jejuni*) with a lag period between the end of illness and neuropathy of around 11 days. Clinically, GBS involves hospitalisation of the patient as onset and exacerbation of disease symptoms can be rapid, resulting in a possible need for ventilatory support. The duration of the disease is variable, but the greatest severity is reached within four weeks in 94% of cases and then resolution of disease lasts from weeks to months.

Pathology

The pathophysiology of GBS is the result of an immune-mediated attack of the Schwann cells. The mechanism of aberrant immune responses is similar to that seen in MS, with 'molecular mimicry' resulting in 'host' Schwann cell ganglioside-surface molecules or myelin structures being targeted.

Current therapies

Treatment regimes used for GBS include early (within first two weeks of disease) plasma exchanges, with up to four or five on alternate days. However, problems involved with this treatment include the lack of plasma-exchange facilities, the high cost and secondary worsening in around 10% of patients, possibly due to persistent active disease or antibody rebound. Alternative therapies include high-dose intravenous immunoglobulin, which carries lower risks, is easier to administer and shows similar efficacy. The common side effects seen are limited relapses in around 10%. Due to the similarities between MS and GBS they share common possibilities for gene therapy strategies, such as those mentioned above.

Parkinson's disease

Aetiology and pathology

Parkinson's disease is a common progressive neurological disorder affecting the areas of the brain controlling voluntary movement. The prevalence rate is 1% in the population above 65 years of age. The underlying cause of Parkinson's disease remains elusive, however it is known to be associated with a degeneration of dopaminergic nigro-striatal neurons within the CNS.

Parkinsonism is characterised by a resting tremor, slow initiation of movement (bradykinesia) and muscle rigidity. Patients exhibit a shuffling gait with short paces, a blank 'mask-like' facial expression, speech impairment and an inability to perform learned tasks. Symptoms of the disease do not manifest themselves until at least 80% of the dopaminergic neurons of the substantia nigra are lost. While the aetiology is unknown environmental factors are thought to be involved. Severe Parkinson's-like symptoms are seen in people who have taken an illegal drug contaminated with the chemical MPTP (1-methyl-4-phenyl-1,2,3,6-tetrahydropyridine) and were also seen in people following infection by a severe form of influenza during an epidemic in the early 1900s.

Current treatments

Current pharmacological strategies have involved maximising the effectiveness of the remaining, ever-depleting number of dopaminergic neurons. Levodopa is the immediate precursor of dopamine and is administered orally, it is transported across the BBB and converted to dopamine, leading to a substantial improvement in motor function. Other drugs employed include dopamine receptor agonists (bromocriptine) and inhibitors of dopamine breakdown (selegiline).

All drug strategies, however are ineffective in treating the neuronal death, and as time passes the progressive neuronal degeneration continues, and in the majority of patients within 5 years there is 'end-of-dose deterioration', which is caused by the inability of the remaining neurons to buffer fluctuating levodopa levels. The capacity of the basal ganglia to 'cushion' this substantial loss of dopaminergic neurons is possibly due to a naturally high reserve facility in order to counteract age-related neurodegeneration and/or the susceptibility of nigrostriatal neurons to damage. Mechanisms of buffering include a compensatory increase in dopamine biosynthesis and release from the surviving neurons and a reduction in the capacity of inactivation systems, such as reuptake carriers at the synaptic space.

Gene therapy

Two gene therapy strategies have been investigated as possible mechanisms to compensate for the loss of dopaminergic neurons. Tyrosine hydroxylase (TH) is the cytosolic rate-limiting step in dopamine biosynthesis *in vivo* and by enhancing the expression levels of the enzyme in the remaining dopaminergic neurons it may be possible to increase the production of dopamine in the nigrostriatal pathway. Methodologies used for the *in vivo* transfer of TH to the nigrostriatal pathway include viral vectors (Horellou *et al.*, 1994), transplantation of *ex vivo* TH-transduced cells (Lundberg *et al.*, 1996) and administration of TH-encoding liposomes (Cao *et al.*, 1995; Imaoka *et al.*, 1998). Optimisation of this strategy has involved the gene transfer of the complete dopamine synthetic pathway by the incorporation of the enzyme GTP-cyclohydrolase-1 (GTPCH) to generate the TH co-factor tetrahydrobiopterine (Leff *et al.*, 1998) and aromatic amino acid decarboxylase (Fan *et al.*, 1998).

The second gene therapy strategy investigated in Parkinson's disease has been the introduction of neuroprotective genes, such as endogenous nerve growth factors which inhibit cell loss and enhance recovery of damaged dopaminergic neurons. Glial cell line-derived neurotrophic factor (GDNF) *in vitro* promotes survival, high-affinity dopamine uptake and neurite outgrowth of embryonic neurons (Lin *et al.*, 1993). It is the most potent neurotrophic factor and is specific, with no effects on CNS astrocytes. Intracerebral injection of GDNF has been shown to protect the substantia nigra and prevent neuronal death and atrophy in the rhesus monkey, rat and mouse animal models of Parkinson's disease. GDNF is a disulfide-bonded homodimer protein that is heterogeneously glycosylated and unable to cross the BBB, therefore gene transfer may allow continuous biosynthesis without the need for repeated intracerebral administration. Adenovirus-mediated GDNF-transgene delivery into the substantia nigra has been reported to protect dopaminergic neurons from progressive degeneration in the 6-hydroxydopamine (6-OHDA) animal model of Parkinson's disease (Choi-Lundberg *et al.*, 1997; Bilang-Bleuel *et al.*, 1997). Brain-derived neurotrophic factor (BDNF) is a member of the neurotrophin family of growth factors and is expressed in low levels in the substantia nigra and striatum. Supranigral implants of fibroblasts engineered to secrete human BDNF have been shown to protect dopaminergic neurons from 1-methyl-4-phenylpyridinium (MPTP)-induced toxicity (Frim *et al.*, 1994). NT4/5 is another member of the neurotrophin family of growth factors with a lower level of expression than BDNF. A problem encountered with adenovirus-mediated vectors is the destruction of dopaminergic neurons seen with both therapeutic and control vectors. The mechanism of toxicity remains unknown, but a positive aspect of the Ad-GDNF vector was that it compensated for the adenovirus-mediated neuronal death *in vivo*.

Motor neuron disease and amyotrophic lateral sclerosis

Aetiology

Motor neuron disease (MND)/amyotrophic lateral sclerosis (ALS) is a neurodegenerative disorder (prevalence around 5 per 100 000) characterised by progressive loss of primarily motor neurons in spinal cord, brainstem and motor cortex.

ALS occurs in sporadic, familial and Western Pacific forms. Both the sporadic and familial ALS (age-dependent autosomal dominant) have a mean onset at 50 years, followed by a 3-year rapid progression. During this period mortality rates are approximately 50%, although in a proportion of patients the disease course may continue over decades. The Western Pacific form of the disease is probably related to environmental factors, and clusters of high incidence are seen within West New Guinea, Guam and the Kii peninsula.

Pathology

The initial neuropathology is characterised by shrinkage of motor neurons followed by extensive motor neuron loss in the spinal cord and degeneration of the corticospinal tract. Common clinical features seen with ALS are inextricably linked to the underlying neurodegeneration and include muscle weakness and wasting, principally in the limbs, face, throat and tongue, muscle cramps and fasciculations. Symptoms result in an increasing inability to walk, to use hands and arms, to speak and to swallow.

Increasing evidence via linkage analysis on chromosome 21 has identified mutations in the enzyme superoxide dismutase 1 (SOD-1) as a possible cause of the degeneration of motor neurons. SOD-1 is a ubiquitous cytosolic copper/zinc-dependent enzyme with high concentrations in the liver and CNS. It has a homodimer structure with 153 amino acids that is highly conserved between species. Currently there are over 30 reported SOD-1 mutations in the familial form of ALS (deBelleroche *et al.*, 1995).

Therapies

Protection of susceptible neurons by neurotrophic factors has been suggested as a potential therapy for ALS/MND although systemic administration of the proteins has yielded poor clinical trials data due to the low levels reaching the CNS. Candidate neurotrophic factors showing the greatest potential include neurotrophin 3 (NT3), ciliary neurotrophic factor (CNTF) and glial cell line-derived neurotrophic factor (GDNF). NT3 has been reported to increase the lifespan of progressive motor neuropathy (*pmn*) mice by 50%, with reduced loss of motor axons and improved neuromuscular function (Haase *et al.*, 1999). GDNF prolonged the onset of disease, delayed deterioration of motor behaviour and slowed muscle atrophy (Sagot *et al.*, 1996) and CNTF reduced motor neuron cell death in rodent models of ALS (Sagot *et al.*, 1995). Due to a lack of possible pharmacological interventions in MND/ALS, current therapeutic strategies are based on support facilities and the use of dedicated carers. At present a clinical trial using intrathecal mini-pump administration of the neurotrophic factor BDNF is underway.

Huntington's chorea

Huntington's disease is an autosomal dominant genetic disorder that results in a progressive loss of gamma-aminobutyric acid (GABA)-containing neurons of the striatum and then later in the cerebral cortex. Clinically, the symptoms of Huntington's disease first become manifest in middle age, leading to progressive dementia and severe involuntary sudden jerky movements, resulting in loss of speech and ability to feed. Huntington's disease is linked to an increase in the number of CAG repeats from 11–34 to greater than 40 in the *HD* gene found on chromosome 4q16.3. The gene product from this increase in CAG repeats results in an elongated huntingtin protein with 40–150 glutamine residues.

Huntingtin protein is degraded intracellularly via a process that first requires conjugation with ubiquitin followed by proteolytic cleavage to amino acid constituents by proteasome. During Huntington's disease there is thought to be aberrant processing of proteins resulting in transport and aggregation of huntingtin, ubiquitin and other proteasome components within the neuronal nucleus, leading to cell death via apoptosis.

Therapies

Current therapies for Huntington's disease are ineffective and do not affect the underlying cause of the disease. Pharmacological intervention is based on antagonising dopaminergic neurotransmission and thus reducing the involuntary movements.

Ciliary neurotrophic factor (CNTF) protein promotes the growth and survival of striatal neurons *in vivo* and has been speculated as a possible therapeutic agent in Huntington's disease. Implantation of CNTF-secreting cells into a primate model of Huntington's disease have been shown to be neuroprotective on several populations of striatal cells, including GABAergic, cholinergic and diaphorase-positive neurons which would normally perish during the animal model (Emerich *et al.*, 1997). Therapy utilising CNTF gene insertion into striatal neurons by a viral or plasmid-mediated mechanism or transplantation of genetically modified cells into the damaged areas may have a beneficial effect on the pathophysiology of Huntington's disease by enhancing neuronal survival.

Alzheimer's disease

Alzheimer's disease (AD) occurs in both familial and sporadic forms. It is generally characterised by impairments of memory, language and judgement and other 'higher order' cognitive functions. Although affected by escalating psychological dysfunction, AD sufferers are usually spared basic motor and sensory abilities. At present, Alzheimer's disease accounts for up to 70% of dementia cases, equating to 1% of the population.

AD is associated with general brain tissue shrinkage without large-scale loss of cortical neurons. Measurement of post-mortem brain tissue has shown reduced levels of numerous neurotransmitters, but the deficits in learning and memory are closely associated with a selective loss of cholinergic neurons in the basal forebrain nuclei. The classical extracellular lesion associated with AD is the presence of senile (dense core, neuritic) plaques. Senile plaques (SP) are spherical deposits, consisting principally of a central core of amyloid protein. Furthermore, the abundance of SPs is linked with dystrophic axons and dendrites allied to activated microglia and reactive astrocytes.

Therapies

Pharmacological research into a therapy for AD has primarily concentrated on redressing the balance of cholinergic transmission within the brain. Two drugs that have recently entered the clinic for mild to moderate Alzheimer's disease are donepezil and rivastigmine, both of which inhibit the metabolising enzyme (acetylcholinesterase) of the neurotransmitter acetylcholine, thereby enhancing cholinergic transmission, particularly within the basal forebrain.

Neurotrophic gene therapy strategies investigated in animal models of cholinergic neurodegeneration have involved NGF and BDNF gene delivery directly into the medial septum via recombinant adeno-associated viral vector (Mandel *et al.*, 1999). These systems resulted in attenuation of cholinergic cell loss with a BDNF-derived effect persisting for six months post treatment (Klein *et al.*, 1999).

Gene therapy in other neurological diseases

Epilepsy

Epilepsy is a disease characterised by seizures resulting from episodic, high-frequency discharge of cerebral neurons. It affects approximately 0.5% of the population. Epileptic seizures are classified according to the focus and spread of the seizure area and the symptoms that are produced.

Partial (focal) seizures result from an abnormal charge that originates from a specific locus and does not spread to other cortical areas. Generalised seizures are caused by the spread of the abnormal discharge from a focus (particularly in the temporal lobe) and then spread to other areas.

The aetiology of epilepsy is unknown in 60–70% of cases, however damage to the brain via head injury, tumours and cerebrovascular accident may result in epilepsy. The basis of epilepsy is not known, although an imbalance between excitatory glutamate and inhibitory GABA neurons is speculated.

Therapies

Treatment of epilepsy is based on pharmacological intervention by reducing the electrical excitability of the cell membrane and enhancing GABA-mediated synaptic inhibition. Currently, pharmacological intervention is effective in 70–80% of patients, with the main aim of the therapies to control seizures with the minimum of adverse side effects.

Gene therapy strategies for epilepsy are still relatively early in development, however initial reports using HSV and adenovirus vectors have been encouraging. Gene transfer of the GABA-synthesising enzyme glutamic acid decarboxylase (GAD67) *in vitro* resulted in increased GABA production in neuronal and glial cell cultures (Robert *et al.*, 1997). Another approach has been the insertion of heat shock protein 72 (HSP72) in rat models of epilepsy, which increased the survival of neurons after excitotoxin-induced seizures (Yenari *et al.*, 1998).

Stroke/ischaemia

Stroke is the largest single cause of severe disability in England and Wales, with over 300 000 people being affected at any one time, and is the third most common cause of death, after heart disease and cancer (see also Chapter 6). Annually, over 100 000 people in England and Wales experience a first stroke. A stroke occurs when the artery supplying an area of the brain becomes occluded and, due to the reduced oxygen availability, the tissue supplied by that vessel becomes ischaemic. Some strokes are caused by bleeding within or around the brain from a burst blood vessel. Some strokes are fatal, while others cause permanent or temporary disabilities. Around a third of people who have a stroke die within a year, a third are left with serious disabilities and the remainder make a good recovery.

Pathology

Neuronal death following an impairment of blood flow in the brain is not simply due to cells dying because of a lack of oxygen supply and the resultant anaerobic glycolysis-dependent energy depletion. Complex cascade events are initiated that develop in the subsequent hours, including alterations in ion homeostasis, generation of inflammatory mediators, production of free radicals and cerebral oedema formation. Experimental evidence from animal models has implied a mechanism of excessive glutamate-mediated Ca^{2+} influx (excitotoxicity) into the neurons, resulting in functional impairment and morphological damage.

Therapy

Current therapies for stroke patients are based on removal of the blood clot and re-establishing a normal blood supply to the affected area.

Treatment includes daily low-dose aspirin to prevent further blood coagulation and reduction of risk factors such as high blood pressure and diet (see Chapter 6 for further details).

Gene therapy strategies have concentrated on inhibiting the final part of the apoptosis cascade. Gene transfection of *bcl-2* via an HSV vector has been shown to increase neuronal survival in an ischaemic injury model (Linnik *et al.*, 1995). The *bcl-2* gene is part of a family of genes that encode proteins which inhibit apoptosis induced by damage or trophic factor withdrawal. Supporting evidence for this strategy comes from a neuronal apoptosis inhibitory protein (NAIP) vector, which has been reported to reduce neuronal damage *in vivo* (Xu *et al.*, 1997). Inhibition of the cerebral oedema formation and reduction in inflammatory response has been achieved by adenovirus vector-mediated administration of IL-1 receptor antagonist (Betz *et al.*, 1995).

Neurotrophic therapy using *ex vivo* implanted modified fibroblasts that secreted NGF in a rat model of ischaemic damage were reported to protect neurons in the CA1 and CA2 regions of the brain (Pechan *et al.*, 1995).

The future of gene therapy for neurological diseases

Further investigations to fully dissect the underlying pathological mechanisms of neurological disease and continued improvements in vector delivery systems are necessary before therapy and repair strategies can be taken to the clinic. Nevertheless, some of the strategies have already been implemented for experimental systems of human disease and brain tumours, and it is hoped that further advances in gene therapy and identification of genes related to neurological disorders will lead to the treatment of other incurable chronic and progressive neurological disorders in the not too distant future.

Acknowledgements

The authors' research is supported by the Multiple Sclerosis Society of Great Britain and Northern Ireland, the Stichting Vrienden Multiple Sclerosis Research of the Netherlands and the European Commission shared cost programme 'Biosafety of vaccines based on self-replicating recombinant alphaviruses'.

References

Bankiewicz K S, Leff S E, Nagy D, *et al.* (1997) Practical aspects of the development of *ex vivo* and *in vivo* gene therapy for Parkinson's disease. *Exp Neurol* 144: 147–156.

Betz A, Yang G, Davidson B (1995) Attenuation of stroke size in rats using an adenoviral vector to induce overexpression of interleukin-1 receptor antagonist. *J Cereb Blood Flow Metab* 15: 547–551.

Bilang-Bleuel A, Revah F, Colin P, *et al.* (1997) Intrastriatal injection of an adenoviral vector expressing glial-cell-line-derived neurotrophic factor prevents dopaminergic neuron degeneration and behavioral impairment in a rat model of Parkinson disease. *Proc Natl Acad Sci USA* 4: 8818–8823.

Blömer U, Naldini L, Kafri T, *et al.* (1997) Highly efficient and sustained gene transfer in adult neurons with a lentivirus vector. *J Virol* 71: 6641–6649.

Bode W, Fernandez-Catalan C, Tschesche H, *et al.* (1999) Structural properties of matrix metalloproteinases. *Cell Mol Life Sci* 55: 639–652.

Byrnes A P, Rusby J E, Wood M J A, Charlton H M (1995) Adenovirus gene transfer causes inflammation in the brain. *Neuroscience* 66: 1015–1024.

Cannella B, Hoban C J, Gao Y L, *et al.* (1998) The neuregulin, glial growth factor 2, diminishes autoimmune demyelination and enhances remyelination in a chronic relapsing model for multiple sclerosis. *Proc Natl Acad Sci USA* 95: 10100–10105.

Cao L, Zheng Z C, Zhao Y C, *et al.* (1995) Gene therapy of Parkinson disease model rat by direct injection of plasmid DNA-lipofectin complex. *Hum Gene Ther* 6: 1497–1501.

Choi-Lundberg D L, Lin Q, Chang Y N, *et al.* (1997) Dopaminergic neurons protected from degeneration by GDNF gene therapy. *Science* 275: 838–841.

Constantini L C, Bakowska J C, Breakfield X O, Isacson O (2000) Gene therapy in the CNS. *Gene Ther* 7: 93–109.

Croxford J L, Triantaphyllopoulos K, Podhajcer O L, *et al.* (1998) Cytokine gene therapy in experimental allergic encephalomyelitis by injection of plasmid DNA-cationic liposome complex into the central nervous system. *J Immunol* 160: 5181–5187.

DeBelleroche J, Orrell R, King A (1995) Familial amyotrophic lateral sclerosis/motor neuron disease (FALS): a review of current developments. *J Med Genet* 32: 841–847.

Doering L C (1994) Nervous system modification by transplants and gene transfer. *Bioessays* 16: 825–831.

Emerich D F, Winn S R, Hantraye P M, *et al.* (1997) Protective effect of encapsulated cells producing neurotrophic factor CNTF in a monkey model of Huntington's disease. *Nature* 386: 395–399.

Fan DS, Ogawa M, Fujimoto KI, *et al.* (1998) Behavioral recovery in 6-hydroxy-dopamine-lesioned rats by cotransduction of striatum with tyrosine hydroxylase and aromatic L-amino acid decarboxylase genes using two separate adeno-associated virus vectors. *Hum Gene Ther* 9: 2527–2535.

Federco M (1999) Lentiviruses as gene delivery vectors. *Curr Opin Biotechnol* 10: 448–453.

Frim DM, Uhler TA, Galpern WR, *et al.* (1994) Implanted fibroblasts genetically engineered to produce brain-derived neurotrophic factor prevent 1-methyl-4-phenylpyridinium toxicity to dopaminergic neurons in the rat. *Proc Natl Acad Sci USA* 91: 5104–5108.

Glasgow G M, McGee M M, Tarbatt C J, *et al.* (1998) The Semliki Forest virus vector induces p53-independent apoptosis. *J Gen Virol* 79: 2405–2410.

Guy J, Qi X, Hauswirth W W (1998) Adeno-associated viral mediated catalase expression suppresses optic neuritis in experimental allergic encephalomyelitis. *Proc Natl Acad Sci USA* 95: 13847–13852.

Haase G, Pettmann B, Vigne E, *et al.* (1998) Adenovirus-mediated transfer of the neurotrophin-3 gene into skeletal muscle of pmn mice: therapeutic effects and mechanisms of action. *J Neurol Sci* 160 (Suppl. 1): S97–105.

Hahn A F (1998) Guillain-Barré syndrome. *Lancet* 352: 635–641.

Hermens W T J M C, Verhaagen J (1998) Viral vectors, tools for gene transfer in the nervous system. *Prog Neurobiol* 55: 399–432.

Horellou P, Vigne E, Castel M N, *et al.* (1994) Direct intracerebral gene transfer of an adenoviral vector expressing tyrosine hydroxylase in a rat model of Parkinson's disease. *Neuroreport* 6: 49–53.

Imaoka T, Date I, Ohmoto T, Nagatsu T (1998) Significant behavioral recovery in Parkinson's disease model by direct intracerebral gene transfer using continuous injection of a plasmid DNA-liposome complex. *Hum Gene Ther* 9: 1093–1102.

Klein R L, Muir D, King M A, *et al.* (1999) Long-term actions of vector-derived nerve growth factor or brain-derived neurotrophic factor choline acetyltransferase and Trk receptor levels in the adult rat basal forebrain. *Neuroscience* 90: 815–821.

Lachmann R H, Efstathiou S (1999) Use of herpes simplex virus type 1 for transgene expression within the nervous system. *Clin Sci* 96: 533–541.

Le Gal La Salle G, Robert J J, Berrard S, *et al.* (1993) An adenovirus vector for gene transfer into neurons and glia in the brain. *Science* 259: 988–990.

Leff S E, Rendahl K G, Spratt S K, *et al.* (1998) *In vivo* L-DOPA production by genetically modified primary rat fibroblast or 9L gliosarcoma cell grafts via coexpression of GTP cyclohydrolase I with tyrosine hydroxylase. *Exp Neurol* 151: 249–264.

Lin L-F, Doherty D, Lile J, *et al.* (1993) A glial cell lined-derived neurotrophic factor for the mid-brain dopaminergic neurons. *Science* 260: 113–132.

Linnik M, Zahos M, Geschwind M, Federoff H (1995) Expression of bcl-2 from a defective herpes simplex virus-1 vector limits neuronal death in focal cerebral ischaemia. *Stroke* 26: 1670–1675.

Lisak R P (1998) Intravenous immunoglobulins in multiple sclerosis. *Neurology* 51: 25–29.

Lundberg C, Horellou P, Mallet J, Bjorklund A (1996) Generation of dopa-producing astrocytes by retroviral transduction of the human tyrosine hydroxylase gene – *in vitro* characterisation and *in vivo* effects in the rat Parkinson model. *Exp Neurol* 139: 39–53.

Lundstrom K (1997) Alphaviruses as expression vectors. *Curr Opin Biotechnol* 8: 578–582.

Maidment N T, Tan A M, Bloom D C, *et al.* (1996) Expression of the lacZ reporter gene in the rat basal forebrain, hippocampus, and nigrostriatal pathway using a nonreplicating herpes simplex vector. *Exp Neurol* 199: 107–114.

Mandel R J, Gage F H, Clevenger D G, *et al.* (1999) Nerve growth factor expressed in the medial septum following *in vivo* gene delivery using a recombinant adeno-associated viral vector protects cholinergic neurons from fimbria-fornix lesion-induced degeneration. *Exp Neurol* 155: 59–64.

Martínez-Serrano A, Björklund A (1997) Immortalised neural progenitor cells for CNS gene transfer and repair. *Trends Neurosci* 20: 530–538.

Martino G, Poliani P L, Marconi P C, Comi G, Furlan R (2000) Cytokine gene therapy of autoimmune demyelination revisited using herpes simplex virus type-1-derived vectors. *Gene Ther* 7: 1087–1093.

Mincera A, Vigneti E, Aloe L (1998) Changes of NGF presence in non-neuronal cells in response to experimental allergic encephalomyelitis in Lewis rat. *Exp Neurol* 154: 41–46.

Mossman S P, Bex F, Berglund P, *et al.* (1996) Protection against lethal simian immunodeficiency virus SIVsmmPBj14 disease by a recombinant Semliki Forest virus gp160 vaccine and by a gp120 subunit vaccine. *J Virol* 70: 1953–1960.

Pechan P A, Yoshida T, Panahian N, *et al.* (1995) Genetically modified fibroblasts producing NGF protect hippocampal neurons after ischemia in the rat. *Neuroreport* 6: 669–672.

Peltékian E, Parrish E, Bouchard C, *et al.* (1997) Adenovirus-mediated gene transfer to the brain: methodological assessment. *J Neurosci Methods* 71: 77–84.

Princen F, Lechanteur C, Lopez M, *et al.* (2000) Similar efficiency of DNA–liposome complexes and retrovirus-producing cells for HSV-tk suicide gene therapy of peritoneal carcinomatosis. *J Drug Target* 8: 79–89.

Raymon H K, Those S, Gage F H (1997) Application of *ex vivo* gene therapy in the treatment of Parkinson's disease. *Exp Neurol* 144: 82–91.

Robert J J, Bouilleret V, Ridoux V, *et al.* (1997) Adenovirus-mediated transfer of a functional GAD gene into nerve cells: potential for the treatment of neurological diseases. *Gene Ther* 4: 1237–1245.

Sagot Y, Tan S A, Baetge E, *et al.* (1995) Polymer encapsulated cell lines genetically engineered to release ciliary neurotrophic factor can slow down progressive motor neuronopathy in the mouse. *Eur J Neurosci* 7: 1313–1322.

Sagot Y, Tan S A, Hammang J P, *et al.* (1996) GDNF slows loss of motoneurons but not axonal degeneration or premature death of pmn/pmn mice. *J Neurosci* 16: 2335–2341.

Saito T (1998) Negative regulation of T cell activation. *Curr Opin Immunol* 10: 313–321.

Siegal T, Rubinstein R, Bokstein F, *et al.* (2000) *In vivo* assessment of the window of barrier opening after osmotic blood–brain barrier disruption in humans. *J Neurosurg* 92: 599–605.

Shi N, Pardridge W M (2000) Noninvasive gene targeting to the brain. *Proc Natl Acad Sci USA* 97: 7567–7572.

Singh V K, Mehrotra S, Agarwal S S (1999) The paradigm of Th1 and Th2 cytokines: its relevance to autoimmunity and allergy. *Immunol Res* 20: 147–161.

Simonato M, Manservigi R, Marconi P, Glorioso J (2000) Gene transfer into neurons for the molecular analysis of behaviour: focus on herpes simplex vectors. *Trends Neurosci* 23: 183–190.

Wood M J A, Charlton H M, Wood K J, *et al.* (1996) Immune responses to adenovirus vectors in the nervous system. *Trends Neurosci* 19: 497–501.

Xu D G, Crocker S J, Doucet J P, *et al.* (1997) Elevation of neuronal NAIP reduces ischemic damage in the rat hippocampus. *Nat Med* 3: 997–1004.

Yenari M A, Fink S L, Sun G H, *et al.* (1998) Gene therapy with HSP72 is neuro-protective in rat models of stroke and epilepsy. *Ann Neurol* 44: 584–591.

Zhou X, Berglund P, Zhao H, *et al.* (1995) Generation of cytotoxic and humoral immune responses by nonreplicative recombinant Semliki Forest virus. *Proc Natl Acad Sci USA* 92: 3009–3013.

10

Xenotransplantation: promise and problems

Robin A Weiss

A technique in its infancy, xenotransplantation is raising concerns similar to those voiced about DNA manipulation at its birth. A quarter of a century ago molecular biologists met at Asilomar in California to discuss the imposition of a temporary ban on recombinant DNA technology, then known as genetic engineering. The moratorium, designed to allow time for potential biohazards of inserting DNA from one organism into another to be investigated, proved to be short-lived. Despite the current controversy surrounding genetically modified food plants, recombinant DNA technology has not led to any known damage to the environment or to human health. We now have a substantial portfolio of pharmaceutical proteins manufactured through recombinant DNA technology, as well as gene therapy and the potential for DNA-based vaccines, as illustrated in this volume and its predecessor (Brooks, 1998).

'Uncertain peril and certain promise' was how Joshua Lederberg described recombinant DNA technology at Asilomar. Today, the same epithet applies to xenotransplantation, the grafting of animal cells, tissues and organs into humans. As with genetic engineering in 1975, xenotransplantation has also led to calls for a moratorium (Bach *et al.*, 1998; Butler, 1998), so that the safety and ethical issues can be discussed. In particular, the potential biohazard of cross-species virus infection through xenotransplantation procedures needs to be thoroughly explored.

Xenotransplantation is a type of cellular therapy, and as with all transfer of living cells into patients from extraneous sources, human or animal, those cells of course contain genetic material. Moreover, in xenotransplantation of whole organs, genetically modified source animals will invariably be used. Thus because it involves cell and DNA transfer, xenotransplantation merits a brief review here.

Curiously, some of the earliest examples of clinical xenotransplantation have been conducted as gene therapy trials for the treatment of glioblastoma. The therapeutic genes were to be delivered via a retroviral vector but because the vector titre was insufficient, the murine packaging cells producing the vector were inserted directly into patients' brains (Oldfield *et al.*, 1993; Ram *et al.*, 1997; Palu *et al.*, 1999). Although the gene therapists have not commented upon it, this procedure constitutes a form of xenotransplantation. One of the reasons that it is difficult to achieve high-titre delivery of retroviral vectors of gene therapy *in vivo* is that naturally occurring human antibodies destroy the vector envelope by complement-mediated inactivation. The human antibodies recognise carbohydrate antigens expressed on most animal cells used as packaging cells and they become incorporated into the glycolipids and glyco-proteins of the lipid envelope of the vector. The major antigen, galactose-alpha(1–3)-galactose (αGal), is the same moiety that triggers hyperacute rejection of non-primate xenografts transplanted into simians or humans (Rother and Squinto, 1996; Takeuchi *et al.*, 1996). Thus a clearer understanding of early events in xenograft rejection have helped to elucidate problems in gene therapy, and have encouraged the generation of high-titre vector packaging cells (Cosset *et al.*, 1995) derived from human or simian cell lines suitable for the production of other biopharmaceuticals. Moreover the high-titre natural human anti-bodies to αGal (Galili, 1993) make the transfer of the porcine alpha(1–3)-galactosyltransferase gene an attractive approach to cancer gene therapy (Jäger *et al.*, 1999).

Meeting the demand for transplantation

Organ transplantation from human to human has moved over the past 30 years from being an experimental control to a routine clinical procedure. However, immunosuppressive drug treatment is needed for the majority of genetically mismatched donor–recipient allografts and this creates conditions for opportunistic infections to arise. These may arise from latent infections in the recipient or as *de novo* infections from the donor or from the environment. Infectious disease then, is a major complication of allotransplantation, as it will be for xenotransplantation. Nevertheless, allotransplantation of kidneys, liver, heart, combined heart and lung and, more recently, pancreas has proved to be such a success as replacement therapy for failed organs that there are now long waiting lists for organ transplants.

With a falling number of cadaveric organs and tissues available, thanks to improved road safety and other accident prevention policies, the imbalance between supply and demand for organ transplants is increasing. Moreover the usefulness of organs will continue to rise as more patients and more disease entities are deemed eligible for treatment by transplantation. Even if 'opt out' policies were adopted, so that people were assumed to consent unless they specifically stated otherwise, the availability of organs could not match the need. It is the hope that xenografts could bridge this gap between supply and demand that has spurred a number of biotechnology and pharmaceutical companies to invest in research and development in xenotransplantation.

In fact, the first applications of xenotransplantation are beginning to emerge in cellular and tissue grafting rather than whole organ transplantation. As described later, intact animal organs require the integrity of the donor vasculature and are subject to rapid rejection, whereas dispersed cells and tissues survive longer. Thus fetal pig neurons have been tested to treat Parkinson's disease (Deacon *et al.*, 1997); porcine islets of Langerhans have been engrafted into patients with insulin-dependent diabetes mellitus (Groth *et al.*, 1994); and there is interest in the *ex vivo* use of animal hepatocytes for short-term treatment by extracorporeal transfusion of patients with acute liver failure.

Several groups have developed 'bioartificial livers' using porcine hepatocytes. These include flat membrane bioreactors, hollow fibre devices (Gerlach *et al.*, 1994) and other culture systems (Rozga *et al.*, 1993). It is therefore likely that the initial advances in clinical xenotransplantation will come from cellular and tissue therapies, generating new sets of treatable disease and new demands for supply. Here, the main competition will come from new techniques in human cellular therapies, including redirecting the differentiation of specialist cells, which may eventually replace the use of animal cells.

The challenge to find suitable animal sources

There are four distinct problems to consider in xenotransplantation – ethical, physiological, immunological and microbiological. The favoured solutions to each of these issues do not necessarily coincide, but together they have led to specially bred, genetically modified, domestic pigs being considered most appropriate for the development of xenotransplantation.

From the physiological and immunological points of view, animals closest to our phylogeny, the apes and Old World monkeys, would be the most promising sources of tissue, but their use raises serious ethical, safety and practical concerns. All apes are seriously endangered species, and their slow breeding in captivity could not keep pace with medical demand. Monkeys such as macaques and baboons raise similar problems, as there are ethical issues in using our near relatives as an 'organ and tissue farm'. In order to provide primates that are not contaminated by the numerous viruses that are potentially pathogenic for humans, infant monkeys would need to be born by Caesarean section and reared in isolation. This would deprive them of the parental care and behavioural development that is crucial for all primates. Primates take a long time to mature, and few species would yield organs of appropriate size for xenotransplantation to adult humans.

For these considerations, domestic species are the only animals under serious consideration as a future source of whole organs for xenotransplantation. While there has been some discussion over the potential use of ruminants or dogs, pigs are the only species currently under xenograft development. Pigs can be reared in specific pathogen-free conditions via hysterotomy, they produce large litters, and they grow quickly to an appropriate size. Pigs can also be genetically manipulated to produce organs less likely to be rejected by humans. The ethical issues over pigs seem to be less than those about primates. They are routinely reared and slaughtered for human consumption, and non-living pig heart valves have been successfully used surgically for many years. Those religions that prohibit or disapprove of the consumption of pork have not raised serious objections to the medical use of pig heart valves and are unlikely to do so over cell or organ xenotransplantation if it is life-saving.

Xenotransplantation across wide phylogenetic groups, however, raises questions of physiological compatibility. Pig insulin functions in humans, so pancreatic islet cell xenotransplantation for insulin-dependent diabetes mellitus has already undergone a phase I trial (Groth *et al.*, 1994). Pig fetal neurons secreting dopamine have been used to treat patients with Parkinson's disease (Deacon *et al.*, 1997) and similar xenotransplantation is proposed for stroke, Huntington's disease and some forms of epilepsy. Although a pig heart may perform its pumping function and pig kidneys should function in humans diuretically, pig erythropoietin produced by kidneys does not bind to human erythropoietin receptors. Therefore recombinant human hormone would be required to treat kidney xenograft recipients, as for dialysis patients, unless transgenic pigs expressing human erythropoietin could be used.

A pig liver is unlikely to provide all the correct metabolic and biochemical functions of a human liver. Nevertheless, perfusion or dialysis of human blood across porcine hepatocytes extracorporeally is being proposed for clinical trial to treat acute liver failure. Such treatment has been performed with an intact pig liver (Chari *et al.*, 1994) and is useful to bridge a patient until a human liver allograft becomes available, or until the patient's own liver has regenerated. Ironically, successful xeno-perfusion or the successful use of short-term bridging xenotransplants may serve to increase the waiting list for human allografts by tem-porarily saving patients' lives.

Immunological aspects of xenotransplantation

Rejection remains a major hurdle to successful xenotransplantation (Dorling *et al.*, 1997; Weiss, 1998a; Auchincloss and Sachs, 1998; Platt, 2000a). There are three main mechanisms of rejection: hyperacute rejec-tion (HAR), acute vascular rejection (AVR) and delayed, cell-mediated rejection.

Hyperacute rejection of xenografted organs represents a comple-ment-mediated destruction of the vascular endothelium of a discordant graft, such as one from a pig. It occurs within minutes of transplanta-tion or perfusion, and is analogous to a human allograft mismatched for the ABO blood groups. Like ABO, hypercute rejection results from the recognition of carbohydrate antigens, in particular the major porcine antigen already mentioned, galactose-alpha(1–3)-galactose, known as αGal (Rother and Squinto, 1996; Platt, 2000b). Most mammals, including pigs, place αGal as a terminal sugar on membrane glycolipids and glycoproteins, but Old World primates, including humans, lack the gene encoding the α(1–3)-galactosyltransferase which catalyses this reaction. Because gut bacteria express αGal, humans make αGal antibodies, just as Group O individuals make anti-A and anti-B antibodies. Some 5% or more of IgM in human plasma is directed to αGal antigen (Galili, 1993).

Acute vascular rejection is also triggered by recognition of αGal antigens on the endothelial surface (Platt, 2000b). Antibody deposition leads to inflammatory cytokine responses, adhesion of leukocytes and extravasation. Both hyperacute rejection and acute vascular rejection occur because humans are pre-immunised against αGal and other xenoantigens. On the other hand, cell-mediated rejection is an acquired immunity, just like cytotoxic T-cell rejection of mismatched or partially matched allografts. This type of delayed rejection may be abrogated by immunosuppressive drugs, such as ciclosporin A, but it is not yet clear whether immunosuppressive regimes even more powerful than those used in allografts will be required for xenografts.

If pigs that lacked the $\alpha(1-3)$-galactosyltransferase gene could be bred, that might reduce hyperacute and acute vascular rejection. However genetic 'knockout' technology for pigs is only just becoming possible through cloning of this species (Polejaeva *et al.*, 2000), though 'knockin' transgenesis is well established. A promising solution to acute and hyperacute xenograft rejection has been to breed transgenic pigs that express human complement-modulating membrane proteins on vascular surfaces. Pigs have been bred that express the complement-regulating proteins CD55 (DAF), CD46 and CD59. Using baboons or macaques as surrogate human recipients, pig hearts from CD55 transgenic pigs have survived up to 40 days rather than a few minutes (Cozzi and White, 1995; Byrne *et al.*, 1997; Schmoeckel *et al.*, 1998). Cellular and small tissue grafts, however, are much less sensitive to acute and hyperacute rejection than are organs requiring an intact porcine vasculature. Less αGal antigen is expressed on pancreatic islet cells and brain cells, and these cells may survive by switching off αGal expression. This is another reason why cellular xenografts have already undergone human clinical trials, while whole organ xenotransplantation remains premature.

Infection hazards of xenotransplantation

Concern that the practice of xenotransplantation might lead to novel infectious diseases in humans has been the topic of much debate in recent years. Known pathogens of animals can readily be detected so it should be possible to eliminate them from colonies of source animals. Thus it would be most unlikely that pathogens, such as influenza viruses or the recently identified paramyxovirus Nipah virus, would colonise pigs destined for xenotransplantation. However, it is not possible to screen for agents that have not yet been discovered, although general procedures such as Caesarean delivery and physical isolation of the founding animals should preclude the majority of microbes that are transmitted postnatally. There are a number of porcine viruses, such as herpesviruses and rotaviruses, that ought to be excludable by appropriate screening. Others, such as parvovirus and circovirus, might re-contaminate the herd because they are ubiquitous on food or footwear. Parvovirus may be controlled by immunisation.

When a virus crosses from its natural reservoir species to a new host, it is not easy to predict whether it will become more or less pathogenic

(Weiss, 2001). Yaba monkey-pox virus, a relative of variola (smallpox) virus causes severe disease in both monkeys and humans. On the other hand, cow-pox behaves in an attenuated manner in humans, which allowed the development of vaccination by Jenner 200 years ago. More troublesome could be the viruses that often show few pathogenic signs or symptoms in their natural animal host yet cause serious disease in humans. The hantaviruses of rodents, responsible for the outbreak of Sin Nombre virus infection in Southwest USA (Nichol *et al.*, 1993), as well as the haemorrhagic viruses causing Ebola, Marburg and Lassa fever, may be less pathogenic in their natural animal hosts. Herpesvirus B, related to Human herpes simplex virus, causes nothing worse than cold sores in immunocompetent monkeys but causes lethal encephalitis in humans. Simian immunodeficiency viruses (SIV) appear to have low if any pathogenicity in their natural African primate hosts, but lead to fatal acquired immune deficiency syndrome (AIDS) in Asian macaques and, sadly, in humans after the transfer of SIVcpz from chimpanzees to become HIV-1 (Weiss and Wrangham, 1999).

Accordingly, despite being given a 'clean bill of health' by veterinarians, we may still not be sure whether source animals such as pigs might harbour potential human pathogens. Moreover, new microbes are coming to light all the time. In pigs, for example, several viruses have been discovered within the last 5 years. These include human-tropic pig endogenous retroviruses (Patience *et al.*, 1997a; Le Tissier *et al.*, 1997) discussed below; a virus related to human hepatitis E virus which may also infect humans (Meng *et al.*, 1998); a torovirus (Kroneman *et al.*, 1998); paramyxoviruses in Australia (Menangle and Hendra virus) (Philbey *et al.*, 1998) and Malaysia (Nipah virus) (Chua *et al.*, 1999), which have caused deaths in both pigs and people and which have spread to abattoir workers in Singapore (Paton *et al.*, 1999).

Thus zoonoses are a major area of concern for clinical xenotransplantation (Allan, 1996; Weiss, 1998a). While the benefit of the xenograft to the individual patient might well outweigh the risk of infection, it is the fear of setting off a new epidemic in the human population that distinguishes the infection hazards of xenotransplantation from the well-known infection hazards of allografts and of blood transfusion.

Of course, animals have transmitted viruses and other infectious pathogens to humans ever since we learnt to hunt or husband them. Some infections do not transmit onwards from person to person (e.g. rabies) whereas others are maintained as human epidemics with their animal origin forgotten (e.g. measles) (Weiss, 2001). We continue to encounter unpleasant surprises. The AIDS pandemic is caused by viruses that have only recently jumped host species from chimpanzees (HIV-1) and sooty mangabey monkeys (HIV-2) (Weiss and Wrangham, 1999). Variant Creutzfeldt–Jakob disease (vCJD) is linked to bovine spongiform encephalopathy which in turn resulted from unnatural feeding practices imposed by humans. The recent epidemic of Nipah virus probably had a reservoir in fruit-bats, but was spread by pigs (Philbey *et al.*, 1998). The lack of onward human-to-human transmission of chicken H5N1 influenza virus was a fortunate, but unforeseen feature of a zoonosis that killed 6 of 18 infected individuals. Zoonotic infections with a short incubation period, such as influenza, Ebola and Nipah should be identified and contained soon after their emergence. But slow persistent infections like HIV and CJD could be much more insidious if they emerged via xenotransplantation because the delay in recognising them would allow them to spread.

Considering that zoonoses happen spontaneously, some proponents of xenotransplantation question its added risk. P Herrling of Novartis Pharmaceuticals was quoted as saying: 'Domestic animals have transmitted infections to humans throughout history. The additional risk of a successful xenotransplantation might be minimal' (Butler, 1998). In fact, natural zoonoses are quite rare events, and xenotransplantation could significantly increase the risk of occurrence for three reasons:

1 The physical barrier is breached by implanting the tissues of one species into another.
2 The recipient patients will be severely immunosuppressed, allowing the infectious agent to become well established.
3 The transgenic animals providing the tissues will be expressing human genes that serve as virus receptors; these may also protect enveloped viruses from complement attack.

Thus source animals will need to be rigorously screened for microbes and potential pathogens. Not all such infections, however, can be readily eliminated. As discussed below, endogenous retroviruses have attracted special concern.

Porcine endogenous retroviruses (PERV)

Retroviruses are classified into several different subfamilies (Figure 10.1) and are well known to switch host species. The primate origins of HIV-1 and HIV-2 (Weiss and Wrangham, 1999) and of some strains of HTLV-I

(Gessain and Mahieux, 1999) demonstrate the potential danger of retroviral zoonoses. Exposed humans can become infected with animal retroviruses, as found for simian foamy viruses following injury, though they have not spread beyond the index persons (Heneine *et al.*, 1998a).

Of particular relevance to gene therapy, the murine retroviral vectors used clinically can also pose a risk if recovered in infectious form. Replication-competent recombinant vectors able to infect human cells were found to be pathogenic in monkeys used in gene therapy trials (Donahue *et al.*, 1992). They also transferred endogenous genetic elements that became packaged in the vector particles (Purcell *et al.*, 1996). Retroviral vectors derived from human packaging cells do not present this technical problem (Patience *et al.*, 1998b).

The DNA genome of retroviruses made by reverse transcriptase integrates into chromosomal DNA to form the provirus. This is why they are such useful vectors for stable gene expression in gene therapy (see Chapter 2). During the evolution of vertebrate hosts, DNA proviruses of retroviruses have become integrated into germ cells, the precursors of eggs and sperm. In consequence, such proviruses become host Mendelian genetic traits and gain vertical passage through host generations without needing to undergo further viral replication. These genomes are called endogenous retroviruses to distinguish them from

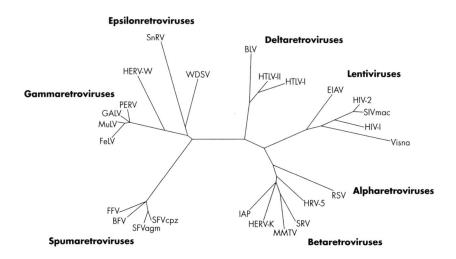

Figure 10.1   Unrooted phylogenetic tree of the major groups of retroviruses. PERV is a gammaretrovirus, also known as C-type viruses.

exogenous, infectiously transmitted retroviruses (Boeke and Stoye, 1997). Most vertebrate species carry multiple copies of endogenous proviruses. For example, over 5% of human DNA may be of retroviral origin, though none are known to give rise to infectious virus (Patience *et al.*, 1997b). Most endogenous retroviruses belong to the betaretrovirus subfamily, resembling Murine mammary tumour virus, and to the gammaretrovirus subfamily, related to murine leukaemia viruses (MLV). Neither lentiviruses related to HIV nor deltaretroviruses related to human T-cell lymphotropic virus (HTLV) have been found as endogenous genomes.

Many endogenous retroviral genomes are defective, but some, including those that have been endogenous in the germ line for a relatively short evolutionary time, can give rise to infectious particles containing RNA genomes with functional genes. These potentially infectious endogenous retroviruses are frequently xenotropic, that is they grow better in cells of foreign host species. Thus they are poised to infect neighbouring, foreign cells when living tissues of two species are juxtaposed in xenotransplantation. This is exemplified by the frequent infection of human tumour tissue by xenotropic endogenous MLV strains after xenotransplantation into immunodeficient mice, known for over 20 years (Achong *et al.*, 1976).

Like mice, pigs carry MLV-related porcine endogenous retroviruses (PERV). These viruses were originally detected as virions released from cell lines derived from porcine kidneys and from lymphoma (Armstrong *et al.*, 1971; Moennig *et al.*, 1974; Todaro *et al.*, 1974). They are C-type, gammaretrovirus genomes with many copies in porcine DNA (Benveniste and Todaro, 1975; Patience *et al.*, 1997a; Le Tissier *et al.*, 1997). Recently, further sets of endogenous retroviral genome have been detected in porcine DNA, representing both beta- and gammaretroviral taxonomic groups (Patience *et al.*, 2001). Since these new sequences appear to be defective, they may pose less of a problem for xenotransplantation. However, the gammaretrovirus particles released from porcine cells are replication-competent, can infect human cells in culture (Patience *et al.*, 1997a), and thus pose a risk in xenotransplantation.

When the host range of PERV was first examined it was shown that PERV released from the PK-15 kidney cell line replicated both in porcine cells (the ST-Iowa testis cell line) and in human cells (293 kidney cells and some other human cell types) (Patience *et al.*, 1997a). In fact, PK-15 cells release a mixture of two PERV strains with distinct envelope sequences, designated PERV-A and PERV-B (Le Tissier *et al.*, 1997). The virus released by another porcine kidney cell line, MPK, was infectious for pig cells but not for human 293 cells (Patience *et al.*, 1997a). This PERV strain, designated PERV-C, has an envelope sequence of PERV-C similar to a PERV genome originally cloned from a pig lymphoma (Akiyoshi *et al.*, 1998). Even PERV-C can infect certain human cells at low efficacy (Takeuchi *et al.*, 1998).

More extensive studies using MLV vectors with a reporter gene and PERV envelopes indicated that many human cells but few simian cells are permissive for PERV-A and PERV-B entry (Takeuchi *et al.*, 1998). Not all human cells are fully permissive for PERV replication, yet they may take up and integrate the PERV provirus (Patience *et al.*, 1997a). Even in human cell lines such as 293 and HeLa, which are among the most permissive for PERV replication, the levels of infectious PERV released are low compared with other human-tropic C-type viruses such as MLV (Takeuchi *et al.*, 1998). PERV-A, PERV-B and PERV-C have virtually indistinguishable protease and reverse transcriptase sequences, but diverge in the outer envelope glycoprotein (Le Tissier *et al.*, 1997; Akiyoshi *et al.*, 1998). Receptor-blocking studies show that PERV-A, -B and -C utilise different cell surface receptors from each other on porcine and human cells, which are also distinct from the receptors for MLV, cat, baboon and gibbon retroviruses (Takeuchi *et al.*, 1998).

Primary, short-term cultures of porcine cells spontaneously release PERV infectious for human cells. This has been reported for porcine lymphocytes (Wilson *et al.*, 1998) and endothelial cells (Martin *et al.*, 1998). It therefore appeared likely that some porcine cells or tissues xenotransplanted *in vivo* will also release PERV. This has recently been exemplified with porcine islets cells xenografted into immunodeficient mice (van der Laan *et al.*, 2000). PERV is also spontaneously released from tissues in pigs, and has been detected in porcine plasma and porcine factor VIII (Takefman *et al.*, 2001).

Southern blotting indicates that most strains of domestic pig carry multiple copies of PERV proviral genomes, dispersed among pig chromosomes, approximately 30 specific to PERV-A and 15 to PERV-B (Le Tissier *et al.*, 1997), as well as numerous other PERV genomes (Patience *et al.*, 2001). Many of these might be defective and incapable of giving rise to infectious virus. The endogenous proviruses will need to be mapped, cloned and sequenced to determine which of them can give rise to infectious virus particles. Thus it will not be simple to develop PERV-negative herds of pig, either by conventional breeding or by knockout technology when it becomes available.

Monitoring clinical infection by PERV

The demonstration that some strains of PERV can infect human cells in culture has led the Federal Drug Administration in USA and the UK Xenotransplantation Interim Regulatory Authority to draw up stringent guidelines for the conduct of xenotransplantation trials and the subsequent monitoring of PERV infection. In the USA, some experts have called for a moratorium on all clinical xenoperfusion and xenotransplantation (Bach *et al.*, 1998; Butler, 1998), whereas in Japan and in Russia (Paradis *et al.*, 1999) the decision seems to lie with local ethical research committees. Although virus infections do not respect political borders, international guidelines on safety in xenotransplantation lag behind its practice.

Before proceeding with clinical trials of porcine tissue, it seemed wise to investigate by retrospective surveillance whether humans already exposed to pig cells and tissues have become infected by PERV. This has been examined in four studies: in ten diabetes patients xenografted with porcine pancreatic islet cells (Heneine *et al.*, 1998b); in two renal dialysis patients whose extracorporeal circulation was perfused through porcine kidneys (Patience *et al.*, 1998a); in 24 neurological patients who were implanted with fetal pig neurons (Dinsmore *et al.*, 2000); and in 160 patients exposed in various ways to living porcine tissue (Paradis *et al.*, 1999), including those previously reported. No evidence was found of PERV infection in any of these cases.

These attempts to detect PERV infection used several approaches, reverse transcriptase activity, PCR and RT-PCR detection of PERV genomes and serological tests for PERV-specific antibodies in recipients (Weiss, 1999). The PCR-based assays in particular are highly sensitive, being based on primers and sequences specific to PERV that do not cross-react with human endogenous retrovirus sequences. However, a careful distinction must be made between PERV infection and microchimaerism of surviving porcine cells in the human body. Among the patients studied in the Novartis/CDC survey (Paradis *et al.*, 1999) were 100 Russian individuals who had been subjected to 'immunotherapy' by extracorporeal blood perfusion through pig spleens. Nearly 25% of these patients showed evidence of porcine cell microchimaerism following the perfusion, some of them several years after a single, one-hour exposure. The microchimaerism was initially identified by PCR detection of PERV sequences. Because mitochondrial or centromeric porcine DNA sequences were also detected, it was assumed that the detection of PERV sequences resulted from the survival of porcine cells rather than from infection of human cells by PERV.

Overall, the surveys conducted to date indicate that PERV is not highly contagious to humans, and that very few xenotransplant recipients are likely to become infected. These findings are consistent with the low titre of PERV replication in porcine or human cells in culture (Patience *et al.*, 1997a; Takeuchi *et al.*, 1998; Wilson *et al.*, 1998). It will be important, nonetheless, to monitor whether PERV can adapt to grow to high titres, or might recombine with other retroviral genomes to yield a more human-tropic retrovirus.

If a patient were to become infected by PERV, it would be wise to be equipped with anti-PERV therapy. Some anti-retroviral drugs active against HIV, but not others, inhibit PERV replication *in vitro* (Qari *et al.*, 2001).

Transgenic pigs and human infection

A potential problem seldom raised by transplant surgeons and immunologists or by biotechnology companies is that the genetic modification of pigs designed to prevent hyperacute rejection (Cozzi and White, 1995; Byrne *et al.*, 1997) might permit porcine viruses to become pre-adapted for human infection. The human complement-modulating genes that have been bred into transgenic pigs could have a direct impact on viruses infection (Weiss, 1998b): CD55/DAF acts as a receptor for human picornaviruses such as echo and coxsackie B myocarditis viruses, and CD46 acts as a receptor for measles virus. Therefore related viruses of pigs might adapt to utilise the human receptor homologues in transgenic pigs. In addition, human complement acts on enveloped viruses budding from animal cells in the same way as in hyperacute rejection. Antibodies to αGal and other carbohydrate xenoantigens bind to virus envelopes bearing these sugar antigens and this leads to complement inactivation, a sort of hyperacute lysis of virus particles (Takeuchi *et al.*, 1996; Rother and Squinto, 1996). For example, PERV released by wild-type porcine cells expressing αGal is rapidly inactivated by fresh human serum, whereas the same virus after one passage through αGal-negative human 293 cells is completely resistant (Patience *et al.*, 1997a). If the virus particles budding from transgenic porcine cells also incorporated human CD46, CD55 or CD59 into their envelopes, complement-mediated lysis may be abrogated. Indeed, the genetic modification of pigs designed to make organ xenotransplantation possible could also result in 'humanising' porcine viruses (Weiss, 1998b) to increase the risk of infection.

Clinical applications of xenotransplantation

Given the need to develop and test genetically modified pigs for whole organ transplantation, cellular and tissue therapies are the first to be considered for clinical trial. The use of fetal porcine brain cells will be expanded from Parkinson's disease to the treatment of Huntington's disease, stroke and possibly certain forms of epilepsy. Extracorporeal perfusion over porcine hepatocyte cultures separated by a semi-permeable membrane is being advocated for acute, fulminant liver failure. Since even extracorporeal exposure to human blood induces hyperacute 'rejection' or lysis of the animal cells, genetically modified pig cells will be used which express human membrane proteins that downmodulate the complement cascade (CD55/DAF, CD46 and/or CD59). If xeno-transplantation of porcine beta cells or whole islets of Langerhans from the pancreas prove successful in the treatment of insulin-dependent diabetes mellitus, it would create a huge market for xenotransplantation in this disease alone. Long-surviving whole organ xenotransplantation of the heart and kidney will require considerable further development and refinement. However, such progress will not be possible without initially using non-human primates as surrogate human recipients, and then engaging in small-scale human clinical trials.

In the mean time, the infection hazards need to be explored more deeply, including a long-term programme to seek pigs that do not release infectious porcine endogenous retroviruses from their cells and tissues. International standards for monitoring infection and for follow-up of xenotransplantation need to be established. Whereas some nations, such as the United Kingdom and Scandinavian countries, have set up such licensing and monitoring systems, others, e.g. Russia, India and USA, have until recently allowed individual physicians and surgeons to engage in what is, in practice, xenotransplantation (Starzl *et al.*, 1993) sometimes under the guise of immunotherapy (Paradis *et al.*, 1999) or gene therapy (Ram *et al.*, 1997). It is in the interests of multinational pharmaceutical companies to endorse international standards of safety and clinical practice.

Conclusions and prospects

Cellular therapies using animal sources has already arrived in clinical trials. Tissue and organ xenotransplantation needs more research but is an area of active inquiry involving multimillion dollar pharmaceutical investment. Therefore the infection hazards of xenotransplantation need to be balanced with the substantial benefit that is likely to accrue when the physiological and immunological problems are resolved. Individual benefit should be weighed against the more remote, yet potentially more devastating longer term risk to the human population.

Acknowledgement

The author's research into porcine retroviruses is supported by the Medical Research Council.

References

Achong B G, Trumper P A, Giovanella B C (1976) C-type virus particles in human tumours transplanted into nude mice. *Br J Cancer* 34: 203–206.

Akiyoshi D E, Denaro M, Zhu H, *et al.* (1998) Identification of a full-length cDNA for an endogenous retrovirus of miniature swine. *J Virol* 72: 4503–4507.

Allan J S (1996) Xenotransplantation at a crossroads: prevention versus progress. *Nat Med* 2: 18–21.

Armstrong J A, Porterfield J S, De Madrid A T (1971) C-type virus particles in pig kidney cell lines. *J Gen Virol* 10: 195–198.

Auchincloss H, Jr, Sachs D H (1998) Xenogeneic transplantation. *Annu Rev Immunol* 16: 433–470.

Bach F H, Fishman J A., Daniels N, *et al.* (1998) Uncertainty in xenotransplantation: individual benefit versus collective risk. *Nat Med* 4: 141–144.

Benveniste R E, Todaro G J (1975) Evolution of type C viral genes: preservation of ancestral murine type C viral sequences in pig cellular DNA. *Proc Natl Acad Sci USA* 72: 4090–4094.

Boeke J D, Stoye J P (1997) Retrotransposons, endogenous retroviruses, and the evolution of retroelements. In: Coffin J M, Hughes S H, Varmus H E, eds. *Retroviruses.* New York: Cold Spring Harbor Laboratory Press, 343–435.

Brooks G, ed. (1998) *Biotechnology in Healthcare. An Introduction to Biopharmaceuticals.* London: Pharmaceutical Press.

Butler D (1998) Last chance to stop and think on risks of xenotransplants. *Nature* 391: 320–325.

Byrne G W, McCurry K R, Martin M J, *et al.* (1997) Transgenic pigs expressing human CD59 and decay-accelerating factor produce an intrinsic barrier to complement-mediated damage. *Transplantation* 63: 149–155.

Chari R S, Collins B H, Magee, J C, *et al.* (1994) Treatment of hepatic failure with *ex vivo* pig-liver perfusion followed by liver transplantation. *N Engl J Med* 331: 234–237.

Chua K B, Goh K J, Wong K T, *et al.* (1999) Fatal encephalitis due to Nipah virus among pig-farmers in Malaysia. *Lancet* 354: 1257–1259.

Cosset F L, Takeuchi Y, Battini J L, *et al.* (1995) High-titer packaging cells producing recombinant retroviruses resistant to human serum. *J Virol* 69: 7430–7436.

Cozzi E, White D J (1995) The generation of transgenic pigs as potential organ donors for humans. *Nat Med* 1: 964–966.

Deacon T, Schumacher J, Dinsmore J, *et al.* (1997) Histological evidence of fetal pig neural cell survival after transplantation into a patient with Parkinson's disease. *Nat Med* 3: 350–353.

Dinsmore J H, Manhart C, Raineri R, *et al.* (2000) No evidence for infection of human cells with porcine endogenous retrovirus (PERV) after exposure to porcine fetal neuronal cells. *Transplantation* 70: 1382–1389.

Donahue R E, Kessler S W, Bodine D, *et al.* (1992) Helper virus induced T cell lymphoma in nonhuman primates after retroviral mediated gene transfer. *J Exp Med* 176: 1125–1135.

Dorling A, Riesbeck K, Warrens A, Lechler R (1997) Clinical xenotransplantation of solid organs. *Lancet* 349: 867–871.

Fishman J, Sachs D, Shaikh R, eds (1998) Xenotransplantation: scientific frontiers and public policy. *Ann NY Acad Sci* 862: 1–251.

Galili U (1993) Interaction of the natural anti-Gal antibody with alpha-galactosyl epitopes: a major obstacle for xenotransplantation in humans. *Immunol Today* 14: 480–482.

Gerlach J, Schnoy N, Smith M D, Neuhaus P (1994) Hepatocyte culture between woven capillary networks: a microscopy study. *Artif Organs* 18: 226–230.

Gessain A, Mahieux R (1999) Genetic diversity and molecular epidemiology of primate T cell lymphotropic viruses: human T cell leukaemia/lymphoma viruses types 1 and 2 and related simian retroviruses (STLV-1, STLV-2, PAN-P and PTLV-L). In: Dalgleish A G, Weiss R A, eds. *HIV and the New Viruses.* London: Academic Press, 281–327.

Groth C G, Korsgren O, Tibell A, *et al.* (1994) Transplantation of porcine fetal pancreas to diabetic patients. *Lancet* 344: 1402–1404.

Heneine W, Switzer W M, Sandstrom P, *et al.* (1998a) Identification of a human population infected with simian foamy viruses. *Nat Med* 4: 403–407.

Heneine W, Tibell A, Switzer W M, *et al.* (1998b) No evidence of infection with porcine endogenous retrovirus in recipients of porcine islet-cell xenografts. *Lancet* 352: 695–699.

Jäger U, Takeuchi Y, Porter C (1999) Induction of complement attack on human cells by Gal(alpha1,3)Gal xenoantigen expression as a gene therapy approach to cancer. *Gene Ther* 6: 1073–1083.

Kroneman A, Cornelissen L A, Horzinek M C, *et al.* (1998) Identification and characterisation of a porcine torovirus. *J Virol* 72: 3507–3511.

Le Tissier P, Stoye J P, Takeuchi Y, *et al.* (1997) Two sets of human-tropic pig retrovirus. *Nature* 389: 681–682.

Martin U, Kiessig V, Blusch J H, *et al.* (1998) Expression of pig endogenous retrovirus by primary porcine endothelial cells and infection of human cells. *Lancet* 352: 692–694.

Meng X J, Halbur P G, Shapiro M S, *et al.* (1998) Genetic and experimental evidence for cross-species infection by swine hepatitis E virus. *J Virol* 72: 9714–9721.

Moennig V, Frank H, Hunsmann G, *et al.* (1974) C-type particles produced by a permanent cell line from a leukemic pig. II. Physical, chemical, and serological characterization of the particles. *Virology* 57: 179–188.

Nichol S T, Spiropoulou C F, Morzunov S, *et al.* (1993) Genetic identification of a hantavirus associated with an outbreak of acute respiratory illness. *Science* 262: 914–917.

Oldfield E H, Ram Z, Culver K W, *et al.* (1993) Gene therapy for the treatment of brain tumors using intra-tumoral transduction with the thymidine kinase gene and intravenous ganciclovir. *Hum Gene Ther* 4: 39–69.

Palu G, Cavaggioni A, Calvi P, *et al.* (1999) Gene therapy of glioblastoma multiforme via combined expression of suicide and cytokine genes: a pilot study in humans. *Gene Ther* 6: 330–337.

Paradis K, Langford G, Long Z, *et al.* (1999) Search for cross-species transmission of porcine endogenous retrovirus in patients treated with living pig tissue. *Science* 285: 1236–1241.

Patience C, Takeuchi Y, Weiss R A (1997a) Infection of human cells by an endogenous retrovirus of pigs. *Nat Med* 3: 282–286.

Patience C, Wilkinson D A, Weiss R A (1997b) Our retroviral heritage. *Trends Genet* 13: 116–120.

Patience C, Patton G S, Takeuchi Y, *et al.* (1998a) No evidence of pig DNA or retroviral infection in patients with short-term extracorporeal connection to pig kidneys. *Lancet* 352: 699–701.

Patience C, Takeuchi Y, Cosset F L, Weiss R A (1998b) Packaging of endogenous retroviral sequences in retroviral vectors produced by murine and human packaging cells. *J Virol* 72: 2671–2676.

Patience C, Switzer W M, Takeuchi Y, *et al.* (2001) Multiple groups of novel retroviral genomes in pigs and related species. *J Virol* 75: 2771–2775.

Paton N I, Leo Y S, Zaki S R, *et al.* (1999) Outbreak of Nipah-virus infection among abattoir workers in Singapore. *Lancet* 354: 1253–1256.

Philbey A W, Kirkland P D, Ross A D, *et al.* (1998) An apparently new virus (family *Paramyxoviridae*) infectious for pigs, humans, and fruit bats. *Emerg Infect Dis* 4: 269–271.

Platt J L, ed. (2000a) *Xenotransplantation.* Washington, DC: American Society for Microbiology.

Platt J L (2000b) Xenotransplantation. New risks, new gains. *Nature* 407: 29–30.

Polejaeva I A, Chen S H, Vaught T D, *et al.* (2000) Cloned pigs produced by nuclear transfer from adult somatic cells. *Nature* 407: 86–90.

Purcell D F, Broscius C M, Vanin E F, *et al.* (1996) An array of murine leukemia virus-related elements is transmitted and expressed in a primate recipient of retroviral gene transfer. *J Virol* 70: 887–897.

Qari S H, Magre S, Garcia-Lerma J G, *et al.* (2001) Susceptibility of the porcine endogenous retrovirus to reverse transcriptase and protease inhibitors. *J Virol* 75: 1048–1053.

Ram Z, Culver K W, Oshiro E M, *et al.* (1997) Therapy of malignant brain tumors by intratumoral implantation of retroviral vector-producing cells. *Nat Med* 3: 1354–1361.

Rother R P, Squinto S P (1996) The alpha-galactosyl epitope: a sugar coating that makes viruses and cells unpalatable. *Cell* 86: 185–188.

Rozga J, Podesta L, LePage E, *et al.* (1993) Control of cerebral oedema by total hepatectomy and extracorporeal liver support in fulminant hepatic failure. *Lancet* 342: 898–899.

Schmoeckel M, Bhatti F N, Zaidi A, *et al.* (1998) Orthotopic heart transplantation in a transgenic pig-to-primate model. *Transplantation* 65: 1570–1577.

Starzl T E, Fung J, Tzakis A, *et al.* (1993) Baboon-to-human liver transplantation. *Lancet* 341: 65–71.

Takefman D M, Wong S, Maudru T, *et al.* (2001) Detection and characterization of porcine endogenous retrovirus in porcine plasma and porcine factor VIII. *J Virol* 75: 4551–4557.

Takeuchi Y, Porter C D, Strahan K M, *et al.* (1996) Sensitization of cells and retroviruses to human serum by (alpha 1–3) galactosyltransferase. *Nature* 379: 85–88.

Takeuchi Y, Patience C, Magre S, *et al.* (1998) Host range and interference studies of three classes of pig endogenous retrovirus. *J Virol* 72: 9986–9991.

Todaro G J, Benveniste R E, Lieber M M, Sherr C J (1974) Characterization of a type C virus released from the porcine cell line PK(15). *Virology* 58: 65–74.

van der Laan L J, Lockey C, Griffeth B C, *et al.* (2000) Infection by porcine endogenous retrovirus after islet xenotransplantation in SCID mice. *Nature* 407: 90–94.

Weiss R A (1998a) Science, medicine, and the future – Xenotransplantation. *BMJ* 317: 931–937.

Weiss R A (1998b) Transgenic pigs and virus adaptation. *Nature* 391: 327–328.

Weiss R A (1999) Xenografts and retroviruses. *Science* 285: 1221–1222.

Weiss R A (2001) Animal origins of human infectious disease. *Phil Trans R Soc Lond [Biol]* 356: 957–977.

Weiss R A, Wrangham R W (1999) The origin of HIV-1: From *Pan* to pandemic. *Nature* 397: 385–386.

Wilson C A, Wong S, Muller J, *et al.* (1998) Type C retrovirus released from porcine primary peripheral blood mononuclear cells infects human cells. *J Virol* 72: 3082–3087.

Glossary

Adhesion molecules   Proteins that mediate binding of one cell to another or to the extracellular matrix.

Adjuvant   Substance that enhances the immune response to an antigen with which it is mixed.

Allele   An alternative form of a gene. Alleles of a specific gene occupy the same location on homologous chromosomes. Thus, in a diploid cell, each gene will have two alleles, each occupying the same position on homologous chromosomes.

Altered peptide ligands   Peptides in which one or more of the amino acids in the 'native' peptide has been substituted for another amino acid.

Annealing   The process whereby DNA sequences combine by hydrogen bonding with other complementary sequences as temperatures fall below a critical denaturation or melting temperature.

Antibody   Immunoglobulin molecule, produced by B lymphocytes, with recognition sites specific for a particular structure on an antigen.

Antigen   Molecule that reacts with an antibody to stimulate T cells.

Antigen presentation   Process whereby antigens – usually fragments of proteins – are displayed on the surface of a cell together with molecules (MHC) required for lymphocyte activation.

Antisense RNA   A sequence of RNA that is the base pair complement of an mRNA. Binding of the antisense RNA to the mRNA (also referred to as the sense RNA) blocks translation of the mRNA into protein.

Autoimmune disease   An immune response to self antigens that induces tissue damage and disease.

Bacteriophage   Double-stranded DNA virus that infects bacteria.

Base pairing   The specific association of nucleotides to each other by hydrogen bonding. In DNA, adenine (A) pairs with thymine (T) and guanine (G) pairs with cytosine (C). In RNA, adenine (A) pairs with uracil (U) and guanine (G) pairs with cytosine (C).

Chromatin   A component of chromosomes that comprises DNA complexed with stoichiometric amounts of histones and, to a lesser extent, other DNA-binding proteins.

Chromosome   Strand of tightly compacted DNA containing sequences of DNA (genes) encoding for proteins and their regulation of expression. Chromosomes are present in all cells. In mammals (including humans), all chromosomes are paired except for the sex chromosomes.

Codon   Part of the genetic code. A sequence of three nucleotides in an RNA molecule which encodes for an amino acid. Many amino acids make up a protein.

Complementary DNA (cDNA)   Artificially produced copy of mRNA. Used due to its increased stability compared with mRNA.

cDNA library   A complete copy of all the genes expressed in a particular cell type in the form of cDNA.

Copy number   Number of replications of the DNA sequence

Cytokines   Proteins produced by cells that affect the action of immune cells.

Deletion   Loss of a region of genomic DNA from a chromosome that results in the loss of part of a gene or of a number of genes which can generate pleiotropic phenotypes.

Denaturation   The process whereby double-stranded DNA is heated to a temperature where the hydrogen bonds between complementary DNA strands break to give two single strands of DNA.

Diploid   A cell or organism that contains homologous pairs of each chromosome. Sometimes abbreviated to $2n$.

DNA   Deoxyribonucleic acid.

DNA-dependent DNA polymerase   An enzyme that will add nucleotides to the 3′ end of a DNA strand which already is bound to a complementary DNA strand but which has single-stranded DNA to act as a template.

DNA fingerprinting   Technique to identify DNA sequences that are specific to an individual. The technique involves restriction enzyme digestion of genomic DNA followed by Southern blotting to detect mini-satellite regions in the DNA that are specific for a specific individual's genetic make-up.

DNA replication   The process by which cells copy their genomic DNA before cell division.

Dominant mutation   Mutation of one gene copy (allele) that results in a disease phenotype.

Duplication   Gain of a region of genomic DNA in a chromosome that results in the duplication of a part of a gene or of a number of genes which can generate pleiotropic phenotypes.

Effector T cells   Cells that can remove pathogens from the body.

Epitope   Site on an antigen that stimulates the immune system.

Episomal   Refers to a plasmid or bacteriophage that usually is found as an autonomously replicating genetic element in the cytoplasm of a host cell.

ES cells   Embryonic stem cells. Cells established in tissue culture from explanted blastocysts.

Exon   Region of DNA that is found in the mature mRNA. Derived from the term expressing sequence, exons can be divided into coding and non-coding exons. Coding exons contain sequence that codes for amino acids whereas non-coding exons contain sequence that is found in the untranslated regions of the mRNA. The number of exons in a gene can vary from one to >20.

Expressed sequence tag (EST)   A small part of the active part of a gene, made from cDNA, which can be used to determine the rest of the gene sequence out of the chromosome, by matching base pairs with part of the gene. The EST can be radioactively labelled in order to locate it within a larger segment of DNA.

Founder animal   Animal that has been developed from an injected egg.

Fv (variable fragment)   Variable region/antigen-binding domain of an antibody molecule.

Gene   A sequence of nucleotides that encodes for a protein and its expression in the cell.

Gene therapy (gene transfer)   The treatment of a genetic disease or disorder with a corrective DNA sequence (gene).

Gene transfer   See gene therapy.

Genetic linkage   Genes or DNA markers at two or more loci are inherited together due to their close proximity on a chromosome. When they are physically close together the linkage is said to be tighter and there is less chance that they will be separated during meiosis.

Genetic profiling   See pharmacogenomics.

Genome   The total genetic content of a cell.

Genomics   The study of genes and their regulation.

Genotype   The genetic constitution of an individual cell or organism.

Germ cell   Sperm, egg or early embryo.

Germ line gene therapy   Gene therapy involving the germ cells (sperm and egg), cf. somatic gene therapy.

Haploid   A cell that contains only a single copy of each particular chromosome. In higher eukaryotes, haploid cells are restricted to the gametes. Commonly abbreviated to *n*.

Helicase   The enzyme that disrupts the secondary structure of double-stranded DNA to produce single-stranded DNA so that DNA replication can occur.

Homologous genes   Genes that give rise to proteins with similar function but which have different protein sequences. Often two genes in two related organisms will have the same function but slightly different sequences. They are said to be homologous.

Homologous recombination   Genetic recombination that occurs between DNAs with long stretches of homology (e.g. between homologous chromosomes at meiosis) and which is mediated by enzymes that show no particular sequence specificity. Homologous recombination can be used to target introduced DNA to particular regions of the chromosome, thus disrupting selected genes.

Idiotype   Antigen-binding site of the immunoglobulin expressed on the surface membrane of tumour cells.

Immunoblotting (Western blotting)   Technique of identifying specific proteins following electrophoretic resolution, transfer and immobilisation to a membrane support and incubation with a specific antibody.

Infection (with a retrovirus or adenovirus)   Used as a method of introducing a therapeutic gene into a recipient cell.

Intrabody   Single chain antibody developed by cloning in light and heavy chain genes from a hybridoma that produces an antibody to the peptide of interest. Attached to the endoplasmic reticulum.

Intron   The region(s) of DNA that do not code for gene products and that are removed during the generation of mRNA. Derived from the term intervening sequences, introns are found between the exons of a gene and are sometimes referred to as 'junk DNA' due to the apparent lack of biological function. The number of introns in a gene can vary from zero to >20.

Isoforms   Genes or proteins found in the same organism and often in the same cell with similar but not identical sequences. They may have different functions.

Karyotype   The full set of chromosomes of a cell arranged with respect to size, shape and number.

Knockout   The process of preventing the expression and function of a protein by introducing a DNA sequence that inhibits translation of the messenger RNA encoding the gene.

Locus   The position or location of a gene (or a gene polymorphism) on a given chromosome.

Major histocompatibility complex (MHC)   Cluster of genes encoding for molecules that are able to present antigens to lymphocytes.

Messenger RNA (mRNA)   An RNA molecule that carries the message for protein synthesis.

Microsatellites   Short tracts of tandemly repeated di-, tri- or tetranucleotide sequences dispersed throughout the genome. They are very simple DNA sequences with high mutation rates. These sequences often show variation in length between different genetic lineages. Also known as simple sequence repeats or SSRs.

Mini-satellite DNA   A short sequence of DNA that consists of a tandem repeat. These regions are known to occur in regions of DNA that vary greatly between individuals and are used as the basis of an individual's DNA fingerprint.

Monogenic disorder   A disorder where the pathology of the disease is caused by a single gene defect.

Multiple locus probes   DNA fingerprinting probes that have sequence similarity with many repeat regions in the genome and so recognise multiple bands on a Southern blot of genomic DNA and give rise to the classical DNA fingerprint pattern.

Multiplicity of infection (MOI)   A term used in virology to define the ratio of infectious particles to target cells.

Naked DNA   A specific gene sequence inserted into a plasmid vector.

Northern blotting   Technique of identifying specific RNA sequences following electrophoretic resolution, transfer and immobilisation to a membrane support and hybridisation with a specific labelled probe.

Nucleotide   An organic molecule containing a purine (adenine or guanine) or pyrimidine (thymine or cytosine) base, a five carbon ribose or deoxyribose sugar and one or more phosphate groups.

Nucleotide triphosphate   A nucleotide with three phosphate groups, which is the building block of DNA and the energy source for many chemical reactions.

Oligodendrocyte   Cell responsible for producing central nervous system myelin.

Oligonucleotide   A short sequence of nucleotides (usually <30).

Packaging cell line   Cell line that provides retro- (adeno-)viral genes necessary for viral replication, assembly and packaging.

Peptide   Short fragment of a protein comprising a number (usually <20) amino acids.

Pharmacogenomics (pharmacogenetics)   The use of the genetic profile of a patient to determine which drug(s) would be most suitable for treating a genetic disease.

Phenotype   The observable character of a cell or organism.

Plasmid   Circularised DNA fragment distinct from genomic DNA, isolated from bacteria, used as a cloning vector.

Poly(A)+ RNA   See messenger RNA.

Polymerase chain reaction (PCR)   The technique where small quantities of specific sequences of DNA can be amplified exponentially to provide analytical quantities of DNA.

Polymorphism   A difference in DNA sequence between individuals. Polmorphisms may give rise to alterations in gene function and can be found in both introns and exons. They are useful for linkage analysis and can be associated with specific diseases and populations.

Primer   A short sequence of DNA or RNA (up to 30 bases) used to prime the elongation of DNA replication.

Primer, degenerate   A mixture of DNA oligonucleotides that vary only by one or two bases.

Promoter   Region of the gene that signals the initiation of transcription (i.e. copying of mRNA from DNA).

Pronucleus   The nucleus of either the unfertilised egg or sperm.

Proteomics   The study of protein expression and protein function.

Pseudopregnant female   A female in oestrus that has been mated with a vasectomised or genetically sterile male.

Recessive mutation   Mutation of both alleles of the gene which gives rise to a disease phenotype.

Replicon   Sequence in the DNA that initiates replication.

Reporter gene   A marker gene which is easy to detect once transfected into cells (e.g. β-galactosidase, which produces a characteristic blue colour in those cells which have taken up and expressed the gene). Used to study the levels and efficiency of expression of the transfected gene.

Restriction enzyme   Enzyme that cuts (digests) DNA at specific sequences.

Ribozymes   RNA molecules that possess enzymatic activity and have potential as therapeutic agents since they can cleave mRNA molecules or affect the repair of mutant RNAs.

RNA   Ribonucleic acid.

RNA decoy   Positive-stranded sense oligonucleotide that mimics essential regulatory sequences and prevents RNA transcription.

RNase   An enzyme that cleaves and destroys RNA molecules.

RNA primase   An enzyme which lays down a 10-base strand of RNA using single-stranded DNA as a template.

RT-PCR   Reverse transcription polymerase chain reaction. Semi-quantitative measure of mRNA expression.

Sequence   The order of nucleotides or amino acids found along a strand of DNA or a protein respectively.

Short tandem repeat polymorphisms (STRPs)   Small repetitive nucleotide sequences that exist in tandem arrays of varying repeat numbers.

Single locus probes   Highly specific repetitive element probes that recognise a single repeat element in genomic DNA. Southern blots probed with a single locus probe generate two distinct bands and give rise to a DNA profile rather than a DNA fingerprint.

Somatic cell   All cells except germ cells.

Somatic gene therapy   Gene therapy involving any cell other than germ cells, cf. germ line gene therapy.

Southern blotting Technique of identifying specific regions of DNA following restriction enzyme digestion, electrophoretic resolution, transfer and immobilisation to a membrane support and hybridisation with a specific labelled probe.

Sticky ends Protruding, cohesive 5′ termini that are produced in DNA strands cut with certain restriction enzymes.

Stringency The degree of selectivity used to anneal a DNA sequence to its complementary strand, decided either by temperature or buffer composition.

T-cell receptor (TCR) Cell surface-related molecule on T lymphocytes that recognises peptide antigen in association with an MHC molecule.

TAQ polymerase A heat-stable version of DNA-dependent DNA polymerase obtained from the bacterium *Thermus aquaticus*.

Transfection The insertion of genes into cells (mammalian).

Transformation The insertion of genes into cells (bacterial).

Transgene The foreign DNA that is transferred to and expressed in the recipient animal.

Transgenic The introduction of a gene from one species into the germ line of another, distantly related, species.

Transcription The process of synthesising an mRNA strand from a DNA template (the gene).

Transcription factor A protein that binds to a specific sequence in the promoter region of a gene to initiate transcription of that gene.

Translation The process of synthesising a protein product from an mRNA transcript.

Vector A circular self-replicating DNA molecule into which the gene of interest is inserted prior to transfection into mammalian cells or transformed into bacteria.

Viral load The number of viral RNA copies per millilitre of plasma.

Western blotting See immunoblotting.

Xenotransplantation The transfer of an organ or cell from one species to another, unrelated, species.

Yeast artificial chromosome (YAC) Vector that is able to propagate segments of human DNA over a megabase in size.

Zygote A fertilised egg.

Index